Is Human Nature Obsolete?

Basic Bioethics
Glenn McGee and Arthur Caplan, editors

Pricing Life: Why It's Time for Health Care Rationing, Peter A. Ubel

Bioethics: Ancient Themes in Contemporary Issues, edited by Mark G. Kuczewski and Ronald Polansky

The Human Embryonic Stem Cell Debate: Science, Ethics, and Public Policy, edited by Suzanne Holland, Karen Lebacqz, and Laurie Zoloth

Engendering International Health: The Challenge of Equity, edited by Gita Sen, Asha George, and Piroska Östlin

Self-Trust and Reproductive Autonomy, Carolyn McLeod

What Genes Can't *Do*, Lenny Moss

In the Wake of Terror: Medicine and Morality in a Time of Crisis, edited by Jonathan D. Moreno

Pragmatic Bioethics, 2d edition, edited by Glenn McGee

Case Studies in Biomedical Research Ethics, Timothy F. Murphy

Genetics and Life Insurance: Medical Underwriting and Social Policy, edited by Mark A. Rothstein

Ethics and the Metaphysics of Medicine: Reflections on Health and Beneficence, Kenneth A. Richman

DNA and the Criminal Justice System: The Technology of Justice, edited by David Lazer

Is Human Nature Obsolete? Genetics, Bioengineering, and the Future of the Human Condition, edited by Harold W. Baillie and Timothy K. Casey

Is Human Nature Obsolete?

Genetics, Bioengineering, and the Future of the Human Condition

edited by Harold W. Baillie and Timothy K. Casey

The MIT Press
Cambridge, Massachusetts
London, England

MIT Press books may be purchased at special quantity discounts for business or sales promotional use. For information, please e-mail special_sales@mitpress. mit.edu or write to Special Sales Department, The MIT Press, 5 Cambridge Center, Cambridge, MA 02142.

This book was set in Sabon by SNP Best-set Typesetter Ltd., Hong Kong. Printed and bound in the United States of America. Printed on recycled paper.

Library of Congress Cataloging-in-Publication Data
Is human nature obsolete? genetics, bioengineering, and the future of the
  human condition / edited by Harold W. Baillie and Timothy K. Casey.
      p.   cm.—(Basic bioethics)
      Papers from a conference held in spring 2001 at the University of Scranton.
      Includes bibliographical references and index.
      ISBN (invalid) 0-262-02569-9 (alk. paper)—ISBN 0-262-52428-7 (pbk. :
  alk. paper)
      1. Genetic engineering—Moral and ethical aspects. 2. Philosophical
  anthropology. I. Baillie, Harold W., 1950– II. Casey, Timothy. III. Series.
QH438.7.I8 2005
174′.957–dc22

                                                                2004040298

10   9   8   7   6   5   4   3   2   1

Contents

Series Foreword   vii

Acknowledgments   ix

1 Introduction   1
   Harold W. Baillie
   Timothy K. Casey

I Historical Perspectives   33

2 Nature, Technology, and the Emergence of Cybernetic
   Humanity   35
   Timothy K. Casey

3 Nature and Human Nature   67
   Mark Sagoff

4 Life Sciences: Discontents and Consolations   99
   Paul Rabinow

5 Genetic Engineering and Eugenics: The Uses of History   123
   Diane B. Paul

II Embodiment and Self-Identity   153

6 The Body and the Quest for Control   155
   Jean Bethke Elshtain

7 Visions and Re-visions: Life and the Accident of Birth   177
   Richard M. Zaner

8 Aristotle and Genetic Engineering: The Uncertainty of
   Excellence   209
   Harold W. Baillie

III Freedom and Telos   233

9   Human Recency and Race: Molecular Anthropology, the
    Refigured Acheulean, and the UNESCO Response to
    Auschwitz   235
    Robert N. Proctor

10 Human Nature in a Post–Human Genome Project World   269
    Thomas A. Shannon

11 Telos, Value, and Genetic Engineering   317
    Bernard E. Rollin

IV Social and Political Critiques   337

12 Nature, Sin, and Society   339
    Lisa Sowle Cahill

13 Human Genetic Intervention: Past, Present, and Future   367
    LeRoy Walters

14 Resistance Is Futile: The Posthuman Condition and Its
    Advocates   385
    Langdon Winner

Contributors   413
Index   415

Series Foreword

We are pleased to present the thirteenth book in the series Basic Bioethics. The series presents innovative works in bioethics to a broad audience and introduces seminal scholarly manuscripts, state-of-the-art references works, and textbooks. Such broad areas as the philosophy of medicine, advancing genetics and biotechnology, end-of-life care, health and social policy, and the empirical study of biomedical life are engaged.

Glenn McGee
Arthur Caplan

Basic Bioethics Series Editorial Board
Tod S. Chambers
Susan Dorr Goold
Mark Kuczewski
Herman Saatkamp

Acknowledgments

Without our contributing authors, this volume would simply not exist. Their willingness to take the risk of joining the original conference and their commitment to the exchange of ideas that gave rise to the final versions of their chapters, places them first on our list of those to be acknowledged and thanked. The conference and the work on this volume were supported by a subgrant from the Northeast Regional Cancer Institute, which had received support from a U.S. Department of Energy Grant, DE–FG02–98ER62592. We wish to thank the Northeast Regional Cancer Institute, its then president, Susan Belin, and the chair of its board of directors, Dr. Harmar Brereton, for giving us the opportunity to gather together these scholars. We would also like to thank our colleagues Professors William Rowe and Charles Pinches, directors of the Center for Ethics Studies at the University of Scranton, for their encouragement and suggestions for our efforts. Clay Morgan, senior acquisitions editor at the MIT Press, was a constant source of advice and direction. Eleanore Harrington provided tireless secretarial support and good humor, which kept us going when the task seemed endless. And at the last minute, our colleague Crina Geschwandtner added crucial editorial support.

Thomas A. Shannon's essay is excerpted from *The New Genetic Medicine: Theological and Ethical Reflections* (2003), by Thomas A. Shannon and James J. Walter. Reprinted with the permission of Sheed and Ward, an imprint of Rowman and Littlefield Publishers.

Paul Rabinow's essay is excerpted from *Anthropos Today: Reflections on Modern Equipment* (2003), by Paul Rabinow. Reprinted with the permission of Princeton University Press.

Robert N. Proctor's essay is reprinted from *Current Anthropology* (44.2, April 2003), with the permission of the author.

1
Introduction

Harold W. Baillie and Timothy K. Casey

Ours is the age of technology. What this means exactly has for some time now been the subject of intense debate that spans the entire spectrum of opinion from Luddism to the most unabashed technophilia. Technology, in one form or another, has always been a significant element of the human condition, but never has it been so ubiquitous and determinative of who and what we think we are. Cyborgs, artificial intelligence, cloning, and genetic engineering—all are indicative of a swiftly moving reality we struggle to make sense of in the absence of traditional signposts and historical precedents. What distinguishes modern technology from all other types, both premodern and non-Western, is its exclusive focus on the perfection of technical procedures and processes that had historically been subordinate to supratechnical norms and standards, usually of a moral, political, and religious nature. The underlying assumption in this revolutionary shift in orientation is the radical separation of technical and humanistic concerns. This divorce expresses itself in the widely held belief that technology is a neutral tool whose internal operations fall under a kind of immunity from the judgmental gaze of ethicists and metaphysicians, reducing their role, with few exceptions, to commentary on what is essentially a fait accompli. Environmental and medical ethics in particular rarely, if ever, get to question ongoing scientific research and its technological applications, but instead have been limited to reacting to discoveries and products and their possible ramifications on the natural and human worlds.

The power and unpredictability of modern technology outstrip traditional ways of thinking and judging at every turn. The reasons for this novel situation are too many and complex to be examined here, but a few remarks are in order to shed light on the problems presented by bioengineering and genetic research. The most obvious difficulty we face is the degree of specialization now characteristic of the pursuit of scientific and technological knowledge that when coupled with the rapidity with which this knowledge is developed and disseminated, makes it extremely difficult to construct the kind of overview necessary for effective assessment and evaluation. In addition, the calculative kind of thinking employed in the constant improvement and refinement of methodology and technique simply does not lend itself to—though it does not necessarily preclude—a reflective or self-critical turn of mind. When the focus is on results and cost-benefit analyses, it would be naive, perhaps even otherworldly, to expect technicians and scientists to think like traditional humanists. All of which tells us that there exists a culture that has grown up around a class of intellectual elites whose progressive mores, values, and goals go unquestioned, if they are considered at all. The best description of this culture remains Francis Bacon's visionary *New Atlantis*, which already in the seventeenth century outlines the kind of research community best suited to the development of a systematic scientific knowledge that lends itself to technological exploitation and application. Guided by the goal of the "relief of man's estate" and the emerging modern principle of the division of labor where every researcher has a function to perform much like factory workers on an assembly line, Bacon foresaw an enterprise whose collective wisdom would be ensured by the goodness of its intentions and the triumph of its techniques. What is more, the communal aspect of "Solomon's House," Bacon's somewhat presumptuous though revealing name for this enterprise, would, he believed, transform the nature of scientific endeavor from the empirical groping of isolated individuals into a vast, intricate project requiring large amounts of financial and technical support that could be made available only by a civilization that sees and defines itself in terms of that project. And he was right.

The obstacles confronting a critical assessment of this project, which has been in full swing for centuries now, are thus formidable. But they are not insurmountable. Indeed, in the case of genetics and its various technological applications, something new has occurred. While it is true that the cloning of nonhuman animals and the engineering of agricultural products have gone forward without much serious public reflection or debate (at least in the United States) about their desirability or chances of success, the very real possibility of applying these techniques to humans in the not-too-distant future seems finally to have caused many in the political community and some in the scientific professions to step back and ask whether we really want to go down this road. Already in most of Europe, the cloning of humans is banned for reproductive—though not, as in the case of England, for therapeutic—purposes, and support for similar legislation is growing in North America as well. This suggests that cracks may be appearing in the collective will to subject ourselves and future generations to changes whose inalterability is matched only by their profundity. To be sure, the compromises and shifts in popular and scientific opinion that undoubtedly lie on the horizon are unknown and impossible to predict. One can legitimately wonder whether this is merely a pause in a process that no human or group of humans can hinder or stop in the long run. But what is becoming clearer to many through the public voice of environmentalism and the high profile of many bioethical issues such as stem cell research is the unprecedented character of our technologies in their temporal and geographic impact on the planet. The effects of genetic enhancement, like the consequences of atomic fission, will last far into the future and will not be limited to localities or even large regions. Dealing with this sobering fact has recently taken on a new sense of urgency, since the distinction between somatic and germ line therapies has become increasingly difficult to maintain in light of a variety of new techniques as simple as preimplantation genetic diagnosis that blur the demarcation of what is presently permissible in genetic research and application.

The chapters in this book should be seen against this background. Specifically, they arose out of a conference in spring 2001 at the University of Scranton dedicated to posing two questions: (1) does genetic engineering of humans require a new understanding of what it means to be human, and (2) does what we already know suggest that there should be (and can be) effective limits to what can be done? With these considerations in mind, we brought together thinkers from a variety of disciplines for three days of intense discussion and exchange of ideas. (Jean Bethke Elshtain was unable to attend, but graciously agreed to write a chapter especially for this volume.) Papers were not read but briefly summarized, having been distributed several weeks beforehand. This of course allowed for advance preparation, and so for a longer and more sustained conversation. In planning the conference, we were acutely aware that most of our participants had not met one another—a result no doubt of the narrow disciplinary character of conference-going today. Nor, we knew, were they of one mind about the issues we laid out before them. In fact, the group as a whole represents a diversity of views: some in the group are very much concerned with the impact of biotechnology on humans and on the role the concept of the human condition should play in determining genetic research and application, while others contend that such concerns may be obsolete and, at the very least, are not a necessary condition for moral reflection on the refashioning of our genetic constitution. What these scholars do have in common are national and international reputations for their astuteness in these matters and the sobriety of their reflections. Most important for us was the public nature of their work, ranging from publishing books for the general populace and writing for popular journals and magazines to testifying before Congress and even advising the president. Their ability to speak in nuanced and sophisticated ways to an educated audience outside their own disciplines and beyond the walls of academe, we believe, is reflected in the chapters published here.

Still, the quality of the conversation, not to mention the genuine bonhomie that quickly emerged in the group, exceeded our most optimistic expectations. Rather than getting bogged down in questions of medical or scientific practice, everyone focused on questions of fundamental, ontological importance. And instead of rushing to the practical side of the debate, where all too many believe the real "action" is, the group was eager to explore the humanistic implications of a technology that promises not just to add a trait here or subtract a defect there but to alter radically our very being. The results of this interaction, which have been incorporated into these published papers, were exciting to the participants and will be to readers as well.

Summary of Chapters

It is the philosophical nature of these issues and chapters that make this volume unique. The substance of each chapter remains philosophical, or at times theological, rather than technical. The issues discussed may touch on cloning, reproductive choices, or economic justice, but as examples and not as the purpose of the argument. Throughout, the focus remains on the question of what it is to be human and how just thinking about bioengineering alters our self-understanding. Clearly, if the success of the conference is any indication, there exists today an intellectual hunger to address in a public way the array of ontological and human issues clustered around bioengineering. The potential impact of these powerful technologies on humans whom we will never and can never know is so profound and far-reaching that the old disciplinary constraints can now only be seen as archaic and counterproductive. It is our hope that this collection will help to establish a model for addressing bioethical issues that finally razes these traditional barriers, and in doing so, moves the academy into the space of public discourse where the decisions about these vital matters will ultimately be made.

Tim Casey introduces this collection by laying out what he sees as the historical and philosophical context within which we can make sense of genetic engineering as the ultimate chapter in the ongoing Western project of subduing nature for human ends. "Nature, Technology, and the Emergence of Cybernetic Humanity" argues that despite the novelty of genetic enhancement, this new technology remains part of a tradition whose arc is discernible in certain key events over the last millennium. In particular, he focuses our attention on the metaphysical dualism arising out of modern science and its roots in a medieval technological revolution informed by both increasing mechanization and an underlying Christian anthropocentrism that initiated a new feel for matter. Here the seeds were sown for both the Galilean mathematicization of nature and the technological rationale for Galileo's new physics. Casey reminds us that the Cartesian reaction to this science resulted in a dualism intended to preserve human freedom in the face of a mechanistic determinism inherent in a clockwork universe. But more than this, he argues that out of the Cartesian compromise with Galilean science arose a productionist metaphysics whose scientific and technological hallmark was and remains the suppression of spontaneity, choice, and ultimately, any hint of indeterminacy in the natural world. The radical sense of displacement ushered in by this suppression can be gauged by more recent attempts to move beyond what are perceived as antiquated conceptions of human nature.

With this in mind, Casey discusses at some length the responses of Karl Marx and Martin Heidegger to our emerging technological age and the concomitant problem of world alienation it poses. For Marx, humans are no longer the rational animal of the Aristotelian tradition nor the thinking spectator of Western philosophical idealism. Instead, humanity is recast as the *animal laborans*, the toolmaker who has incorporated nature into human history in the historically necessary pursuit of the abolition of scarcity. As the producer of its own existence, the modern proletariat exemplifies the productionist metaphysics initiated by René Descartes and developed further by such thinkers as David Hume and Immanuel Kant. In this metaphysics, humanity has become the measure of being and the creator, quite literally, of a new reality amenable to the satisfaction of basic material needs. Hence, for Marx, production is not a mere means to human life but is in fact the expression of humanity's "species-essence," insofar as such production finally overcomes humanity's historical alienation from nature and the worst aspects of Cartesian dualism. Heidegger's take on this metaphysical situation is remarkably similar, but in the end he is not as sanguine about what this portends for the human condition. The Heideggerian account of modern technology is to view it ontologically as a mode of revealing that challenges humans to assault nature with the intent of reducing it to a standing reserve of energy and information subject to our control and manipulation. The deeper question posed by this analysis is whether such an assault threatens not only nature but humanity in its very essence.

Of particular concern to Casey is whether the human body itself is to be taken up into the standing reserve and treated as just so much raw material. His central argument is that such reductionism is leading us to the final technological frontier where we ourselves will become material to be shaped and reinvented through feedback mechanisms that jibe with the Darwinian emphasis on adaptive behavior as part of evolutionary progress. Utilizing the critique of cybernetics by Hans Jonas, Casey contends that the danger of a cybernetic humanity, armed with the powerful new tool of genetic enhancement, is in truth a more radical displacement than Cartesian dualism and that such a threat can be countered, not by attempts to restore what is left of more traditional concepts of human nature but rather through a reconsideration of our humanness that takes seriously our technological power and prowess without, however, granting it ontological supremacy. Such a reconfiguration of the human condition, he concludes, must begin with the recognition of our essential historicity, and thus of those limitations placed on our power by the inherent indeterminacy and hence elusiveness of beings encountered in time—including that most baffling entity of all, the human body itself.

Mark Sagoff's "Nature and Human Nature" suggests that neither nature nor history is any longer sufficient as a moral force to restrain us from pursuing the technological transformation of our genetic constitution. Such restraint, Sagoff argues, has depended on maintaining a fundamental difference between the natural and the artifactual—a difference placed in question by modern technology. The impact of this fact on the question of human nature becomes most apparent in the area of biotechnology, where the line between the human as a product of nature and the human as a fabrication of technology is already becoming blurred. Sagoff makes a strong case for the view that whatever moral limits we might wish to impose on genetic engineering have been, at least traditionally, rooted in the natural as a nonhuman sphere to which we must ultimately submit. Theologians such as Paul Ramsey, for example, have appealed to this sphere not only to put the breaks on "man's limitless self-modification" but to salvage the very concept of human nature itself. Sagoff, then, wisely points us toward the nexus of nature and human nature, and the revolution brought about by the prospects of genetic therapy and enhancement in how we are to understand this relationship. Already, he maintains, biology has opened the door to these prospects by demonstrating that humanity no longer resides near the trunk of the tree of life but rather occupies an "undistinguished spot at the periphery of evolution," thus making us genomically indistinguishable from, say, yeast. Sagoff is therefore concerned with those kinds of arguments (which he takes quite seriously) against genetic engineering that rely on a demonstrable connection between the human genome and a natural and ecological order moral in its import.

To his credit, the chapter explores fairly and openly the various facets of such arguments. Sagoff begins by noting that genetic inheritance in particular lies at the heart of the moral dimension of nature since what is passed down in our genes binds us to our natural heritage as a limit to what we might become. To fool with this inheritance is to play with an ethical norm that has guided humanity, for better or worse, down through the ages. When opponents of genetic engineering point to the danger of obscuring, if not obliterating, human nature, they are appealing, Sagoff says, to the distinction between a child that is born and one that is "made." In the former case, the child remains part of a natural lineage that connects it to family and the heritage of the species. A fabricated human, on the other hand, is severed from its history and natural lineage, and so is reduced to a mere means lacking in the dignity of a full-fledged person. Theologians like Karl Rahner argue in this fashion, presupposing that the givenness of nature and the human genome forbids the kind of self-determination that results in the manufacture of humans. Here we see quite clearly the moral status of the natural lying precisely in its independence from ultimate human control and intervention. From this it follows that human nature is also a given that while it might admit of minor alterations, should never, for any reason, be tampered with in its essentials. But there are other Christian theologians, Sagoff informs us, who maintain that as cocreators with God, we are entitled to transform our genome as long as our purposes for doing so are in accord with God's. And Jewish theologians are even more open to such activity because, unlike their Christian counterparts, they are not indebted to Aristotelian form and function as essential and unchangeable. If there is an argument against genetic engineering to made here, it will point to the potential arrogance of modern technology and not to the harm it might inflict on nature and the human gene pool.

Sagoff concludes by considering two senses of nature delineated by John Stuart Mill in the nineteenth century. One specifically applies in modern science and encompasses everything that exists. In this view of nature, everything humans do is natural, including technology. The second sense is narrower and includes only what is not made by human hands. Such a notion is of course nonsensical to a scientist, but it provides a basis for normative questions concerning the fabrication and use of technology. This is the nature that until recently has provided humans with a discernible set of limits, and hence an ethical basis for reining in certain kinds of manufacture and bioengineering. But once technology has invaded the processes of life itself, such a notion becomes questionable at best and outdated at worst, as does the very notion of human nature. Clearly, then, since the moral worth of the larger natural world is a concept that is increasingly unsupportable, appeals to a fixed human nature, in Sagoff's view, have become irrelevant. Instead, the problem facing us is not whether engineering of the human genome will alienate us from our nature—for, as he tells us, nature in fact became hostile and lost its moral resonance when we were evicted from the Garden of Eden—but whether we can bear the coming moral burden of responsibility for the creation of a "second nature," including our own.

Paul Rabinow is likewise opposed to turning our backs on genetic intervention out of a misplaced allegiance to human nature. His argument in "Life Sciences: Discontents and Consolations" is that romanticism about a fixed human essence is not only impossible in the face of modern scientific development and its disenchantment of the world but constitutes an all-too-familiar cultural immaturity and even narcissism that can lead to the kind of dire political consequences that littered much of the twentieth century. Applying the Freudian analysis of civilization and its modern discontents, Rabinow challenges us to strip away any lingering illusions about occupying a privileged place in the cosmos and finally to accept the scientific demystification of the natural world. The lessons of the Copernican, Darwinian, and Freudian revolutions have combined to deflate humanity's pride and tendency toward a megalomania. A twentieth-century heir to the Enlightenment, Sigmund Freud regarded his own work as embodying a scientific wisdom that counsels pursuit of the truth wherever it leads, however subversive such knowledge may be to our reigning self-image or however uneasy it may make us feel. Max Weber expresses similar sentiments in his essay "Science as a Vocation," one of the great statements, according to Rabinow, of the scientific ethos as a model of maturity and sober realism. But unlike Freud, Weber rejects the Enlightenment equation of science with wisdom, restricting knowledge to the rarified sphere of specialization and calculative reason. Today, the knowledge business is an exclusively technical affair with no pretensions to wisdom or meaning. Indeed, the idea that science could or should submit to the guidance of the cultural sciences is as futile as it would no doubt be harmful to the *Geisteswissenschaften* themselves. As Rabinow puts it, the value of science is simply "to invent concepts and conduct rational experiments," not to judge its usefulness for mastering the world or for producing the greatest happiness for the greatest number (a goal Rabinow scornfully dismisses as suitable for

Friedrich Nietzsche's "last men"). On ultimate philosophical matters science is therefore mute, though as a training in disciplined thought it does contribute to the ideal of clarification, which for Rabinow, underpins the primary virtue of an ethos of maturity: responsibility.

Rabinow does not flinch from recognizing the complicity of modern science and scientists in the "gravest betrayals," as Jürgen Habermas puts it, of reason and responsibility over the last hundred years. But, he warns, this should not tempt us to an irrationalism or rejection of the scientific ethos. Science, as Freud and Weber made clear even in the midst of last century's horrors, remains a vocation and an inspiration for a humanity devoted to peace and the overcoming of the Thanatos instinct. In our own time, molecular biology and biochemistry have emerged as new and fresh challenges to the remnants of a universal narcissism in contemporary human beings. And though these sciences are ineluctably intertwined with the state and increasingly dependent on the largesse of multinationals, this calls not for rolling back research but for serious reflection on the moral and political consequences of this situation. More important, Rabinow contends, is what we have learned from biology over the past decade or so—namely, that at the genetic level, all forms of life are materially the same, and that the technology central to this discovery demands "further intervention into that materiality." In the shift in the 1990s from a focus on genes to the production, mapping, and sequencing of DNA, a "new industrial mode of operation" has been instituted in molecular biology, which in turn has led to a rethinking of the gene as the locus of a DNA sequence as opposed to its reification in classical genetics. The next exciting step will entail seeing when genes are switched on and off, and for what duration, since we now know, as the geneticist Sydney Brenner observes, that evolution proceeds "by modulating the expression of genes" and not by "enlarging the protein inventory."

Thus, while genetic mapping and sequencing have neither yielded the meaning of life (such metanarratives are in Rabinow's view alien to science and hence unsuitable for our time) nor ushered in eugenics, biology today does raise the question of human nature by demonstrating our similarities with all living things (recall Sagoff's point about how little we differ genetically from yeast). The inevitable intervention into our genetic constitution therefore requires rigorous reflection on the meaning of a gene and the human genome, rather than on whether we should go forward with mapping and subsequent engineering. A realistic ethics of science will avoid both sociobiology as just another meta-narrative and moral hand-wringing as juvenile self-denial. Instead, it will address the moral, political, and material conditions of this new advance in knowledge and its claims to power. And it will recognize that Western humanity has been engaged in its own self-production through labor, language, and, for some time now, genetic manipulation. While there is, of course, a justifiable discontent with the kind of power that science has given humans over other humans, there is a consolation, Rabinow argues, in the recognition of both the limits of science and its role in fostering our growing maturity. Indeed, herein lies a more consoling thought than the illusory belief in a static human nature. True enlightenment, harsh as it may be, is an authentically adult consolation. In daring to know, Rabinow writes, science gives us real hope, not in an ultimate technical mastery of nature but in finally arriving at the awareness that we are not the center of existence or a higher kind of being free to wield our immense power, without scruple, over the rest of life.

In "Genetic Engineering and Eugenics: The Uses of History," Diane Paul explores the ways both advocates and critics of human genetic engineering turn the history of eugenics to disparate ends. Optimists and pessimists alike have adopted a narrative that emphasizes brutal measures of state control, such as the compulsory sterilization of those considered defective and the Nazi murder of mental patients. The similarity of their narratives is not a simple reflection of fixity to historical facts. On the contrary, much eugenics was voluntary, not coercive. "Positive" eugenics, which relies on the cooperation of its subjects, is necessarily so, and as an effort at improvement, much closer in spirit to human genetic engineering, with its promise (or threat) of human enhancements, including a wholesale transformation of human nature. Thus Paul asks, If one looks to history for lessons, why focus on sterilization and murder to the exclusion of other, utopian projects whose goals are much closer to contemporary aspirations to improve humanity?

As a start toward constructing a history more germane to issues arising from human genetic engineering, Paul analyzes the utopian strain in eugenics, including works by Francis Galton (in some of his moods), Alfred Russel Wallace, and such scientific socialists of the 1920s and

1930s as J. B. S. Haldane, J. D. Bernal, and H. J. Muller. She notes that Bernal's *The World, the Flesh, and the Devil: An Inquiry into the Three Enemies of the Human Soul,* which envisioned a sci-fi future of the human race divided into the masses and their scientific masters, anticipates a recent raft of similar prophecies—for example, one by German philosopher Peter Sloterdijk, who even employs Bernal's metaphor of a "human zoo," and another by U.S. biologist Lee Silver, who predicts an ultimate splitting of humanity into the "normals" and the "gen-rich." Paul looks in particular detail at Haldane's 1923 *Daedalus,* which prefigures almost every aspect of the contemporary debate over human genetic engineering, including the famous "wisdom of repugnance" argument associated with bioethicist Leon Kass. She also notes that as Marxists, Haldane, Bernal, Muller, and Trotsky emphasized the human capacity for self-transformation, rejecting the idea that there was an immutable human nature exempt in its sacredness from genetic intervention. Paul extends the analysis of arguments about improving human nature through the 1960s and 1970s, when the morality of genetic engineering was first hotly contested.

Given the rich history of projects to redesign humanity, why do both the celebrants of human genetic engineering and those more impressed by its dangers constantly invoke a history of eugenics told as a story of brutal state action to cull the unfit, and thus maintain the status quo? Paul argues that enthusiasts savor the evident libertarian moral: If a central wrong of eugenics was the use of coercion, then leaving people free to make their own reproductive decisions seems an obvious way to avoid the mistakes of the past. But the nightmare of those who worry about where human genetic engineering may lead is hardly an authoritarian state intent on forcing parents to design their offspring. Quite to the contrary, it is a world in which those parents demand the right to use the available reproductive technologies. Thus it is a privatized, consumer-oriented eugenics they fear, a eugenics directed by the market and not by the state. Given the perceived source of danger, the solution cannot be a laissez-faire approach toward the new technologies. Yet this is the direction in which the standard narratives point.

Critics favor oversight of human genetic engineering because they believe that even libertarian eugenics has consequences that should concern us all. Invoking Nazis lends an emotional charge to their claims, but it also misleads in ways that are counterproductive to the larger agenda. Critics favor some kind of regulatory oversight out of misgivings detailed by Paul in her essay; they include the impact of genetic manipulations on parent-child relationships, assumptions about human worth, and attitudes toward individuals with disabilities. Notwithstanding these and other worries, Paul notes that the exigencies of abortion politics have made it difficult for those on the political Left to call for curbs on consumer sovereignty in the realm of reproduction. In her view, some oversight (along the lines proposed by LeRoy Walters elsewhere in this volume) is badly needed. Yet to establish a degree of social control over genetic engineering, it will first be necessary to acknowledge that the principle of respect for autonomy is not absolute.

For a theologically based thinker like Jean Bethke Elshtain, abandonment of the idea of an unalterable human nature presents serious ethical difficulties. In "The Body and the Quest for Control," Elshtain argues for a moral standard rooted in our bodily nature and the order of creation itself. While she is not opposed to gene therapy or medical attempts to alleviate suffering where reasonably possible, genetic engineering and cloning are from the standpoint of one committed to a Christian anthropology merely the latest manifestations of a "messianic project" to perfect the human body and overcome human finitude. This project, moreover, is based on a false sense of freedom and a misconception of the self as radically autonomous. Indeed, all signs, as Elshtain reads them, point to a culture that has reduced the body to a commodity malleable in the hands of modern technique and constructable by a technocratic elite. Citing Martin Luther, she traces this reductionism to a rebellious willfulness that separates us from God, the "source of undistorted love," and from a natural order given in advance as a moral and theological compass whose dismissal is now apparent in a number of technological projects such as genetic screening, prenatal testing, abortion on demand, and cloning. Such projects, she writes, have at their core an ideal of bodily perfection demeaning to the disabled and the "developmentally different" among us. Thus, the flight from finitude results in a slippery slope that ultimately narrows our concept of humanness in light of culturally fleeting notions of normality.

Tying these various projects together, in Elshtain's view, is a fundamental rejection of the sphere of the "unchosen" and a concomitant enlargement of the sphere of "control-over" (her example here is the elimination of Down syndrome as an acceptable human type). But even more important is what underlies this urge to dominate the corporeal world—namely, the unstated though powerful theological presumption that nothing in God's original creation is good, but rather that everything must be redeemed and transformed according to images that reinforce the dominant cultural ideals, most especially the notion that it is culture itself (and not nature) that now generates our moral ideals and projects. It is for this reason that Elshtain believes it impossible to overstate the significance of the technocratic mentality of our time and, in particular, the growing sense that we are duty bound to exercise control over our descendants, including deciding which culturally determined types of humans should be allowed to exist at all. The goal in all this is the elimination of imperfection, inconvenience, and risk; and the danger of this denial of our essential finitude is a moral one, since it goes to the heart of human nature as well as to the very meaning and being of such a thing as nature at all.

What is lacking in this denial is an appropriate ontological understanding of the human body and its centrality to our humanness and genuine exercise of freedom. Specifically, an ontology grounded in our Jewish and Christian traditions teaches us that embodiment is a given, not a construction or cultural product, of human being itself, and that any conception of human freedom grows out of the basic indeterminacy of this embodiment as an image but not a replication of God's perfection. What is more, this limited freedom exists only in relationship, not in a radical autonomy disconnected from the creation and its existential demands. Sin is thus understood by Elshtain as the abuse of this freedom, and its expression today is to be found in the enhancement of human power over the creaturely world—an enhancement that predicates itself on the rejection of a natural order of things and the situatedness of the human being in the world through its body. But the proper use of this freedom, Elshtain maintains, arises from a moral understanding of nature where the very givenness of creation serves as a standard against which we might measure the claims and pretensions of whatever Platonic cave we happen to inhabit. The freedom of finitude, in other words, can bring us back from our absorption in the world, providing a perspective on our culture and history from which we might imagine alternative possibilities; whereas its denial can only result in our incapacity to effect change within the boundaries of our situation.

Clearly, Elshtain sees a threat to our humanness in the notion that "creation itself must be put right." Remove the idea that nature is a given and you destroy the time-honored belief that moral norms and standards exist outside of cultural prejudice and power plays. Eliminate the fact of a natural order, with all its imperfection and disappointment, and you erode what tolerance we have left for difference and unpredictability. Elshtain singles out the technology of cloning as indicative of our desire for control and sameness, and hence of our fear of the Other. As a significant part of the eugenics project to exert full authority over human reproductive material, cloning represents an anthropocentrism antithetical to natural diversity and, even more disturbing, to the Judeo-Christian ontology of creation that underpins our conviction that nature is good regardless of whether it serves our needs or not. As Genesis shows, such an ontology provides us with a story of our origins, a story that roots human freedom in the body and human will in the creation. An unbounded will is thus a will that respects neither life nor the givenness of our humanity. The will toward the unnatural, Elshtain argues, is in the end what connects genetic engineering and cloning to euthanasia, abortion, physician-assisted suicide, capital punishment, and even slavery, torture, and deportations. Needed, then, in our "world of rootless wills" is a Christian theological anthropology that can at once revivify the categories of nature and human finitude, and debunk the constructs of a culture that denies that naturalness in the name of ontological sameness and the prideful idea of human perfectibility.

Richard Zaner's "Visions and Re-visions: Life and the Accident of Birth" also explores the potential impact of genetic engineering and cloning on our understanding of the human body, particularly the body's role in the constitution of self-identity. Echoing Elshtain, Zaner reminds us that even today, most of the world remains a given and not a construction of modern technology or social theorists. Moreover, he cautions that many technological deeds, especially in the area of biomedical research, have gone awry, confounding the best of intentions. Zaner thus points to the thorny problems of chance and control as well as to the questionableness of culturally constructed notions of normalcy and illness as keys to an understanding of the underlying difficulties genetic engineering poses. Since such an understanding requires an act of imagination concerning our future, Zaner turns to a recent novel, Simon Mawer's *Mendel's Dwarf*, and the story of Ben, a geneticist and descendant of Gregor Mendel who happens to be a dwarf and the father (through in vitro fertilization) of eight embryos, four of which he determines to be protodwarfs. Ben is faced with the decision of whether to remove the "dwarf gene" from the four "mutants" (in effect denying his own selfhood) or to buck the reigning social yardstick of normalcy and affirm his own embodiment as central to who he is. At issue here is the philosophical concern with self-identity and whatever role the body plays in resolving this question.

As Zaner rightly observes, because traditional medicine has almost always recognized restoration as an inherent limit, it therefore cannot judge Ben to be defective and in need of improvement. And yet, at the same time, Ben himself knows that he is different and suffers his otherness acutely, for he now exists in a world where the boundaries of restorative medicine have been stretched by the mapping of the human genome to include genetic enhancement as measured against socially defined norms and ideals. Thus have molecular biology and the technique of cloning already brought into question the meaning of health and disease, not to mention medicine itself, precisely through a blurring of the formerly unassailable distinction between culture and nature. Indeed, in the world of post-Mendelian genetics, nothing is unthinkable, and everything now seems possible, if not desirable. The venerable adage "Do no harm" increasingly fails to measure up to the brave new reality we find ourselves in, as evidenced, for example, by the disturbing need for patient consent in most scientific experimentation on human subjects. The result, Zaner fears, is a situation where we now deem the handicapped to be certifiable freaks and hence, not being fully human, in need of a medical fix. And lurking in the background, if this were not troubling enough, is the very real possibility of a technocratic elite who, under the cloak of treating disease, will in fact be tempted to institute a political agenda through a eugenics aimed at redirecting nothing less than human evolution itself. As a philosopher, Zaner wants to direct our attention to the heart of this scandal, namely, the paucity of wisdom so characteristic of the technocratic mind, an appalling ignorance, moreover, which is the direct result of the naturalization of consciousness inherent in any reduction of our humanness to DNA. Here, he concludes, theory and practice will inevitably reinforce one another in a downward spiral into the nightmare of nihilism.

Underlying these moral and political consequences is the even more difficult problem of human identity, of "whether there is a self at all" or simply "genetic information encoded in and on strands of DNA/RNA nestled within any individual's body cells." In wrestling with this question, Zaner appeals to the attempt by the twentieth-century phenomenologist Alfred Schutz to ground our humanity in our sociality, and to further ground that sociality in the "primal . . . we-relationship" of mother and fetus and the experience shared by all human beings of being born. Zaner interprets Schutz to mean here that humanness is a gift, perhaps the "originary gift," since we are brought into this world through the love of a woman and not through any choice of our own. The very mystery of being born—and hence, the lack of any apparent reason for our existence—returns Zaner's meditation on embodiment to Ben's dilemma and the threat genetic control poses to that mystery, that is, to the gratuitous character of our being as the very source of our humanity. Zaner is thus led to the conclusion that one's uniqueness as a person, grounded in the accident of birth and in particular birth by a woman, has been placed in question by both the control promised by the imminent technology of human cloning and the bewildering choices it now presents to us. To be sure, Zaner admits, this technique is in essence no different than in vitro fertilization. Thus, the real question becomes whether the cloned embryo is implanted in an actual human womb or an artificial uterus. The issue of our humanness, in other words, is one of development: "to be human is to become human." And that means to be socialized by the primal other—one's mother. Clearly, for Zaner, socialization (and by implication humanization) is primordially a bodily experience. To contravene this biological attachment of the fetus to its mother is to thwart the givenness of who and what we are. Significantly, it is only on these grounds that Zaner parts company with thinkers like Elshtain and their blanket rejection of human cloning. The danger of this looming technology is thus not so much to the uniqueness of the clone but more profoundly to its biological link to a primal other constitutive of its identity as a person.

Nonetheless, Zaner urges caution and vigilance regarding cloning, and argues that the asymmetrical power now placed in the hands of the medical establishment ought to transform the definition of medical wisdom into one of judicious restraint. Such humility, he believes, can be fostered primarily by serious reflection on the fact of being born and borne by woman, and the relevance of that to our humanness. Seen in this light, one's world—that is to say, the culture into which one is born—is also gifted in the form of an existence unconditionally bequeathed to one by one's mother. To preserve, then, both the idea and the reality of the gift and givenness is in the end to save the mystery of being born at this time, in this place, to this particular mother, family, society, and so on. By inscribing our self-identity in embodiment, Zaner seeks to delimit the human condition precisely in our being subject to chance and an inability to find a "firmer footing" in existence. In doing so, he throws up a metaphysical and perhaps even religious challenge to the current technological impetus toward control and the elimination of randomness and indeterminacy. More positively, he argues for a recognition of finitude as the first step in the affirmation of embodiment as the essential link to others—a link that with all its imperfection and uncertainty, is ignored at the expense of our selfhood and whatever meaning the human condition might have in a world where traditional metaphysical answers no longer pack the force they once had before the advent of the technological imperative.

Harold Baillie's chapter "Aristotle and Genetic Engineering: The Uncertainty of Excellence" raises the question of uncertainty in discussions of both genetic engineering and human nature. He begins by noting that ethics is in a sense tragic, as it reflects on past events with only a slight ability to anticipate or predict. Particularly with genetic engineering, the pace of change and the newness of the results threaten to leave ethics, at least in the sense developed by Lisa Sowle Cahill and LeRoy Walters later in this volume, reflecting on a series of fait accompli. Given this implicit criticism of social theory and utilitarianism as approaches to the evaluation of genetic engineering, Baillie turns to the traditional distinction between genetic therapy and genetic enhancement, which he suggests is inadequate to establish any clear understanding of, much less limits to, the possibilities of genetic engineering. The slippery slope he sees linking therapy and enhancement can only be avoided by a refocusing of the discussion of genetics as engineering—that is, of the possibilities of technology and control—to an examination of the metaphysical roots of personhood.

He argues that two traditional understandings of the person cast no light directly on the ethics of genetic science. Descartes' dualism, as in the second and sixth of his *Meditations on First Philosophy*, fails to be useful in addressing genetics because it suggests that the soul, or res cogitans, exists utterly independently of the body. Thus, modifications of the body (for example, the improvements in the health of the body called for in the *Discourse on Method*) can improve the situation of the soul, even its wisdom, without altering its nature. Second, Jean-Jacques Rousseau's sense of freedom as the ability to imitate and change leaves open the questions of limits to that change. Fundamental to Rousseau's position is the suggestion that we have already significantly altered our nature simply by joining society, so there is no inherent objection to further changes. Freedom does not in principle suffer from genetic engineering, nor does it offer any guidance to a discussion of the appropriateness of genetic change in general or specific forms of it.

Baillie then attempts a more positive discussion of the issue by turning to Aristotle's hylomorphism. Like Tom Shannon's effort in this volume at ressourcement, Baillie suggests that a rereading of hylomorphism may help in the discussion of embodiment and the impact that genetic engineering can have on the person. He identifies *person* with the actuality of a body with organs, a "possession" of the body by its own being. This actuality is both the cause of the unity of the parts of the body and the result of this unity. As such, the position avoids the freedom-materialism distinction, or the soul/body distinction, by seeing the relationship as a vertical one of potentiality and actuality. What the person is, is identified by what the person consists of, and what the person does with that what. This is the ground for Baillie's distinction between freedom and serendipity. Freedom tends to be understood as unidirectional. Rousseau, for example, orients freedom to the possibilities opened by imitation, and neglects the material source of those possibilities. In contrast, serendipity is the response of the person to his or her embodiment, a response made possible by the body itself. Thus, the person goes beyond the body by making more of the body than it is. The life activity of a body always comes as a surprise, in essence, a discovery.

Baillie uses this sense of life as a discovery to argue against any position that presents life as a plan, something that is "known and recognized," or at least whose basic capabilities are known and recognized. For example, John Rawls's suggestion that because of the natural lottery people can be unfairly disadvantaged, presumes a given collection of natural abilities, the absence or degradation of which is a problem of nature that society has an obligation to correct. This position encourages genetic therapy, as well perhaps as genetic engineering, as a likely extension of this social obligation. Rawlsian limits on this would be due to other problems of social justice—that is, the equal protection of rights or a fair distribution of resources—not because of any interference with human nature.

Baillie argues against this abandonment of the discussion of human nature in favor of issues of social justice. His hylomorphic view of human nature does generate adequate content to critique genetic engineering before later limiting conditions of social justice appear. As a critique, he claims "the focus of genetic engineering is the body actualized. . . . [I]t seeks to eliminate the need for a soul by substituting a developed genetic code for the serendipity of the soul." Genetic engineering, whether in the form of therapy or enhancement, seeks to substitute control of the body for surprise by the soul. This substitution of controlled genetic code for the soul makes impossible the discovery of the self by taking away the only means by which the self is discovered: a life in which serendipity (no matter what the occasion) can occur. It is not that we know the person and know the effects that genetic engineering will have; it is rather that genetic engineering will make it impossible to be a person. The substitution of control for spontaneity is ultimately the basis of his critique of genetic engineering.

Robert Proctor is a historian of science and technology. His approach to the question of the future of human nature reflects a historian's preference: he looks back. Specifically, he looks back at the paleontological record of human diversity to illustrate the difficulties in arriving at a clear sense of what is "fully human." His reflection on this record leads to several observations. Humanness is a recent phenomenon (dating back between 150,000 and 50,000 years), and in general the attribution of humanness is a bit faddish—or at least influenced by the concerns of the times. For the purposes of his discussion, Proctor equates humanness with language and culture, attributes that do not require a fixed human essence but do seem to argue for an identifiable human condition—that is, for a set of limits within which human life has historically functioned. But his concern is not to define humanness so much as to observe the disputes that have altered the dating of the attribution of humanness. This dating has recently gone through three crises, in archaeology, paleontology, and molecular anthropology, and the core of Proctor's chapter is a review of each.

In archaeology, the crisis has been over the interpretation of the oldest tools, those found in the Oldowan Gorge in Kenya and, of particular interest to Proctor, in St. Acheul, northwest of Paris. These tools tend to be uniform in style and manufacture for vast stretches of time, and their use seems to cross different hominid species during that time. This suggests that these tools are not necessarily the indicators of human culture they have been taken for since their endurance does not seem to depend on the transmission of knowledge of their use by symbolic language. The second crisis is in paleontology, where it has been discovered "that more than one species of hominid must have coexisted at many points in the course of hominid evolution." The recognition of this diversity has implications for our understanding of the politics of doing science since this question of diversity was submerged in our concern to deny the category of race, as in, for example, the 1952 United Nations Educational, Scientific, and Culture Organization (UNESCO) "Statement on Race." Finally, there is the crisis in molecular anthropology, arising from the discovery that all living humans share a common ancestor from Africa approximately 135,000 years ago. This not only points to human recency, but it also emphasizes the unity of the surviving species.

Proctor suggests that "if evolution has taught us anything, it is that there is no essence of humanity, no fixed form." But he is also concerned to point out that political goodwill can stifle science, which points to the larger issue of whether the ethics and politics of genetic engineering can be considered in isolation from the question of what constitutes our humanness. The UNESCO "Statement on Race" denounced racial theory and racial prejudice, but it accomplished this political good on the basis of a conception of the unity of hominid development—the only significant diversity was the hominid split from apes, perhaps eleven or twelve million years ago—that slowed the recognition both of hominid diversity and human recency. Proctor's conclusion is to endorse "hominid bushiness," a recognition of the variation in the evolution of hominids, and that "the prehistory of tools, bodies, and beliefs will forever remain a fertile field for projection and wishful thinking." In a concluding note, Proctor suggests that humanness is a linguistic concept, opening the possibility that other language-using creature or machines might be considered human. But at this stage in the development of our understanding of the relationship between human nature and genetic knowledge, the tale of hominid bushiness is primarily a cautionary one about exclusion.

While Proctor's chapter is a call to caution about bold claims regarding the nature of our physical inheritance, Tom Shannon's is a more aggressive argument against using materialist reductionism to limit the range of discussion about human nature. He finds this error in two of the major voices in the current literature on genetics and human nature: Richard Dawkins and E. O. Wilson. A theologian, Shannon's contention is that reality itself is ambiguous enough to be open to the possibilities of transcendence that go beyond the arguments of scientific materialism, but do not stand independent of contemporary genetic information. There are three foundation stones for his argument. He is concerned with scientific reductionism and its contrast with the larger question of the relationship between the parts and the whole. He uses the method of ressourcement, part of the Roman Catholic tradition of reappropriating concepts and ideas from the tradition for contemporary discussions. Finally, he is concerned with the limitations of our current genetic knowledge and the temptation to overestimate the clarity our limited knowledge has provided us, a point of significant concern with regard to sociobiology. In particular, Shannon focuses on John Duns Scotus's distinction between *affectio commodi* and *affectio justitiae* to illustrate the openness of human nature to transcendence, particularly its ability to transcend itself as part of nature. Shannon contrasts this approach to the difficulties Dawkins and Wilson experience when attempting to explain altruistic behavior and, more generally, our ability to resist the apparent genetic-based tendencies of our nature.

For Duns Scotus, *affectio commodi* is a drive rooted in the nature of the individual entity "to seek his perfection and happiness in all he does." Shannon identifies this with Dawkins's and Wilson's "genetic selfishness," and points out that for Duns Scotus this self-interest of a divine creation was good, while Dawkins and Wilson are ambivalent about this wellspring of evolutionary development. Duns Scotus's conception of *affectio justitiae* refers to an "inclination to seek the good in itself"; it is, in other words, "the means by which we can transcend nature and go beyond our individually defined good and ourselves to see the value of another being." While Duns Scotus sees this as a fundamental human inclination, Wilson and Dawkins struggle with the phenomenon and find no clear explanation. Duns Scotus is able to speak of the human will as free and as oriented to a transcendent good that allows it to act unnaturally—that is, to transcend its own nature. The materialism of the sociobiological position must find a purely naturalistic position and, Shannon argues, stumbles in the effort. This added dimension of Duns Scotus's account is a central example of the advantages of ressourcement for Shannon. It also illustrates the larger philosophical problem at stake here: Is there a need to understand the larger phenomena, that is, understand what they are, before we begin to locate the phenomena's material conditions? For example, we need to understand in some sense what memory is before we go looking for its "place" in the brain, or we need to understand what altruism is before we look to see its genetic basis.

The discussion is, in essence, about the contrast between materialism and freedom, and the adequacy of each in explaining the phenomenon of human life. But our knowledge of genetics reinvigorates another traditional discussion, that of nature and grace. Genetics reminds us that nature is not abandoned, and thus cannot be ignored, in the full expression of a human life. Shannon quotes Lindon Eaves and Lora Gross to sum up the theological implications of his argument: "Genetics provides *a basis for grace within the structure of life itself.*" Matter must be taken seriously even while it cannot be taken as providing the entire explanation.

Clearly, for Shannon, the discussion of freedom illuminates the orientation of human nature toward the transcendent, leaving unanswered the question of the relationship between transcendence and genetic engineering. Genetic engineering can be seen as an expression of transcendence and freedom, one that should be tempered by the inconsistent rhetoric of materialist explanations of human life and existence. Bernard

Rollin addresses this question of transcendence and materialism by introducing the notion of telos as a starting point for parsing out acceptable and unacceptable genetic manipulation. In his chapter *"Telos*, Value, and Genetic Engineering," Rollin starts with Aristotelian insights regarding telos, and argues for a distinction between "is" and "ought" that would reveal ethically acceptable and unacceptable forms of genetic engineering. His chapter falls into two sections. The first deals with establishing a contemporary understanding of telos, rooted in Aristotle's metaphysical concern with individuals, while the second uses this understanding to tease apart two sets of concerns with human nature: the biological and the social.

A short introductory section endorses the Aristotelian love of the world we live in and suggests that Aristotle's understanding of biology as the master science avoids many of the difficulties to which the Cartesian mechanistic view of the world, with physics as the master science, falls prey. He echoes Shannon and several others in his more traditional sense that we have an access to nature that can guide us (somewhat) in these discussions. But as his analysis of animal telos makes clear, nature can be surprisingly flexible.

In the first section of his chapter, Rollin notes that telos refers to a thing's nature, particularly its needs and interests that constitute its nature. Articulating these needs and interests allows us to see how each living thing responds to the challenges of living. Aristotle developed telos into the ground for an ethic for human beings, but did not extend this to the animal world. Yet Aristotle did see continuity between the animal and the human worlds, particularly with regard to the similarities in the use of slaves and domesticated animals. Rollin ties this similarity to the issue of husbandry, the practical obligations humans have to their animals because "domestic animals existed in a state of symbiotic unity with their human owners." For animals to survive, thrive, and fulfill their domestic function, owners had serious responsibilities to care for their animals, as in the biblical notion of the shepherd. The nature of animals required a connection between their well-being and their successful domesticated use. When the notion of husbandry was replaced by industry, the connection between animals' well-being and their successful use was severed. Industry is able to use a variety of technologies to ensure that animals are successfully manipulated to meet human needs, but these technologies and their results are independent of, and generally insensitive to, the telos of animals.

The use of the concept of telos with regard to human beings creates difficulties for the obvious reason that the "plasticity" in human nature, its rationality and sociality, dramatically overshadow the relatively focused biological component. Rollin examines this plasticity and concludes that "rationality and sociality are highly variegated in their instantiation, and to attempt to create a descriptive account that does justice to all of their differing manifestations would seem to be impossible. For this reason, the notions of 'is' and 'ought' seem to be much more closely connected in a teleological worldview than in a mechanistic one." Rollin's argument rests on this sharp distinction between biological or animal telos and human telos. Animal telos functions as a basis for husbandry and for a critique of current industrial practices. This extends to humans, with regard to our principally biological functions. Thus, the general practice of medicine and future possibilities of genetic therapy are acceptable to Rollin, as they focus on the biology of the human telos. But human telos, properly speaking, involves "rationality, sociality, moral concern, and so forth," issues about which no precise description of "what we ought to strive for" can be provided. Here, we cannot change what is without altering what ought to be. "Efficiency, productivity, wealth—none of these trump reason and autonomy, and thus the *Brave New World* scenario is deemed unacceptable." That is, we should never accept any form of genetic engineering that would alter these central human concerns.

One implication of this distinction is that it would be allowable to genetically alter an animal to change its (biological) telos and, in so doing, make it more productive or more suited to an efficient environment. We could engineer a legless, blind chicken that would not suffer if raised in a battery cage. But we ought not fundamentally alter the human telos of a human being in any analogous way. Rollin argues that the key unalterable elements in human beings are "traits in people that would radically separate them from the companionship of other humans," such as immortality, living underwater, or abnormal size. Only therapeutic interventions, including both somatic and (preferably) genomic efforts, would be acceptable. Rollin is aware that there would be difficulties at the boundaries between a human's biological telos (and what might count as a disease or correctable condition) and a human telos (and thus what counts as suitable for companionship). He thinks that these ambiguities should be settled politically.

Lisa Cahill's "Nature, Sin, and Society" is an exploration of the concerns regarding genetic research and engineering from the perspective of theological ethics. Echoing Elshtain, she asserts that traditional, theological understandings of human nature carry the resources to respond to current concerns with genetic work, and in particular these resources call for serious limitations. Her argument, however, is not an intrinsicist or essentialist one; rather, it springs from the focus of Catholic social teaching on the social and political nature of human beings. Thus, her primary concern is with social justice and the social context within which the results of genetic work will be expressed and manipulated. Like Rollin, she is optimistic that not only are limits on genetic work necessary and desirable but indeed they are possible.

Cahill's starting point is Catholic social teaching, particularly that tradition that began with Pope Leo XIII's encyclical *Rerum Novarum* (*On the Condition of Labor*), and that has been developed and expanded in a variety of encyclicals by Pope John Paul II. The well-known elements of that position include an appeal to objective and universal standards of behavior, human solidarity, a trust in the "human propensity for cooperative social living," and "imaginative empathy with our fellow human beings" enlivened by biblical symbols and commands. Generally speaking, there is a common good that draws human beings together, both in individual societies and ultimately in a global community.

Important to Cahill's ultimate position is the moderation of Catholic social "optimism" by a discussion of Reinhold Niebuhr's "Christian realism." Neibuhr suggests that in the tension between human freedom and human finitude resides human sin, a problem less manageable on the social level than it is for the individual. The pride and sensuality that arises from sin is structuralized in society, and acts much more powerfully as a force for division and conflict. For Neibuhr, coercion is a necessary element of social ethics, enforcing reasonableness on society and its members. Cahill finds this darker picture a needed corrective to the "encyclical tradition's nonconflictual social optimism."

Cahill then concludes her argument with a critique of global capitalism, particularly the waning power of the liberal welfare state in the face of international capital and the impact of international patents that exacerbate differences between the rich and the poor. Her chapter ends on an optimistic note, as she cites the examples of a variety of international organizations working to establish hedges against international capital in favor of a renewed sense of the common good. She suggests that these efforts, such as those by Oxfam or the pharmaceutical company Cipla, Ltd., or even China's State Council, are limitations on foreign-funded genetic research, and are hopeful indications that genetic research and engineering can be limited and guided by an internationally shared sense of the common human good. Thus, Cahill, like Rollin and Langdon Winner, looks to a political and institutional solution to the questions of genetic engineering. Insights offered by the tradition may be helpful in such discussions, but those insights are not metaphysically compelling and cannot be relied on to answer practical questions in a pluralistic world. Only a shift in discussion to the social conditions of humans can provide the resources to work out acceptable principles of guidance for the opportunities offered by genetic engineering.

LeRoy Walters's "Human Genetic Intervention: Past, Present, and Future" is a review and analysis of the fortunes of federal oversight of human-gene-transfer research by the Recombinant DNA Advisory Committee (RAC) within the National Institutes for Health (NIH). Walters summarizes the past, present, and future prospects of the RAC, tracking its bureaucratic fortunes and the parallel problems of oversight regarding cutting-edge—and dangerous-human-gene-transfer research. He then gives an account of the degeneration of the RAC, originally formed as a proactive group of research academics to foster the public transparency of research and standards of evaluation, to provide anticipatory oversight for researchers, and to develop clear and current research guidelines. He argues that when policy makers at the NIH and the Food and Drug Administration (FDA) weakened the RAC in 1996–97, genetic researchers and their financial backers began to operate with increasing secrecy. The loss of transparency led to a refusal to disclose adverse results, a loss of objectivity in planning research projects, self-interested manipulation of results, a failure to submit full and timely reports of progress and difficulties, and ultimately to the death of a patient.

Walters is well aware that the RAC was not without its detractors and inherent difficulties. Indeed, the difficulties inspired the attention from policy makers that led to the changes in the size and functioning of the RAC and in its relations with the NIH and the FDA. Yet when he turns his attention to the future of human-gene-transfer research, Walters endorses several steps that perhaps do not require a RAC but nevertheless call for procedures and duties that were very much like the RAC's original tasks. His recommendations are in response to both the changes in research funding and the now tragically obvious insufficiencies regarding oversight of clinical research. These are reforms that must occur at both the local and the national levels, and call for greater cooperation and integration of these two levels. Walters remains convinced that the regulatory opportunities of government can adequately identify limits for genetic research and protect both research subjects and scientific integrity. Much like Cahill, he relies on the fundamental authority and goodness of the social nature of human beings to protect us from not only the excesses of research process but also the vainglory of research ambition.

Like Cahill and Winner, Walters is concerned primarily with the social structures that will limit and guide genetic research. He seems confident that proper procedures will allow for both adequate public discussion of the direction such research should take and high ethical standards to protect research subjects and the integrity of the research itself. Ideally, science should be allowed to pursue its own research agenda, and to ensure this, science must be protected from such nonscientific factors as the market concerns of funding sources and the unabashed enthusiasm of researchers.

Langdon Winner writes from a humanistic tradition suspicious of the technological domination of nature and its more recent attempts to turn modern techniques against humanity itself. His chapter "Resistance Is Futile: The Posthuman Condition and Its Advocates" marvels not so much at the fact that the dire predictions of the Jacques Elluls and Lewis Mumfords concerning technology might still come to pass but that their fulfillment is embraced by some with such enthusiasm and fascination. While Winner admits that most of us have yet to join the chorus singing the praises of a posthuman future, he is nonetheless troubled by the potential influence the "scientific enthusiasts of posthumanism" might wield in the not-too-distant future. With this in mind, he reviews for us the latest literature in this genre, subjecting it to a searching critique. Of particular interest are the predictions of such futurists as Gregory Stock, Lee Silver, and Hans Moravec of a posthuman, Nietzschean world where humans have either been divided into "superior and inferior genetic classes" or, what is perhaps more probable, surpassed and made obsolete by "robotic decision makers." But more important here than the actual predictions is the prevailing view of human nature among these prognosticators. As Winner makes clear, their extrapolations stem from a commonly held belief that our "stone-age biology," to cite Moravec, has already been superseded in the information age. The idea, then, that humans might be technologically reconstructed or pushed aside has already moved from the realm of science fiction into a world where the appeal of a posthuman future runs the gamut from profit to fame to simple adventurousness. At the forefront of such thinking are groups like The World Transhumanist Association, The Extropy Institute, and, of course, the Raelians, all of which advocate the transformation of humans from organic to mechanical beings for the purposes of abolishing death and illness and of ushering in an age where everyone has been cosmetically refashioned and groomed for success.

The rejection of the givenness of our biological makeup, Winner correctly notes, finds its apotheosis today in the idea of the cyborg: that amalgam of human biology and technological hardware now so familiar to us from a slew of movies and pulp fiction. Winner points out that the desirability of this posthuman creature is in fact gaining traction in academic circles and especially in the social sciences. For it is there that the hoary concept of a "stable, coherent" human nature (and all its ethical and political implications) has finally given way to all forms of theoretical and social constructionism. In short, among our university elites, nothing now stands in the way of seriously considering the merging of our bodies with technical devices. Winner traces the breakdown in this metaphysical belief in a fixed human essence to the Marxist definition of humans as the toolmaking animal and, later, to the engineering-inspired notion that our technologies are really nothing more than "powerful extensions" of our organs. Over the last century, both ideas have come together to argue for technology as the central fact of human existence, elevating the goals of dominating nature and removing biological limitations to a status unknown in the premodern world. The emergence, then, of the ideal of a cyborg, a hybrid of the human and the technological, is not surprising. And yet, with this hybrid we have moved beyond both Marxist and engineering kinds of humanism. For in creating cyborgs, we will not just make technology, we will become it. Technology will no longer function as an extension of our physical capabilities but will actually constitute them. Here, Winner observes, the tendency in the social sciences to no longer recognize the traditional distance between culture/artifice and nature/biology serves as a powerful underpinning to the desirability of replacing humans with manufactured hybrids.

While applauding the undoubtedly positive ethical and political aspects of social constructionism in helping us detect the strategies of domination and marginalization in many appeals to the "natural," Winner admonishes against a too hasty embrace of these entities. Citing the work of Donna Haraway, he observes that proponents of hybridization are more prone "to generate a collection of moral sentiments" than arguments that lead to "explicit ethical commitments." Moreover, their attempts to denigrate the supposed integrity of natural things, while clothed in progressive sensibilities and liberal convictions, fail in the end to address the challenge of biotechnology and its possible violation of a natural order that exists beyond human influence or control. And finally, Winner worries over the conflation of a leftist social constructionism with "the work of radical reconstruction and recapitalization at stake in today's technical and corporate realms." In effect, Winner reaffirms Zaner's and Elshtain's essential presupposition: that most of the world remains a place, not of human making, but of things—including humans—that are simply given. But in doing so, he extends their arguments by raising the question of whether genetic engineering is the appropriate tool to address the injustice that always accompanies the world in its imperfect givenness. Might, he asks, an engineering approach to all our problems actually subvert the claims of justice by refusing to simply let beings be?

Winner is thus anxious to expand the question of human nature and genetic engineering to include its moral and political aspects. Progressives have traditionally focused on institutional change and a critique of political life. But this template is now being challenged by the seemingly more rational prospect of biological transformation, especially at the genetic level. Aside from the disturbing question of the justice of employing such means, Winner leaves us with the practical fear concerning the untold consequences that will follow from our abandonment of a political theory and praxis focused on social structures and their capacity for oppression, including those that result from modern technoscience itself.

And so we are left to contemplate a paradox. There is little doubt that humans as humans—whatever in the traditional sense that means—have a long and storied history of wondering and tinkering with our understanding of our abilities and place in the world. This history has brought us astonishing accomplishments, and now has brought us even to the brink of altering our own nature. Yet, at what many see to be the moment of our highest accomplishments, we find animating the turn toward hybrids and cyborgs an impatience with the merely human—that is, with a being whose biological limitations seem to be at the root of so much violence, suffering, and unhappiness. In the final analysis, the challenge raised by the question of this book is quite possibly a weariness with the human condition itself.

I
Historical Perspectives

2

Nature, Technology, and the Emergence of Cybernetic Humanity

Timothy K. Casey

We have modified our environment so radically that we must now modify ourselves in order to exist in this new environment.
—Norbert Wiener

Even as we stand on the threshold of the permanent alteration of the human genome and what many consider to be the final chapter in the Western subjugation of nature for human ends, the problem of the natural and our relation to it is far from settled. Admittedly, there are many who think it has been settled, whether from philosophical complacency or a positivism that simply refuses to entertain anything that smacks of metaphysics. But the questions ultimately raised by genetic engineering itself and the prospect of constructing our bodies and the bodies of future human beings are ones that go to the heart of our humanness and place in the larger scheme of things, and thus can be ignored only at our peril. And yet, what are we to make of a rethinking of such perennial philosophical questions that hardly seems able to keep pace with the discoveries and technical advances we read about daily in newspapers and magazines? How are we to ponder a living phenomenon that is being invented as we think? Caught up as we unavoidably are in the swirl of events, it becomes apparent that any chance of discerning the meaning and direction of it all requires a perspective and hence a distance that perhaps only history can provide. As radical and novel a concept as genetic engineering is, even in comparison with other forms of genetic manipulation such as gene therapy and cloning, it nevertheless remains part of a tradition whose assumptions about the human and the natural continue to assert themselves and yet are easily overlooked in our fascination with the technical brilliance of this technology.

The most important elements in this tradition—important, that is, for my purposes here—are the early modern quarrel with Aristotle and his anthropomorphic conception of nature, the roots of this quarrel in medieval industrial life, and the subsequent failure of Cartesian dualism to rescue human freedom from the metaphysical determinism Descartes and others quite rightly discerned in Galilean science and its rejection of Aristotle. To keep the plot of this centuries-long story as simple as possible, the philosophical response to this dualism—which will bring us finally to the question of genetic engineering and cybernetic humanity—will be limited for the most part to the works of Karl Marx and Martin Heidegger in their attempts to twist free of Cartesianism and its false choice between a worldless idealism and a physicalism inhospitable to human autonomy and spontaneity. In opposition to the Western philosophical bias against productive praxis, a tendency that persisted even after the modern Industrial Revolution, these two seminal thinkers placed the technological mediation of human experience at the center of their thought and reflected deeply on its implications for a new understanding of our humanness. The deeper affinities existing between Marx and Heidegger, heretofore submerged in their obviously different political orientations and even conceptions of philosophy, have become clearer now that we have entered the ultimate technological frontier where we ourselves become material to be shaped and reinvented through feedback mechanisms echoing and reinscribing the Darwinian world of natural selection and adaptation. Just how we got to this point and what it means for our future is the burden of what follows.

The Medieval Prologue

Surprisingly, the technological side of our story begins in medieval Europe, where an industrial revolution more far-reaching than even that of the eighteenth and nineteenth centuries laid the groundwork for the modern scientific revolution that was soon to follow. At the outset of the Middle Ages, technology in the West lagged behind its counterpart in the East and in fact looked to it for such essential items as ivories and silks, glasswork and metalwork, and various mechanical devices like the spinning wheel. Around 800 A.D., however, there occurred in northern Europe an agricultural revolution most notable for its invention of the heavy plough, the shoulder and the tandem harness, the nailed horse-shoe, and the three-field crop rotation system. Greater agricultural pro-ductivity, as one would expect, soon led to a significant increase in population, freeing up large numbers of peasants for urban, industrial activity. Here, in this burgeoning technological milieu and time that we moderns are so accustomed to writing off as an impractical age of cathe-dral building and Scholasticism, capitalism began to germinate and the mechanization of Western technology started to take hold. Not only did the building of bigger and more durable ships in tandem with such inven-tions as the lateen sail, the magnetic compass, and the astrolabe enable the geographic discoveries and colonizations of early modernity; there also arose a more systematic approach to technological innovation as well as a new feeling for the natural world that, while not as aggressive as modern technology, certainly was indicative, in retrospect, of a coming change in attitude toward nature in the West.

As proof of such change, historians usually point to the large-scale uti-lization of nonhuman power sources such as oxen and horses, water and—with the invention of the windmill—wind power. These in their own way provided an impetus for the development of machinery and machine design in such areas as mining—with its use of geared wheels, revolving fans and bellows, and the suction pump—and the woolen industry—newly dependent on the spinning wheel, the horizontal frameloom, and the fulling mill. But probably the most far-reaching medieval inventions were the crank and the mechanical clock.[1] The crank allowed for the translation of rotary into reciprocal motion and vice versa, doubling, for example, the productivity of the spinning wheel, according to Adam Smith; whereas the clock made possible the emer-gence of a synchronized and disciplined workforce, not to mention the objectivization of time into discretely measurable units that was to prove so useful to modern physics and its mathematicization of nature. The emergence of the metaphor of the clockwork universe as early as the fourteenth century is clearly indebted to this technological development. In sum, power machinery and an increasingly mechanical disposition of nature were prevalent by the thirteen century; and by the fourteenth, the population of Europe was comfortable in the presence of this machin-ery, while the elites looked to it as central to emerging notions of mate-rial and, later, scientific progress.

None of this happened in a vacuum. As early as the seventh century, Benedictine monks initiated a postclassical reevaluation of work, endorsing simple, technological activities through the sanctification of labor as prayer (*laborare est orare*). Indeed, the origin of the mechanical clock can be traced, if Lewis Mumford is correct, to the Benedictine monasteries and the need for more precise and reliable timepieces to regulate their strictly ritualized activities twenty-four hours a day and in every season—a demand that obviously rendered the sundial and water clock insufficient. In monastic life, order and regularity constituted the external manifestation of a devotion to God, in effect raising mechanical routine to the level of a virtue. Nicholas Oresmus, a fourteenth-century philosopher, was the first to employ the clockwork metaphor for the inner workings of the universe—a metaphor that was destined to become a metaphysics that in essential respects is still with us today.

According to Lynn White Jr., the new mechanical technology took on a moral dimension as well. Pointing to the iconography of the late Middle Ages, White observes that mechanization acquired an aura of virtuousness and sacredness. The Italian depiction of temperance in particular worked its way north and became the "icon of Christian life." In one painting, striking in its symbolism, Temperance is shown atop a windmill, wearing a clock for a hat with bit and bridle in mouth and rowel spurs at her feet. In telling contrast to Christendom in the East, Latin Christianity appropriated the mechanical clock as an apt metaphor for God's orderly cosmos and thus permitted, unlike its Byzantine neighbor, the presence of astronomical clocks inside its churches. From this White, himself a Christian, conjectures that "engineering was so creative in Europe partly because it came to be more closely integrated with the ideology and ethical patterns of Latin Christianity than was the case with the technology and the dominant faith of any other major culture."[2] Central to this "ideology" was the idea of a creator-God, an architect-engineer really, who commanded humans, made in His image and likeness, to subdue nature and "complete" the original creation.[3] The necessary corollary to this religious sanction of a more mechanical and hence more powerful technology was a new feel for matter formed or created for a spiritual plan in which humanity now played a key role.[4] Out of these theological assumptions that gave voice to a new understanding of humanity's place in the world, there then grew a positive conviction regarding the dignity and spiritual value of labor, initially manifested, as mentioned earlier, in monastic life. Christian compassion, moreover, demanded the development of labor-saving devices and the cultivation of a mechanistic attitude previously maligned in Western civilization.

But why, one might ask, did this transformation not occur under the auspices of Byzantine Christianity? Why did Western technology turn when it did in a more mechanical and aggressive direction? These questions, so obviously relevant to our understanding of modern science and technology, led White to search for an explanation in the sphere of religion. From the beginning, he argues, Byzantine theology was essentially Greek in its outlook and thus oriented toward contemplation as the highest human activity and toward a conception of sin as ignorance. In contrast, Latin Christianity was born out of the voluntarism of the Roman world, emphasizing good works as a bulwark against moral evil. The voluntaristic tone of Western theology was much more apt, in White's account, to engender a spiritually sanctioned technological approach to the world than was the contemplative religiosity of the East. Although Europe was for much of the Middle Ages dependent on Byzantium (as well as Islam) for much of its technology, what it eventually did with that inheritance is unique in the history of humankind, sparking an epochal change in humanity's relation to and understanding of the natural world. It is true, of course, that by the end of the medieval period, traditional religious and philosophical convictions seemed secure. Aristotelian science in particular had been successfully adapted to a theological triumphalism to which the Stagirite would certainly have objected, but to which his thinking lent itself when placed in the right hands. In its otherworldly directedness, however, the spiritual life of Western Christianity, unlike that of the ancient Greeks, became radically interiorized, permitting medieval society to deal with external things in a secular, more utilitarian fashion. In its relative isolation from theology and science, technology was poised to develop in a more mechanical direction, and thus as a new and more powerful means to spiritual ends posited outside the sphere of its technical concerns.

Galileo and the Mechanical Tradition

The great technological innovations of the fifteenth and sixteenth centuries grew out of this medieval mechanical tradition. Leonardo da Vinci and Johannes Gutenberg were its most prominent heirs, standing on the shoulders of inventors and engineers whose names are lost to history, but whose contributions to Western scientific, technological, and economic progress are now finally being recognized.[5] And it was out of these unique circumstances that modern science emerged as well. Significantly, medieval science played no role in the creation of the new technical order, and small wonder, since as purely speculative it meticulously avoided contact with the mechanical arts. Its spirit and problems were inherited mainly from the Greeks. Galileo, the archetype of the new scientist, would change all that by joining science and the new technology in a way that would transform the West.

Both the separation of natural science from theology after Saint Thomas Aquinas and the basic principles of mechanics developed in the fifteenth century by direct and conscious analogy with machines came to fruition in the work of Galileo. In addition to producing the kind of lasting material prosperity and hence leisure we know to be a precondition for scientific research, the impact of technology on modern science was from the start multifaceted. To begin with, the new mechanical arts provided specific problems for scientists to ponder—for example, in the case of the mariner's compass and William Gilbert's theory of magnetism. The fateful connection for Galileo in this respect was between ballistics and a new understanding of motion.[6] More obviously, modern science from its inception was heavily dependent on sophisticated instruments for more precise observations and experimentation. The use of such aids as the telescope and microscope, a new hydrostatic balance, and the thermoscope and geometric compass helped establish this trend. Finally, the new technology in concert with Christian theology laid the foundation for a more aggressive attitude toward nature that looked for the first time in human history to a *systematic* exploitation of nature's powers through mechanical means. Without this fundamental shift in posture, it is difficult to imagine Galileo's positing of phenomena not found in experienced nature but rather isolated in controlled, technologically manipulated situations.

Clearly, the effect of the medieval industrial revolution on Galileo was profound. His early career, during which practical and mechanical interests predominated, demonstrates most dramatically that prior to 1600 Western technology had surpassed Western science by developing on a separate and, until recently, little noticed path. It is hardly an accident, then, that Galileo opens the *Discourses* of 1638 with an acknowledgment of his debt to the Venice arsenal—and by implication to the mechanical arts—as the source of his fascination with how things function mechanically (one is again reminded of the mechanical clock and its central place in Western culture by this time). Reflecting this essentially technological milieu, Galileo made more explicit the new "feel" for matter and motion that was, as the historian of science Herbert Butterfield puts it, "the result not of any book but of the new texture of human experience in a new age."[7] To reiterate, Galileo embodied a new breed of scientist, one who combined philosophical and mechanical interests in order to move beyond what he and others perceived to be the sterility of the speculative approach of both ancient and medieval science. This new combination, in alliance with developments in astronomy and mathematics, effectively nullified the Aristotelian conception of knowledge and its emphasis on teleological explanations and accounts. Instead, science was now limited to the search for efficient and material causes mechanically construed; and although religious aspirations initially animated the need to demonstrate the mathematical orderliness of the universe (one sees this especially in the work of Johannes Kepler), such ideals soon faded away in favor of more worldly and pragmatic motives.

Freedom and Mechanism: The Cartesian Compromise

Equally, if not more important, was the metaphysics implicit in Galileo's mathematization of nature. It fell immediately to Descartes to flesh out the meaning of this new world of mathematically determinable bodies in motion. Deeply impressed, like his contemporaries, "by lifelike clockwork mechanisms and indeed by all automation," he quickly grasped the significance of machines for a new metaphysics that would reflect and explain a world consonant with the new Galilean science.[8] Butterfield writes that René Descartes "was determined to have a science as closely knit, as regularly ordered, as any piece of mathematics—one which, so far as the material universe is concerned . . . would lay out a perfect piece of mechanism."[9] Descartes' mission was to solidify the new feel for matter in a logically consistent and cogent portrayal of the natural world as a "vast, self-contained mathematical machine, consisting of motions of matter in space and time," initiated and regulated by God, the divine clockmaker.[10] The ideal of a clockwork universe implied, among other things, the denial of any natural teleology as anthropomorphic; the positing of unobservable entities such as corpuscles or atoms as real and the demotion of perceptual qualities to, at best, useful illusions generously provided by nature to aid in our survival; and in general an idea of the natural as dead, mechanical stuff emptied of any religious, aesthetic, or moral qualities.[11] The mind (and with it all the meanings and values not amenable to quantification) was simply locked up in a small part of the brain, surrounded, if not yet engulfed, by an alien and alienating universe that could not but weaken previous convictions concerning the reality of freedom and by implication moral choice. On a theoretical level, Descartes was thus confronted with the rather daunting task of explaining and, even more important, justifying a world both invisible and in principle unlivable in human terms, a "nature," in other words, that simply does not exist from the standpoint of ordinary, perceptual experience, which until this point in time had been the basis of the Western belief in the world and humanity's place in it.

By grounding this new, theoretical nature in the consciousness of the human subject, the famous *res cogitans*, Descartes constructed a dualism between mind and matter that came to define modern philosophy in its obsession with epistemological questions, in contrast to most of ancient and medieval philosophy, which simply accepted the perceptual world as true and proceeded to fashion a whole metaphysics on the basis of this acceptance. To be fair to Descartes and his contemporaries, modern science from the beginning seemed to entail a breach between a mechanistic sphere of efficient causes and a strictly human realm of freedom directed at final causes. Complicating this picture was the inclusion, again scientific in origin, of the human body in the world-machine.[12] For here, Descartes rightly saw, was an immediate threat to human autonomy, but only insofar as knowledge was believed to begin with sense perception and hence with the use of *bodily* faculties, a hoary conviction he was to cast into serious doubt. But his subsequent appeal to innate ideas—whose truth concerning an invisible, mathematicized world could only be guaranteed by a benevolent god, the now-notorious "god of the philosophers"—failed to heal the embarrassing rift between mind and nature even before this ridiculous deity unceremoniously fled the scene. What eventually followed was the predictable flowering of positivism and various reductionistic and scientistic tendencies, all of which merely added to the alarm over the survival of freedom in a mechanistic universe and further heightened the need for an enduring metaphysical solution that took into account the new scientific realities. For beyond the epistemological quandary of the status of John Locke's secondary qualities (color, sound, odor, and so on) lay the more serious danger of a modern kind of moral solipsism and its logical denial of a world shared in common. The ensuing debate over whether the human mind is actually able to make contact with an objective world beyond itself—as if consciousness were a box in which representations come and go with no apparent relation to what we intuitively know, and feel no need to prove, to be the world "out there"—was a sure sign of something seriously gone awry.

And so it was out of this bizarre epistemological and metaphysical cul-de-sac that the so-called real world, the world of matter-in-motion quantifiable in functionally dependent laws, was believed to be less a reality that is given to us and more a mental construct that we can be certain of knowing only because we have produced it in some mysterious fashion. It was Galileo's genius to have seen that the tool for such a construction was mathematics, itself a construction of the human mind. As David Hume was later to grasp, the ancient standard of truth, still quite visible in Descartes, had in fact shifted from intuitive seeing and logical demonstration to the instrumental ability to predict natural occurrences by conceiving of them as a coherence of forces calculable in advance—that is, as causal events whose necessary connections can only be explained by attributing them to the power of the human imagination. It was then but one more step—though a sizable one, at that—to the Kantian realization that we can and do know the world, not in spite of, but precisely because we are deeply implicated in the creation of its causal structure and of the language of mathematics through which it is expressed. And if any doubt remains concerning our central role in constructing such a world, we need only to trace this epistemology to its logical consequence, which now confronts us: the technological creation of a new or "second nature," including the engineering of our bodies toward an earthly perfection that evolution might promise, but like the Christian creator-God, has so far failed to attain without our active intervention. The cultural and political will to create this second nature, a nature made utterly determinate and thus amenable to human desire, was thus, we can now see, born out of a technological imperative religious and metaphysical in origin that gave rise to a scientific revolution as its perfect expression.

As Descartes knew full well when he sought justification for Galilean science in its promise of a "mastery and possession of nature," the mathematical character of this science makes clear what mastery in this context means—namely, the suppression of all ambiguity, spontaneity, and chance.[13] It became imperative, then, to protect the core of our humanity from such a conception of the world, imperative, in short, to construct a self detached from such a world, a self displaced and alienated, yet still free. Prior to modernity, humans were assured of a quite specific place in the world. In Aristotle's physics, the meaning of cosmic place is determined by a conception of motion grounded in the *inner nature* of particular things. Everything in this world moves toward its proper place as the way of actualizing its inherent and permanent ontological possibilities: fire goes up and earth moves down simply because that is where they belong in a hierarchical universe structured along the lines of perfect and less-perfect beings and kinds of motion. But modern science, Sir Isaac Newton in particular, exposed the inadequacy of such explanations by positing the *external* and ontologically neutral forces of gravity and inertia in order to account for all movement in the cosmos, celestial as well as terrestrial. In this overall scheme, places lose their quality of uniqueness and become mere positions in relation to other positions, points on a mathematical grid, thus undermining the natural status of a humanity now cast into a vast homogeneous space where, as Alexandre Koyre slyly observes, "everywhere is nowhere."[14] Even Newton's understanding of this space as the sensorium of God was soon to be discarded in the relentless march of disenchantment, resulting in a vast, empty container that Koyre describes as "the frame of the absence of all being" and depriving humanity of its traditional cosmic home.[15] And, as they say, there is no going back.

Still, it does not follow that the conundrum of home and homecoming, announced as long ago as Homer, simply vanishes into thin air, an unfortunate but necessary fatality of the collapse of Aristotle's finite universe. Indeed, it reappears (as it always will), but now as the question of whether limits ought to be placed on our technological rearrangement of the natural order, which is nothing less than the question of our fate in a scientific-technological civilization. These are the terms for posing the question of the human condition at the end of modernity. Traditional cosmologies, as Stephen Toulmin has eloquently argued, have always revolved around the problem of the human condition, and this is no different today, even if we eschew essentialist categories and philosophical talk of a human nature.[16] Unlike those traditional accounts, however, we are haunted by a Cartesian metaphysics that disconnects us from the world and, apparently, decides the question of our fate in advance by presuming that we have no place in nature even though we exercise immense power over it. Modernity insists that detachment and objectivity are in fact prerequisites for the acquisition of such power, and that any attempt to connect us to the world outside a power relation is pure sentimentality and nostalgia. And it would be partly right, since nostalgia—properly understood as derived from the Greek verb *nosteo*, meaning to return to one's home or country—is indeed the inescapable longing for home—that is, for a world hospitable to, if not always resonant with, human aspirations and possibilities.

In addressing this hunger for some kind of reconnection to what the U.S. writer Saul Bellow calls the "home-world," Marx and Heidegger stand out in the philosophical life of late, European modernity; and though they make for strange bedfellows in many respects, they share one enormously important presupposition: that Cartesian dualism must be dismantled and deposed, but in such a way that neither discredits nor rejects the genuine achievements of the technoscience that first gave rise to it. Nonetheless, both are distinctive in the last century and a half for having highlighted the human and environmental price to be paid for mechanization and its ever-increasing demand for more powerful energy sources and their utilization.

Marx and the Humanization of Nature

Marx was among the first to see through the modern apotheosis of objectivity, arguing that if we turn to real, existing human beings engaged in the production of their material existence, the ideal of the pure spectator is exposed for the sham it really is. What we find instead are laboring individuals who throughout human history have been intimately engaged with nature and its processes, even in the alienated mode of capitalist, industrial production. A human being is a toolmaker, the *animal laborans*, and not the rational animal of ancient "idealists" that Descartes transformed into the disembodied consciousness of one who views the world in detachment from the material activities of real people. For Marx, labor is "a process in which both man and Nature participate," and "the use and fabrication of instruments of labour . . . is specifically characteristic of the human labour-process."[17] The human species-essence, an early expression of Marx's, is technological in character. The "first historical act" of humankind is the production of the means to satisfy the basic needs of food, clothing, and shelter. Humans first distinguish themselves from other animals not through their higher mental powers but by producing the means of their existence, indirectly producing their material life.[18]

But Marx is actually saying more than this. On the one hand, all products of production are real products only when they are consumed in consumption. Consumption, in other words, seems to guide production and provide whatever measure is necessary to restrain and keep it within reasonable limits. On the other hand, products are in fact consumed as either the instruments or raw material of production or simply the means of subsistence of the producers themselves. Production—and not consumption—is in reality the primary factor, and as such always entails both the satisfaction and *creation of new needs*, which in turn call forth new production in a never-ending cycle. This is the secret of capitalism: the satisfaction of human needs evokes nothing but production itself—a secret that Marx believed socialism could harness and put to work in a more just social and political arrangement. Hence his conception of the animal laborans whose activity is production and consumption, but a consumption whose sole justification is further production.

Part of what makes Marx still relevant to our post-Communist world is his quintessentially modern belief that work itself is the satisfaction of our species-essence and not merely the means to bodily gratification. This belief has its origin, we now know, in the reevaluation of labor in medieval monastic life. Marx, however, radicalized this Christian idea by dropping its theological justification (*laborare est orare*) and by limiting it to the human sphere, where it could serve the supreme value of life. "Yet the productive life is the life of the species. It is life engendering."[19] Production in the real world where nature imposes its harsh discipline on us is humanity's active species life. Accordingly, its essential powers are displayed in the history of industry, albeit in alienated forms up to and including the capitalist mode of production. The "rich" human being, who exists more as an idea than a reality for Marx, is "the human being *in need* of a totality of human manifestations of life," life being understood as the material production of more life.[20] In spite of his protestations against idealism and the "poverty of philosophy," Marx was, when all is said and done, a metaphysician, but one who proposed a theory of being intended to undercut all philosophical dualisms—ideal versus real, subject versus object, spiritual versus material—stretching back to Plato and beyond. Inasmuch as the mode in which humans produce the means of their subsistence is a definite form of activity that expresses their life and hence their very being, production must be carried out in a form that corresponds to the true expression of that life, which Marx believed can occur only in socialism.

Clearly, then, Marx's economic humanism was not limited to the material improvement of the worker. The proletariat must appropriate the forces of production both to preserve their existence and "to achieve self-activity," which is to say to actualize their human essence as producers and toolmakers. For "man produces even when he is free from physical need and only truly produces in freedom therefrom."[21] Truly *free* production—and here we come to the heart of the matter—is the human invasion of the object and therefore its dissolution as a thing existing over and against a subject: G. W. F. Hegel's substance become subject, but the subject now correctly identified as the animal laborans. By making nature the reflection of humans' essential powers, Marx believed he had pointed the way to a self-affirmation in and through the world and not merely in the mind or, worse, in some far-off heaven. In fact, this was the only kind of human freedom worth considering: a freedom won through the struggle with natural forces and necessities. Concomitantly, true nature can only be a "humanized" one, a raw material worked over by human hands and made to serve every human need and desire. Such "mastery and possession" is clearly intended as a riposte to idealism, Cartesian or otherwise, as well as to the false dichotomy between theory and productive praxis.

One can plausibly argue that Marx's real—if ironic—accomplishment was to deepen the Cartesian definition of the real by expanding it beyond the theoretical construction of mathematical physics to technological production and creation. As a result, he proposed a radically new equation: to be is to be produced by human labor. Nothing can any longer be said to exist outside the sphere of the human. And though Marx never tired of emphasizing that humans are conditioned by their natural surroundings, he always added that as the sphere of productive freedom expands, they are conditioned by a nature already humanized by technological forces.

Even prior to Friedrich Nietzsche, Marx embodied the fundamental metaphysical thrust of modernity in two distinct but related ways. First, he clarified the telos of the modern subjectivization of being in its reduction of nature to a mere factor in the labor process of the proletariat and modern technology. Here, being is not merely intelligible, as Hegel would have it, but is technologically subsumable into human activity. The real is the producible, and the producible is the real. Second, in his fascination with the seemingly limitless productivity inherent in the new instruments of modern technics and the division of labor they necessitated, Marx brought to the world's attention for the first time the centrality of technology in human existence and what this means for understanding historical humanity and the natural world as inseparable from that history. The prospect of liberating this productivity through a universal, planetary technique thus promises in his view not just the abolition of scarcity but "the actual realization for man of man's essence and of his essence as something real"[22]—that is, as productively engaged with nature and "real, sensuous objects" through which, and only through which, one can autonomously express one's life as animal laborans. Neither intellect nor sense perception—the false and misleading set of choices of a worn-out epistemology blind to the reality and power of productive praxis—can yield nature in a form adequate to humanity's essence.

It is only when nature finally appears as nothing but the result of human labor, and so as a reflection and affirmation of humanity's species-essence, that it can serve as "the visible, irrefutable proof of [man's] *birth through himself, of the process of his creation.*"[23] Here, then, appears a nature transformed into the historical product of human handiwork, now merely the result of human productive forces and dependent from this point forward on the degree of development of these forces. With capitalism, Marx approvingly writes, "nature becomes for the first time simply an object for mankind, purely a matter of utility; it ceases to be recognized as a power in its own right; and the theoretical knowledge of its independent laws appears only as a stratagem to subdue it to human requirements, whether as the object of consumption or as the means of production."[24] But capitalism, because of its internal contradictions, is incapable, according to Marx, of effecting the total humanization of nature. His argument for a scientific socialism rests precisely on its capacity to conclude what capitalism started but could not finish. Putting aside the etiology of Communism's abject failure in the twentieth century, we still must conclude that Marx, no less than Adam Smith, carried forward the inner meaning of modernity as the technoscientific mission to bring nature to her "true anthropological form," and thus into harmony with humanity's species-essence. But beyond this utopian desire, Marx oddly seems never to have reflected much on the further consequences of the humanization of natural processes already well underway, assuming, as does capitalism, its naturalness and desirability. For a more radical probing of modern anthropocentrism, we must turn to Heidegger and his difficult ontologizing of technology and the world it has created.

Heidegger and the Being of Technology

Like Marx, Heidegger rejected philosophical idealism and the Western metaphysical bias toward theory, and located our fundamental engagement with the world in technological praxis. In *Being and Time*, he embarked—evidently with Marx in mind—on a new interpretation of humanity's productive relationship with beings.[25] There, he argues that our ability to make and utilize tools is grounded in a pretheoretical, bodily understanding of an "equipmental context"—for example, a craftsperson's workshop or a factory floor—where every item of equipment is related to every other through a complex set of meanings teleologically ordered by the potential uses of the artifacts to be produced. While this setting and the larger world to which it belongs vary over time and from place to place, Heidegger's historical understanding of the being of work and the materials utilized in it differs quite markedly from Marx's historical materialism. As Heidegger remarks in *The Basic Problems of Phenomenology*, a work that overlaps *Being and Time*, "Productive comportment is not limited just to the producible and the produced but harbors within itself a remarkable breadth of possibility for understanding the being of beings."[26] Implicit in this ontological approach to technology is a critique of Marx's materialist account of productive praxis as incapable in the end of overcoming the world alienation that had become Cartesianism's main legacy.[27] Very simply, what Heidegger offers—and what Marx was unable to deliver—is a satisfactory explanation of and alternative to dualism, which Heidegger eventually accomplishes by tracing Cartesianism's origins to the voluntarism identified by Lynn White as the defining character Western Christianity and, in Heidegger's view, Western philosophy culminating in Nietzsche.

In a much later essay, "The Question Concerning Technology," Heidegger addresses the mode of revealment unique to modern technology and rejects the widely held belief that technology is merely an instrument subject to human control.[28] Indeed, to restrict one's analysis of any kind of technology to a calculus of simple means and ends is to overlook the complex and subtle ways in which it can and does change the way we perceive and value the world. Against this instrumental conception, which presupposes that machines and technical processes are neutral tools whose goodness is solely a function of the virtue of their users, Heidegger argues that in every technology, craft or industrial, high-tech or low-tech, there occurs a historically conditioned mode of revealing or truth, which in the case of the modern technological age sets up and challenges nature to yield its energy sources to be stored for later human use. It is this challenging character that distinguishes modern technology from its predecessors, which in stark contrast "bring forth" artifacts without assaulting things and radically altering natural processes. To clarify this distinction, Heidegger compares the traditional windmill with an electric power plant.[29] Each harnesses an energy source and puts it to work for human ends, yet the windmill remains related to nature in a way that allows the wind to remain itself even as it serves human ends. This is a technology that lets nature reveal itself as an entity independent of all technical processes and planning, though, to be sure, it first *appears* to us never directly but always in a technological context. A coal-fired electric power plant, by contrast, unlocks basic physical energies and then stores them up in an abstract, nonsensuous form. Hence, modern technology places "unreasonable" demands on nature by aggressively setting upon it and refusing to let it be as it is in itself. Driven by the standard of efficiency—that is, the maximum yield at the minimum expense—it is guided by short-term economic considerations that tend to undermine ethical and environmental concerns. The net result of this aggressive mode of revealing is the transformation of the world into a vast stockroom where everything gains its ontological status in terms of its availability and disposability for the endless cycle of production and consumption endorsed earlier by Marx. Modern technology reduces the world to what Heidegger calls *Bestand*—a stock or standing reserve of energy resources. As early as the mid-1930s, he was already formulating this critique, especially in relation to Nietzsche's doctrine of the will to power that Heidegger explicitly links to mechanization and the mastery of beings that are now everywhere "surveyable." But the nature of this mastery cannot merely be equated with mechanization and mass production. Rather, it is to be found in the kind of beings that are mass-produced, beings that as the term Bestand suggests, possess no inherent ontological standing apart from human consumption and production, seemingly subject to the will to power of a new human type in the history of humanity: Nietzsche's superman.

Yet, Heidegger is insistent (and here his divergence from Marx and modern humanism and anthropocentrism becomes most apparent) that the mode of revealing in modern technology eludes human comprehension and control. Unknown to themselves, producers and consumers alike respond to a way of being Heidegger names *Gestell* or "enframing" that, as a "destiny of being," urges humans to challenge forth nature as a mere resource, as standing on reserve for human consumption and production. Gestell, in other words, is the essence of modern technology, and cannot be detected through anthropological investigations like Marx's that tend to focus on instrumental analyses of machines and technical processes such as the division of labor. As a mode of being that illuminates beings of all sorts, Gestell is nothing technological itself, but indicates that "to be" in the age of technology means to be scientifically calculable and technically controllable, creating the illusion that humanity is now "lord of the earth." In attempting to "humanize" nature in its totality, erasing any significant difference between it and ourselves, we quite unexpectedly and paradoxically intensify our alienation from it, and create against all our good intentions a world where environmental devastation becomes an acceptable by-product of progress and the standardization of mass production applies to consumers as well as to consumables. Nature, in effect, withdraws and, even more strangely, hides itself in this mode of revealing (much as God has gone into eclipse, as Martin Buber has argued), concealing from human making and knowing its character as *physis*, by which Heidegger means nature's capacity to bring itself forth from out of itself in ways that remain ultimately impenetrable to Western science and technology.

There is about modern technology, when seen in this way, an air of hubris, a marked tendency on its part to push both humans and nature beyond their limits, to make "unreasonable demands" on them. Specifically, it is with the earth *as earth* that modern science and technology run up against *their* limits, and so become fateful in a historical sense. Concealed from them is the "unnoticeable law of the earth," a "law" of self-preservation in the face of assaults that would deny and suppress nature's character as physis. "Technology drives the earth beyond the developed sphere of its possibility into such things which are no longer a possibility and are thus impossible," doing so in order to secure a stable human order both on and beyond the earth, where, in spite of its acknowledged successes, it will find that the law of the possible—that is, the hidden and inexhaustible ways of being that govern beings—cannot itself be mastered.[30] Simply put, "nature is not to be gotten around," and most insistently when it is theoretically objectified and technologically entrapped.[31]

Marx's hope of overcoming humankind's age-old alienation from being, manifest for him in Cartesian dualism, and finally establishing a realm of freedom by technologically breaking the yoke of necessities imposed by nature on humanity proves to be a cruel illusion. The belief that modern productive forces can "get around" nature signals for Heidegger the "errancy" of modern technology in its disregard for limits, lending it its fateful quality.[32] Whether this illusion is leading to some ultimate catastrophe is an open question and not really Heidegger's point. Instead, he wants to ask, Can humanity continue to feed on this illusion and still remain human? It is in this sense that Heidegger's philosophy can be characterized as the sounding of an alarm regarding a "supreme danger" threatening the human condition, which for Heidegger is to be at once ecstatically and freely beyond ourselves toward the world while keeping both feet firmly planted on the earth. For errancy in its chronic ignorance of this "condition" gives rise today to the intoxicating fantasy that we are now enlightened enough to order the world according to a ground plan projected in the technoscientific securing of complete objectivity and calculability.

To the obvious danger inherent in this fantasy of crowding out other modes of being, and thus other, less power-oriented human possibilities, belongs the risk of including our bodies in the standing reserve in the hope that in subjecting our genetic makeup to radical manipulation, we might gather our destiny into our own hands under the benign, Baconian intention of the "relief of man's estate." Do we realize the momentousness of this occasion? Do we grasp that our treatment of nature cannot be disconnected from the question of our humanness and place in the world? And so Heidegger urges us to ask these and other unsettling queries: Is it possible to overcome the inhuman submission to scarcity in all its hideous forms—poverty, ignorance, sickness—by removing ourselves from the world as the precondition for exercising power over it? Indeed, can we craft a new home or second nature, confident in the technical knowledge and expertise necessary to create and sustain such a nature? And if we answer in the affirmative to these questions, on what basis do we possess that confidence? Unpopular as such questions may be, they cannot simply be dismissed as intending to return us to a nonexistent, premodern idyll. Rather, they are meant to provoke us into thinking about the high stakes we have wagered in the modern project that, although just over four hundred years old, is only now coming into its own.

The Emergence of Cybernetic Humanity

Looking back over the last two centuries, it is clear that Descartes' attempt to safeguard human consciousness from determinism has failed in at least two respects. First, the theoretical detachment from the world for which his res cogitans was constructed has, as Marx and Heidegger predicted, not held up under intense scrutiny. Theory itself, in the hands of modern science, has come to be a powerful form of praxis replete with its own interests and agenda for changing the world. Science has become technoscience. Second, the breakdown of Cartesian dualism has resulted not in the dissolution of its two terms but in the triumph of the res extensa, a nature objectified and disenchanted, leading scientists and many philosophers (at least in the English-speaking world) to conclude that mind or consciousness is reducible to brain functions and the body to a complex mechanism whose workings are no longer the province of philosophy.

And yet, despite the influence of both Marx and Heidegger, the myth of a value-neutral science has continued to assert itself, challenged, with a few exceptions, by only a handful of continental and feminist philosophers of science. In our confusing and at times chaotic world, science and engineering are still looked to as standing above the fray, concerned with matters far from the messiness of human affairs and the contingencies of historical particularity, paradox, and anomaly. We supposedly can take solace in the fact that there still remains the lawful world of nature and the pristine beauty of its expression in mathematical formulas. This has been the dream. But it is beginning to dawn on many, slowly and in different quarters, that even science can no longer claim to progress on a track separate from the rest of human life, that it is, in fact, implicated in nearly everything we know and do, and permeates in known—and unknown—ways the very texture of our being. One has only to point to recombinant DNA research to show that what happens in the laboratory happens to all of us. Stubborn adherence to the neutrality ruse is, as Toulmin observes, "to argue as though a scientific experiment today were still a piece of mere 'spectating' rather than an action performed by a participant in the real world, with actual and possible effects on both Nature and the rest of Humanity."[33] Because modern technoscience in many cases directly and almost immediately affects the world and its inhabitants, it is no longer possible or desirable for researchers to hide behind the veil of objectivity and value neutrality.

But more than that, as progress in both evolutionary and molecular biology increasingly overshadows the achievements of mathematical physics—which since Galileo has set the standard for what counts as scientific knowledge—it is clear that the search for immutable and universal truths is finally giving way to a historical, evolutionary understanding of nature.[34] The inevitable question of humanity's place in such a world consequently reasserts itself—albeit in a somewhat qualified and therefore tentative sense—in the Darwinian garb of adaptation and natural selection. Our natural status now takes on a dynamic character with the very order of the world reduced at best to patterns in a flux, that is, to a kind of order within disorder, to employ a Bergsonian phrase. As Marx so simply and presciently put it, we have now arrived at the point where all that is solid melts into air. We have arrived at the point of *history*. The rules of the game are thus in the process of changing. "Human nature" is suddenly castigated by many as an outmoded, misleading, and politically pernicious concept. Nor is it certain that a hundred years from now we will even be talking about such a thing as "nature" at all. Still, it is more important than ever to remind ourselves that despite the upheaval of the Darwinian revolution, the ineluctable facts of our humanness—natality and mortality, sociality and embodiment, transcendence and facticity—remain, and must be reconsidered, carefully, only now without resort to the kind of ahistorical, preevolutionary picture of the human condition, especially in its Cartesian form, that has defined Western humanity for well over two millennia. This will require as well the revival of cosmology, as Toulmin wisely argues, but one that will align human powers and possibilities with the historical character of nature, exhorting us to work with, and no longer against, those forces that pulse through our bodies and evolution as a species.

But we should be under no illusions about the difficulty involved in such a reorientation of Western thought and life. Such, at least, was the view of the philosopher of biology and technology Hans Jonas, who quite rightly took a more pessimistic view than Toulmin about the chances of achieving such a reconciliation with nature in the near term. For while Jonas, too, proposed an environmental ethic grounded in an appreciation and creative appropriation of Charles Darwin, he also recognized, as others have not, the continuing influence of Cartesianism and its mechanistic ideal on our understanding of evolution and ecology, and so on reconceiving our place in nature.[35] There is, Jonas conceded, no inherent reason why evolutionary theory—or even the science of ecology, for that matter—will not continue to take a manipulative and even aggressive stance toward the natural processes to which we must now adapt. Thus, he made it clear that the question of what is meant by *adaptation* becomes critical, not only in light of Darwin, but also as part of our response to technology in general and the prospect of genetic engineering in particular.

Given the growing dependency of molecular biology on computerization and the metaphysics it embodies, an answer to this question seems to have emerged: cybernetics.[36] Defined in the *Oxford English Dictionary* as the science of systems of control and communication in both organisms and nonliving machines, cybernetics has given new life to the clockwork universe and the growing conviction that the human mind and body are best understood on the model of a mechanistic pas de deux with their surrounding environment. This should come as no surprise. Modern technology, after all, has always been cybernetic to a degree in its concern with an automation and, more recently, roboticization that are believed to render superfluous direct human control over the operation of tools and machinery, freeing us from the drudgery of labor and immediate involvement in the natural world. What is new today is the extension of mechanical techniques and hardware to living things, including, of course, human beings and their bodies—more or less the scenario foreseen by Descartes in his linkage of the mastery of nature with the promise of a new medicine modeled on the success of the mechanical arts.[37] This is important for two reasons, one epistemological, and the other metaphysical. First, and more obviously, this extension makes possible a computerized model of the human brain, the kind of paradigm that artificial intelligence research has been employing for decades. Further, in claiming to overcome Cartesian dualism, while at the same time failing to address the threat of the metaphysical determinism that first gave rise to it, the biologistic appropriation of cybernetic models allows for a questionable and rather surreptitious transference of the notion of telos from the human to the mechanical sphere. And this has led, oddly enough, to a projecting of the mechanical back onto the mental, in effect naturalizing human consciousness.[38]

Evidence for this hidden importation of teleology into the world of machines abounds. Cybernetic devices such as thermostats and computers, for instance, are said to "adapt" to their environments by means of information transfers and the preprogrammed processing of that information. Here a new anthropomorphism appears, but one where human qualities are now projected onto machines, just as Aristotle once read human teleology into nature. The significance—and danger—of this rather novel "humanization" of machinery is that it allows for, even encourages, the subsequent mechanization of humans. True, our absorption in the world has always inclined us to interpret ourselves in the image of whatever we have found there, and this is no different today when we speak of the body as machine, the brain as minicomputer, and so forth. What needs to be recognized is the underlying move that makes this hermeneutics possible, namely, the anthropomorphizing of technological devices (for example, the amusingly garrulous computer HAL in Stanley Kubrick's *2001: A Space Odyssey*) as a way of smoothing the transfer of mechanistic characteristics to human beings.

We are told, of course, that the age of science and disenchantment has left such mythologizing behind, but this is a presumption of which we should be especially suspicious, since the ideology of objectivity remains a human creation, no different in the end from any other cultural product. To illustrate: Jonas has quite shrewdly pointed out that in judging the "success" (itself an anthropomorphism) of servomechanisms, we unthinkingly introduce such human traits as "purpose," "concerns," and "adaptation," tempting us in turn to reinterpret human conduct in terms of the feedback of information and the mechanical processing of messages. But, as Jonas argues, this is "an attempt to account for purposive behavior without purpose," since the use of information in daily life is a means to various human ends and not the goal itself.[39] Humans, in short, are not essentially feedback mechanisms but purposive beings who act ultimately on the basis of contextual meaning and concern for their own being, and not simply in response to raw data. A thermostat has no intrinsic purpose, but one imposed on it externally, so that its feedback helps to regulate a heater or air conditioner in the service to this human purpose. In truth, the messages received by a servomechanism make sense and are therefore taken *as messages* only on the basis of a complex of meaning (what Heidegger called the equipmental context) that transcends the strictly cybernetic circuitry or loop.

Yet it is obvious that such reflections go against the grain. The workings of evolution are, in fact, increasingly understood in cybernetic terms; and feedback models have become a commonplace in biology. Not surprisingly, then, natural selection is interpreted (in essential accord with the Cartesian outlook) as a mechanistic interaction between organism and environment, a play of information exchange whereby organisms "adapt" themselves to their situations solely by means of feedback loops, especially positive feedback. Here life itself is reduced to a stimulus-response mechanism, though one infinitely more complicated than behaviorism could ever comprehend or account for.

Consequently, when the engineering of the human genome is presented as a kind of cybernetic manipulation and, even more important, is justified as merely the next step in evolutionary history, as some will no doubt argue, we should pause and reflect on just what exactly this "merely" means.[40] In the not-too-distant future, it would seem to portend, we will subject the metabolism between humans and nature to our own control, taking on ourselves in a deliberate and willful fashion the process of natural selection.[41] And we will do this primarily in the hope of finally re-creating our place in a second nature (having been ejected from the original four hundred years ago), such placement now understood not in terms of our nature, as Aristotle believed, but as an adaptability based on the knowledge and control of the information exchange between ourselves and the environment we long to call home. In taking charge in such a fundamental way, we will act in the belief that we are exercising a freedom never available to previous generations: the freedom to invent ourselves and subsequent generations by creating a new image of humanity based on sound scientific principles and powerful techniques. It will be the very power to re-create ourselves that we will attempt to image again and again in such re-creation, most likely through the genetic enhancement of intelligence.

But the further, and really more crucial, question of whether human freedom consists simply in the ever-more-sophisticated manipulation of natural processes, including those in our own bodies, is a problem that, quite frankly, exceeds the capabilities of either science or technology to solve, let alone to address in a philosophically adequate way. Echoing Heidegger's warning of the risks inherent in the inclusion of humans in the standing reserve of natural resources, C. S. Lewis in *The Abolition of Man* laments that the modern conquest of nature will lead not to its stated end but instead to the subjugation of one group of humans by another, confounding the unstated, but widely held assumption that technology *eo ipso* results in human liberation and well-being.[42] It is precisely this difficulty, for example, that now faces non-Western nations and peoples as they struggle with the introduction of Western science and technology into their traditional, indigenous ways of life.[43] From a somewhat different perspective, ecofeminists and feminist philosophers of science have made the same point in claiming that the "logic of domination" present in Western science and technology is patriarchal in character, and thus links the environmental and women's movements in ways deeper than was previously realized.[44]

Toward a New Home-World

What, then, are the pitfalls in adopting a cybernetic understanding of biology and evolution as the basis of an engineering of the human genome? There are at least two: (1) adoption of a mechanistic paradigm for explaining adaptation and natural selection, and (2) biologism, or the explanation of human behavior solely through biological processes. The science of ecology, to take an example that both surprises and disappoints, has proven to be vulnerable to both these mistakes, even as it preaches environmental harmony and ecological balance. For in erasing any significant difference between humans and their natural environment—a move, by the way, that ecofeminism bravely calls to task, attributing it to deep ecology as well—it courts the danger of justifying any action, no matter how environmentally destructive it may be, as adaptive and natural. What is more, in the desire to overcome the lingering effects of dualism, the science of ecology runs the risk of abolishing human transcendence and the moral and political responsibility grounded in it. One disturbing sign of just such a possibility is certainly our profound indifference to the autonomy of future human generations as we move closer to altering irrevocably the germ line of our species.

It is therefore not enough to simply declare Cartesianism dead and the "spectatorship" of an objective, value-free science a dinosaur. Nor is it sufficient to announce our kinship with all living things along genetic lines. Quite the contrary, it is only in the aftermath of the failure of Cartesian metaphysics that the real problem emerges: how to think a new relationship to nature without succumbing to a facile naturalism and a new round of mechanism on cybernetic grounds. For surely there is no going back *simpliciter* to anything like Aristotelianism or natural law in the Roman Catholic tradition, that is to say, to any kind of ahistorical conception of nature whose laws and structures are fixed for all time.[45] Ethical appeals to the natural in this sense will simply run aground the modern refutation of Aristotelian and Thomistic science as well as any theological argument made on the basis of that science. In fact, any serious attempt to counter a cybernetic account of human evolution will have to begin by recognizing the complicity of Western metaphysics in a cybernetic agenda, especially the role played by Christian voluntarism and Neoplatonism in historically propagating and sanctioning a dualism that led to and empowered the scientific objectification and technological enframing of nature.

Indeed, if we have learned anything from thinkers like Marx and Heidegger, it is that the demise of the transcendent, neutral observer, so brilliantly articulated and defended by Descartes, signals not only the end of modernity but the commencement of the final, technological stage in the history of Western metaphysics. We are dislodged once again, but in a more radical sense than occurred in the Copernican/Galilean revolution. Disabused of answers given once and for all time to the riddle of our cosmic place, we find ourselves no longer straddling the City of God and the City of Man, but enmeshed, fully and without recourse, in the turbulence of history (James Joyce's nightmare from which he believed we are trying to awake). But rather than despair we can, as Heidegger and Jonas and other thinkers have done, take up the problem of our historicity as the clue to a mature and measured understanding of the human predicament, an understanding that has expressed itself, however inadequately, under a number of names—*Geist*, dialectic, evolution, eternal recurrence, being in the world—as late modernity has struggled with a phenomenon never encountered before in world history: a sense of exile and dislocation in a sea of prosperity and power.

The choice confronting us is therefore clear. Either we acquiesce to a biological determinism crafted along cybernetic lines, much as we have drifted into tacit approval of genetically modified food; or we resist the thoughtless equations of freedom with technical control and wisdom with technical expertise. The second option, if we take it, will not be an easy haul. It will demand a more cautious if not skeptical approach to our technologies, especially those coming under the rubric of bioengineering. And this, in turn, will depend on the cultivation of an epistemological tolerance for the insurmountable indeterminacy and hence mystery of what still stands at the center of our historicity as its ground and stabilizing force: the individual *thing*, both natural and artifactual, in all its particularity and opaque otherness. Above all, we will need to learn, odd as it may sound, what it means to be at home in our homelessness, and so to thrive in a world that despite our best efforts and no matter how powerful our techniques can be made neither wholly comfortable nor ultimately reassuring. The alternative—which admittedly has the upper hand because it has been long prepared for—is the emergence of a cybernetic humanity whose threat, not just to the thingly basis of the world, but to its own spontaneity and the spontaneity of future generations, we now seem unwilling, even unable, to recognize. But ignorance, though constitutive of our human condition, has never been an excuse and, as the Greeks have taught us, is the essence of tragedy itself.

Notes

1. For a discussion of the crank, see Lynn White Jr., *Medieval Technology and Social Change* (New York: Oxford University Press, 1981), 103–117. For a classic account of the clock, see Lewis Mumford, *Technics and Civilization* (New York: Harcourt, Brace, 1963), 12–18.

2. Lynn White, Jr., *Medieval Religion and Technology: Collected Essays* (Berkeley: University of California Press, 1978), ix.

3. John Locke indicates the cultural power of this idea in "Of Property," chapter 5 of *The Second Treatise on Government*, ed. C. B. Macpherson (Indianapolis: Hachett Publishing, 1980). There he appeals to Revelation, "which gives us an account of those grants God made of the world to Adam, and to Noah and his sons" (18), and specifically interprets Psalm 115—where King David sings that God "has given the earth to the children of men" (18)—to mean that God "commanded [man] to subdue the earth—i.e., improve it for the benefit of life and therein lay out something that was his own, his labor" (21), For a more recent

62 Timothy K. Casey

incarnation of this argument, see W. Norris Clarke, "Technology and Man: A Christian View," in *Philosophy and Technology: Readings in the Philosophical Problems of Technology*, ed. Carl Mitcham and Robert Mackey (New York: Free Press, 1983), 247–258.

4. The new attitude toward nature was in part the result of the de-animization of the world accomplished through the Christian cult of the saints, which displaced nature's "spirits" to a supraworldly heaven. See Lynn White Jr., "The Historical Roots of Our Ecologic Crisis," in *Philosophy and Technology: Readings in the Philosophical Problems of Technology*, ed. Carl Mitcham and Robert Mackey (New York: Free Press, 1983), 263.

5. Lynn White argues persuasively that the Industrial Revolution of the eighteenth and nineteenth centuries was in fact a managerial revolution whose major accomplishment was to usher in the presence of large factories. See White, *Medieval Religion and Technology*, 80.

6. The historical connection between technological invention and development and warfare is noted by many commentators. See especially William H. McNeil, *The Pursuit of Power: Technology, Armed Force, and Society since A.D. 1,000* (Chicago: University of Chicago Press, 1982). Everyone, of course, knows that the Pentagon invented and implemented the Internet, though not many are aware that it also created and continues to oversee the Global Positioning System, or GPS, the only space-based satellite system global in reach.

7. Herbert Butterfield, *The Origins of Modern Science* (New York: Free Press, 1957), 130.

8. Lewis Mumford, *The Myth of the Machine: The Pentagon of Power* (New York: Harcourt Brace Jovanovich, 1970), 85.

9. Butterfield, The Origins of Modern Science, 125.

10. E. A. Burtt, *The Metaphysical Foundations of Modern Science* (Garden City, NJ: Anchor Press, 1954), 104.

11. In his *Meditations on First Philosophy*, Descartes argues precisely for the survival, though not the truth value of sense perception: "But the nature here described truly teaches me to flee from things which cause the sensation of pain, and seek after the things which communicate to me the sentiment of pleasure and so forth; but I do not see that beyond this it teaches me that from those diverse sense-perceptions we should ever form any conclusion regarding things outside us, without having [carefully and maturely] mentally examined them beforehand" (Rene Descartes, *The Philosophical Works of Descartes*, trans. Elizabeth S. Haldane and G. R. T. Rose [Cambridge: Cambridge University Press, 1972], 1:193).

12. William Harvey's depiction of the heart as a pump leaps to mind here.

13. Aristotle once said that *techne* loves happy chance, expressing a fundamental orientation toward technology that the early moderns clearly found untenable (*Nicomachean Ethics* 6.2. 1140a19).

14. Alexandre Koyre, *From the Closed World to the Infinite Universe* (Baltimore: Johns Hopkins University Press, 1976), 201.

15. Ibid., 179.

16. Stephen Toulmin, *The Return to Cosmology: Postmodern Science and the Theology of Nature* (Berkeley: University of California Press, 1985).

17. Karl Marx, *Capital* (New York: International Publishers, 1967), 1:183, 179.

18. See especially Karl Marx, *The German Ideology*, ed. C. J. Arthur (New York: International Publishers, 1977), 42.

19. Karl Marx, *The Economic and Philosophic Manuscripts of 1844*, ed. Dirk J. Struik (New York: International Publishers, 1964), 113.

20. Ibid., 144.

21. Ibid., 113.

22. Ibid., 187.

23. Ibid.

24. Karl Marx, *The Grundrisse*, ed. and trans. David McLellan (New York: Harper and Row, 1971), 94.

25. Martin Heidegger, *Being and Time*, trans. John MacQuarrie and Edward Robinson (New York: Harper and Row, 1962).

26. Martin Heidegger, *The Basic Problems of Phenomenology*, trans. Albert Hofstadter (Bloomington: Indiana University Press, 1979), 116.

27. See Hannah Arendt, *The Human Condition* (Chicago: University of Chicago Press, 1958), 248–257.

28. Martin Heidegger, "The Question concerning Technology," in *The Question concerning Technology and Other Essays*, trans. William Lovitt (New York: Harper and Row, 1973), 3–35.

29. Such talk is not as romantic as it first sounds. Wind farms are becoming commonplace around the world. Ireland, for example, has recently constructed one on a sandbar off the coast of County Wicklow that will provide the republic with 10 percent of its current energy needs.

30. Martin Heidegger, *The End of Philosophy*, trans. Joan Stambaugh (New York: Harper and Row, 1973), 109.

31. Martin Heidegger, "Science and Reflection," in *The Question concerning Technology* and Other Essays, trans, William Lovitt (New York: Harper and Row, 1973), 174.

32. The Greek word for fate is *moira*, perhaps best understood as those limits that circumscribe our existence as human.

33. Toulmin, *The Return to Cosmology*, 251.

34. Some in the scientific world are willing to entertain a flux so radical that the permanence and universality of the underlying laws of nature are called into question. Stephen Jay Gould is a case in point. John Horgan, previously a writer for *Scientific American*, reports a conversation with Gould in which the Harvard biologist and historian of science argued that extraterrestrial life may not conform to "Darwinian principles." Horgan then comments: "By liberating

evolutionary biology from Darwin—and from science as a whole, science defined as the search for universal laws—[Gould] has sought to make the quest for knowledge open-ended, even infinite. . . . Whereas most scientists seek to discern the signal underlying nature, Gould keeps drawing attention to the noise." (John Horgan, *The End of Science* [New York: Broadway Books, 1996], 126–127).

35. See Hans Jonas, *The Phenomenon of Life: Towards a Philosophical Biology* (New York: Harper and Row, 1966), *Philosophical Essays: From Ancient Creed to Technological Man* (Chicago: University of Chicago Press, 1974), and *The Imperative of Responsibility: In Search of an Ethics for the Technological Age* (Chicago: University of Chicago Press, 1984).

36. For the argument that computers incline their users to an epistemology and ontology that are perfectly in line with modern atomism and the belief that being, in the end, is nothing but information, see Michael Heim, *The Metaphysics of Virtual Reality* (New York: Oxford University Press, 1993).

37. When Descartes justifies Galilean science in the *Discourse on Method* as enabling us to become the "masters and possessors of nature," he further justifies that mastery by pointing to ensuing technologies that will aid in "the preservation of health, which is without doubt the chief blessing and the foundation of all other blessings in this life" (*The Philosophical Works of Descartes*, 1:119–120).

38. See Hubert Dreyfus, *What Computers Can't Do: The Limits of Artificial Intelligence* (New York: Harper and Row, 1979).

39. Jonas, *The Phenomenon of Life*, 120.

40. An early and instructive example of the claim that technoscience will enable humans to seize control of their own evolution can be found in J. D. Bernal, *The World, the Flesh, and the Devil* (Bloomington: Indiana University Press, 1929), 47.

41. Turning it into "artificial selection" through the usurpation of evolution's mutational agency.

42. C.S. Lewis maintains that "what we call Man's power over Nature turns out to be a power exercised by some men over other men with Nature as its instrument," adding that "all long-term exercises of power, especially in breeding, must mean the power of earlier generations over later ones" (*The Abolition of Man* [New York: Macmillan, 1947], 69). Sigmund Freud as well argues that "the influence exercised upon the social relations of mankind by progressive control over the forces of Nature is unmistakable. For men always put their newly acquired instruments of power at the service of their aggressiveness and use them against one another" (*New Introductory Lectures on Psycho-analysis*, ed. and trans. James Strachey [New York: W. W. Norton, 1989], 219).

43. See Thomas Friedman, *The Lexus and the Olive Tree* (New York: Farrar, Straus and Giroux, 1999), 267–294.

44. See Karen Warren, ed., *Ecofeminism: Women, Nature, Culture* (Bloomington: Indiana University Press, 1997); Carolyn Merchant, *The Death of Nature: Women, Ecology, and the Scientific Revolution* (New York: Harper

and Row, 1980); Sandra Harding, *The Science Question in Feminism* (Ithaca, NY: Cornell University Press, 1986); and Helen Longino, *Science as Social Knowledge: Values and Objectivity in Scientific Inquiry* (Princeton, NJ: Princeton University Press, 1990).

45. I say *simpliciter* because Jonas in fact does draw on the Aristotelian tradition in arguing that teleology does not have to be a concept alien to modern biology, a point that Bernard Rollin confirms elsewhere in this volume.

3

Nature and Human Nature

Mark Sagoff

Eric S. Lander, director of the Whitehead Institute Center for Genome Research, asks, "Will we adopt the image of humans as a product of manufacture, rather than a product of nature? If we cross that fateful threshold, I don't see how we can ever return." In an editorial in the *New York Times*, Lander argues that humanity should stay on this side of the boundary between what one may call "the world of born" and "the world of made." He concludes, "I would support a ban on modifying the human genome."[1]

In his editorial, Lander reflects a view that has found its fullest expression in the literature of theology. In the well-known 1970 book *Fabricated Man: The Ethics of Genetic Control*, theologian Paul Ramsey similarly discussed the logical—not simply the biological—consequences of what he labeled the "fascinating prospect of man's limitless self-modification." Ramsey inquired whether any conception of "human nature" could survive "the possible future technological and biological control and change of the human species."[2]

More recently, another theologian, Sean Fagan, argued that the biological connection between humanity and other creatures constitutes a morally important fact that the Human Genome Project and related projects both underscore and undermine: "One effect of gene research has been to make us more aware of the unity of life, of our rootedness in nature and of our belonging to a wider whole."[3] Another effect is to suggest ways that humanity can free itself of evolutionary constraints by purposefully manipulating the human genome.

The Unity of Life

Concepts that refer to the "unity of life" and our "rootedness in nature" may invoke a historical premise, namely, that all life-forms are descended from a common source, or at least that human beings are related to other life-forms through the long historical processes of evolution. Ironically, however, the results of genomic research suggest that humans are related to the rest of life—or rooted in nature—in unexpected ways.

First, just as the Copernican revolution led humanity to recognize that it did not stand at the center of the universe, so the genomic revolution shows us that we do not reside anywhere near the trunk of the tree of life. Astronomers locate the earth somewhere in a minor galaxy in an undistinguished spot at the periphery of celestial events. Similarly, geneticists locate multicellular eukaryotic organisms, such as human beings, in a most undistinguished spot at the periphery of evolution. For the most part, living nature consists in prokaryotes, bacterial creatures not burdened, as are eukaryotes, with nuclei in their cells. Eukaryotes, and particularly the multicellular eukaryotes of which plants and animals are familiar examples, "form an outlying twig on a tree of life whose trunk and branches are otherwise largely bacterial."[4]

Second, once one manages to locate the outlying twig where multicellular eukaryotes are found, one finds that they resemble each other. Seen in the context of genetic variation across all life, little distinguishes human beings, say, from yeast. Researchers can find only three hundred human genes that have no recognizable counterpart in the mouse.[5] The striking similarities between humans and their close genetic cousins, such as worms, and the differences between them and almost all other living things lead one to ask whether humanity has anything to learn from these relations besides humility.

Third, ethicists have begun to question the extent to which historical concepts, such as the unity of life, can remain meaningful as biotechnology increases its power to alter genomes for instrumental purposes and, eventually, to create genomes artificially. These artificial creatures, after all, would have to count as living—as part of the unity of life—even though they have a different history. The Ethics of Genomics Group, in a thoughtful essay published in *Science*, discuss the ethical and religious issues raised by efforts to build new organisms, beginning with microbial engineering, based on the creation of a "minimum genome."[6] Those issues will become far more urgent when the engineered organism is not a stripped-down, single-cell microbe but an animal.

Living things had always been thought to be rooted in nature, no matter how much humans might tinker with their properties. The advance of biotechnology throws into confusion the settled distinction between nature and artifact. The ability to change humanity through genetic engineering likewise compels us to question the extent to which a common history must tie humanity to the rest of the living world.

The following pages examine the influential and resilient belief that society should maintain the place of humanity in the natural world, and therefore proscribe the deliberate manipulation of the human genome, except, perhaps, for the therapy of well-characterized disease.[7] This view may suppose that the manipulation of the genome could transform people from created to manufactured or "fabricated" beings.[8] This is thought to be a bad thing. Alternatively, one could view nature as a war of each against all—as having no moral purpose, course, or direction— and so believe that by separating itself from nature, culturally and biologically, humanity fulfills its ethical potential.

A Tale of Two Conferences

Twenty-five years ago, at the Asilomar Conference Center near Monterey, California, more than a hundred biologists gathered with lawyers, physicians, and members of the press to discuss the then–novel technology of genetic recombination–"the most monumental power ever handed to us," according to David Baltimore, one of the conference organizers.[9] Amid the urgency surrounding the conference—the appeals for voluntary moratoriums, the fears of microscopic Frankensteins—no one questioned the assumption that genetic engineering offered scientists unprecedented powers over nature. These new powers appeared to require exceptional institutions, regulations, and policies. Molecular biologists called on themselves to exert a self-discipline rarely expected of scientists.

Scientists considered the ability to manipulate the genome to be truly exceptional because it conferred on them a capacity, on the one hand, apparently so general and far-reaching and, on the other, so intimate and personal as to defy comparison with any other technology. A quarter of a century ago, the metaphor of "playing God" seemed appropriate—as did notions of the genome as the "blueprint," "template," or "periodic table" that determines the nature of a person, plant, or animal. Observers argued that once the genetic code had been "cracked," nothing could deter human will and contrivance. Even today—if the April 10, 2000 *Newsweek* cover story, "Decoding the Human Body," is any indication— the public regards DNA technology in itself as particularly alarming, risky, or perverse—a Faustian bargain, a Promethean assault on the natural world.

In February 2000, a group of scientists, including several of the original conferees, met with other experts again at Asilomar to take stock of their concerns about genetic engineering. Their talk was not of awesome power and heroic self-restraint but of regulatory headaches and business opportunities. Within the scientific and professional community, the intervening years, it seemed, had turned genomic research and technology into business as usual (if big business) and normal science. Popular magazines continue to tout the exceptional powers of biotechnology, but twenty-five years after the first Asilomar conference, scientists and those who deal professionally with medical ethics and policy take a far more restrained view and speak not of Promethean possibilities but of particular strategies to deal with specific diseases.

The matter-of-factness, even complacency, on display at the second Asilomar meeting can be traced to two sources. First, and most obviously, the "monumental power" of genetic technology had created exaggerated expectations that it could not possibly fulfill at least in the near term. With stolen fire in hand, Prometheus hadn't burned down the world. Geneticists have been able to isolate a large number of mutations associated with various diseases—many of which were already regarded as hereditary. Pharmaceutical companies have taken genes from one organism and placed them into other organisms to produce great quantities of important proteins, such as erythropoietin. Doctors have engaged in a few expensive and inconclusive attempts at gene therapy. To understand the significance of the "genetic revolution" in medicine is to explore the intricacies of particular maladies and the difficulties of curing them. (It is useful to note, however, that the reverse situation is true in agriculture, where in a short time genetic engineering has indeed led to enormous changes in the production of food and fiber.) The practical yield of genetic research and technology in its human applications has been more modest, more technical, and far more specialized than had been hoped and feared a generation earlier.

Second, twenty-five years of discussion and debate has helped put to rest the more flamboyant fears and monstrous metaphors that greeted the new genetic "alchemy." This interdisciplinary dialogue and commentary explained the comparatively modest results achieved by genomic technology by pointing to the indirect, limited, complex, and synergistic roles genes play in determining phenotypic traits, including those associated with so-called genetic diseases. Commentators argued that genetic technology offered just another, albeit more precise, technology for altering biological traits in plants and animals.

By the 1990s, scholars had thoroughly criticized the assumptions—and the underlying metaphors—that encouraged the anxieties and expectations commonplace twenty years earlier. These commentators explicitly attacked the idea that genetic technology differed in kind from other medical interventions. For example, in 1993, the Task Force on Genetic Information and Insurance coined the term "genetic exceptionalism," as its chair Thomas Murray has written, "to mean roughly the claim that genetic information is sufficiently different from other kinds of health-related information that it deserves special protection or other exceptional measures." The task force found arguments for this claim unconvincing and "concluded that genetic information did not differ substantially from other kinds of health-related information."[10] Broadening this critique, Glenn McGee has asserted that "in no small part, genetic exceptionalism has also licensed hyperbole about 'holy grails' and 'unlocking the key to life,' language that is not only misleading but also damaging to the understanding."[11]

The exaggerated myths and fears surrounding genetic technology were analyzed under a slightly different rubric in an influential book by Dorothy Nelkin and M. S. Lindee, *The DNA Mystique*. These authors showed how images and narratives of the gene in popular culture reflect and convey a message they called "genetic essentialism," which attributes all that is important about people—their basic traits, their moral potential, their general behavior—to the action of their genomes.[12]

In opposition to popular concerns about a Frankensteinian future, scholars argued that the causal connection between genetic characteristics and phenotypic traits remained too obscure, complex, and case specific to warrant any general conclusions—and certainly too contested to justify any large-scale initiatives in law and public policy.[13] If there was a special danger in genetic research and technology, scholars contended, it lay in reinforcing the mystique of the genome. The sequencing of the human genome would not lead to technocratic dystopias; a danger arose, however, from the growing public belief that it might do so. Critics of genetic exceptionalism argued that the principal thing we have to fear is the fear of genetic research itself—a fear born of false assumptions about the centrality of DNA in determining the character and the course of our lives.

The critique of genetic exceptionalism has debunked myths about genetic technology—for example, that our genetic composition, more than many environmental conditions, determines our prospects, character, and actions. The critique of genetic essentialism, though, has not addressed one of the deep convictions about the human genome that lies behind the resistance to bioengineering. According to this widely held view, even if the human genome plays a more contingent, variable, and limited role in directing human traits than analogies to blueprints suggest, it nevertheless connects human beings as individuals and a species to a natural evolutionary and ecological order. One need not favor nature over nurture to believe, with Ramsey and other critics, that the concepts of nature and the natural play a critical role in guiding our moral intuitions.

Many of those who invoke the concept of nature and the natural in this context—such as Lander—are well aware of the complex, oblique, and limited role genes play in producing phenotypic characteristics. These critics need not appeal to discarded metaphors about the genetic blueprint to argue that genetic engineering, by separating people from the course of evolution, threatens to turn them into artifacts. Without being a genetic determinist or essentialist, one can worry that genetic techniques, if used extensively to alter germ lines, would remove a crucially important link that ties human beings to a common evolutionary heritage and other species in the natural world.

The End of Nature

In *The New Genesis: Theology and the Genetic Revolution*, Ronald Cole-Turner aptly states the problem of understanding the normative force of the "natural" in the context of genetic engineering. He notes that previous technologies, for example, in medicine and agriculture, vastly altered nature, but only up to a point, because the genetic inheritance of species, beyond the arduous changes conferred by artificial selection, lay beyond our reach. "Genetic inheritance," Cole-Turner correctly observes, "came to signify nature itself—nature as *natus*, as that which is born, inheriting inward principles that guide its development and set limits, both physical and moral, on our technological alterations." Genetic engineering differs from other technologies because it is directed at this last frontier or citadel that nature occupies. "Genetic engineering will change nature," Cole-Turner observes, "by altering the genetic arrangement inside living things."[14]

One may agree that genetic engineering will change nature, but one can also offer at least three different kinds of arguments to suggest that this may not be such a bad thing. First, appeals to nature—especially to human nature—have had an unprepossessing, indeed, sometimes unsavory, history. Those who have opposed certain practices have too often and without further justification labeled them "unnatural." The term unnatural can be used thoughtlessly and indefensibly simply to denigrate practices or activities that some people may find offensive. These invidious uses of the term do not show, however, that there is no distinction to be drawn between the natural and the artificial, or that no legitimate normative force is to be associated with that distinction.

Second, one may invoke powerful philosophical arguments in the tradition of Hume and G. E. Moore that deny the possibility of inferring "ought" from "is," that is, the impossibility of using statements about nature to infer statements about morality. All kinds of horrible things, alas, are completely natural, such as cancer. One might then concede that the genome ties humanity to nature, but argue that nature itself is of such dubious morality that it would be a good thing to sever that connection.

Third, human beings have already changed nature pervasively; indeed, the point of all technology may be to control and transform the natural world. Through artificial selection, for example, breeders have changed the genomes of crops and livestock. Genetic engineering, being far more precise than conventional methods of plant and animal breeding, changes the genome far less and less often to achieve the desired results. These novel technologies, one may claim, do not threaten to alter nature—including plant and animal genomes—any more extensively than medical, agricultural, and other technologies that have become familiar and that we readily accept.

While there is something to each of these arguments, they cannot gainsay that the concepts of nature and the natural carry enormous moral importance and emotional force. According to the familiar perspective that may draw on the story of Eden, humankind depends on nature but has "fallen" from it. Nature provides goods and services but also sets limits.[15] Nature is the object of responsibility, respect, stewardship, love, rights, and reverence.[16] In the context of environmental ethics, the natural refers primarily to biological communities or systems that result from the spontaneous course of evolution. Of course, environmentalists and others have questioned whether nature in this sense applies to anything that any longer exists.[17] Books with titles like *The Death of Nature* and *The End of Nature* reflect this concern.[18]

Today, the concept of the natural continues to carry enormous moral weight and emotional power. The more deeply technology penetrates nature and "conquers" it, the stronger efforts become to preserve what remains of our evolutionary and ecological heritage. Programs to protect natural biodiversity, for example, have increased greatly at the time when biotechnology has shown its potential to create genetic variability artificially. Calls to protect the human genome from manipulation, at least at first impression, have much in common with arguments environmentalists and others present to protect what is "wild" from human intervention, particularly from genetic engineering. The underlying idea may be that nature is sacred—that its wonderful organization defies our imagination and thus seems to be divine. The prospect of extending longevity as well as changing inherited characteristics adds weight to the metaphor of playing God.

Mill on Nature

An examination of the normative power of appeals to nature or the natural may begin with John Stuart Mill's remarkable essay "On Nature," one of his *Three Essays on Religion*. There, Mill questioned the romantic view that nature exhibits an order or plan. He wanted in part to refute the well-known argument from design, which infers the existence of God from the orderliness of the natural world. Rather than concede this argument for the existence of God, Mill wrote that the violence, arbitrariness, and sheer horror of natural history—parasites, predation, starvation, freezing, fire, and so on—led him to think that principles of beneficent design could not be true of the natural world. Nature is "too clumsily made and capriciously governed," he wrote, to justify the attribution of order, purpose, or design to its spontaneous course.[19]

"In sober truth," Mill declared, "nearly all the things which men are hanged or imprisoned for doing to one another, are nature's every day performances. Killing, the most criminal act recognized by human laws, nature does once to every being that lives; and in a large proportion of cases, after protracted tortures such as only the greatest monsters whom we read of ever purposely inflicted on their living fellow-creatures."[20] How could so vicious an arrangement be thought of as well designed, much less the creation of a beneficent deity?

To make his argument, Mill distinguished between two senses of the term *nature*. First, nature may refer to everything in the universe—that is, everything to which the laws of physics apply. In this context, the natural constitutes the opposite of the supernatural. Everything human beings do, in this sense, is natural. Second, nature may refer to the spontaneous arrangement of things—that is, all that is independent of or unaffected by human agency. In this sense, the idea of the natural is defined in terms of its significant opposite, the artificial or cultural. (This distinction, fundamental in Western culture, harks back to the Greek distinction between *physis* and *nomos*, nature and convention.) Mill asks whether nature in either of these senses possesses a design, an organization, an order, or—as we might say—an integrity. Does nature either in the sense of "everything" or in the sense of "untouched by humankind" obey patterns, embody principles, or display uniformities that humanity should reckon with and respect? In either of these senses, should we design with nature, obey nature, or accept its barriers and bounds?

The answer is plainly affirmative insofar as we refer to nature in the sense of "everything in the world." The laws of nature—for example, of gravitation and motion—apply to human beings as to all objects. In this context, however, the admonition to obey nature or respect nature, while excellent advice, would be unnecessary since no one can do otherwise. By knowing and taking advantage of the laws of physics—such as the principles of Newtonian mechanics—humanity can command nature, as it were, by obeying it. Mill concludes: "To bid people to conform to the laws of nature when they have no power but what the laws of nature give them—when it is a physical impossibility for them to do the smallest thing otherwise than through some law of nature—is an absurdity. The thing they need to be told is, what particular law of nature they should make use of in a particular case."[21]

Now consider the term nature in the sense in which it means not everything that happens but that which takes place without human agency. How may we understand the maxim to respect nature in this sense, that is, to keep ourselves within nature's spontaneous course? This maxim, Mill writes, "is not merely, as it is in the other sense, superfluous and unmeaning, but palpably absurd and contradictory." He explains:

For while human action cannot help conforming to Nature in the one meaning of the term, the very aim and object of action is to alter and improve nature in the other meaning. If the natural course of things were perfectly right and satisfactory, to act at all would be a gratuitous meddling, which as it could not make things better, must make them worse. . . . If the artificial is not better than the natural, to what end are all the arts of life? To dig, to plough, to build, to wear clothes, are direct infringements of the injunction to follow nature.[22]

Mill's argument poses a dilemma for those like Lander who seek to ban the manipulation of the human genome in order to maintain humanity as a product of nature. If one considers the term nature to refer to everything that obeys the laws of nature—in short, all that is not supernatural—then it is clear that whatever humans do is natural, depends entirely on nature, and is completely consistent with nature. If one supposes that terms like nature and the natural refer only to that which has not been altered intentionally by human beings, then humans cannot help but depart and exclude themselves from nature's spontaneous course.

Anything human beings may do—to get a haircut, for instance, much less an education—grossly infringes on the injunction to follow nature's course. All moral behavior may oppose, conflict with, or alter human nature, or why do we socialize children? Why should the genes be off-limits to manipulation when the mind, equally "given" but equally manipulable, is not off-limits to education?

The Medical Humanities and the Naturalness of Medicine

Many philosophers, theologians, and others have searched for ways to show that the manipulation of the genome by novel methods, even if it does not surpass older technologies in the extent of its effects on the natural world, differs from these technologies along important moral dimensions. Within the medical humanities, philosophers and other analysts—Leon Kass is one example—have argued that by engaging in genetic manipulation, doctors at least incrementally will commodify life.[23] Technologists may treat the embryo, say, more as a resource than as an end in itself, the form of which is to be accepted and respected.[24] This concern reflects a centuries-old debate over the role of medicine as either (1) working with nature and within its limits, or (2) overcoming or conquering nature to better serve human desires.

The first view, which holds that the physician must work with nature, draws from a tradition in medicine associated with Plato and Hippocrates that regards the physician as helping, but at the same time constrained by the natural processes by which the body can heal and restore itself.[25] This tradition regards medical science as nature's helpmeet. Guided by a sympathetic understanding of or an intuitive feel for nature's own processes, medicine instructs people how to live healthy lives. It facilitates the body's own ability to restore disturbed balances, heal injuries, and adapt to altered circumstances. In this tradition, the natural is considered normative.

Among the recent studies in the medical humanities that embrace this tradition are those by Leon Kass, *Toward a More Natural Science*, and Daniel Callahan, *Setting Limits* and *What Kind of Life?*[26] These authors, among others, appeal to the importance of the concept of the natural in dealing with decisions about aging and death. They reject what they believe is a kind of technological hubris that denies that there is any natural cause of death or that death is ever a natural event that should be welcomed. The concept of the natural, these authors have argued, helps us to understand what to attempt and what not to attempt in medical intervention, and it grounds the crucial distinction between acts of commission and omission.

The second view draws from a tradition in medicine associated with Lucretius and Francis Bacon that regards the physician as standing apart from, and often in opposition to, nature. The natural is not normative; it is merely the biological status quo, which will frequently be inimical to the patient's health. In order to achieve the goals of medicine, the physician must often treat nature as an adversary. The physician's justification for assisting and interfering with nature is understood in terms of the balance of risks and benefits. With the growth and broad acceptance of modern surgical procedures, particularly organ transplantation, this view, and the tradition it draws from, have become dominant. But the first, more conservative view has made a modest comeback in recent years in bioethics literature, if not in medical practice.[27]

The two opposing views interpret the goals of medicine quite differently. For the first, the goals of medicine are as fixed as our nature; health is linked in crucial ways to the natural and the biologically normal. The idea of improving on nature is a contradiction of sorts. For the second view, the goals of medicine are not fixed by the natural or the biologically normal, and the idea of improving on nature is perfectly intelligible. Proponents of this view exhort us to improve our capacities and performance to the greatest extent possible, sometimes by reinforcing, or, if necessary, by altering or suppressing what may be considered natural processes and limits. In the recent bioethics literature, this Promethean approach has been discussed primarily in the context of various forms of enhancement—surgical, pharmacological, and genetic—and in relation to aging.[28]

Not surprisingly, the two perspectives have different implications for genetic engineering. The first one, drawing on the Hippocratic tradition, counsels greater restraint, but how much and what kind of restraint depends on how it understands the relationship between the genome and nature. In one extreme view, the genome contains the full set of nature's instructions for the individual, and any genetic alteration, whether somatic or germ line, constitutes unacceptable interference with nature.

But one may still regard the genome as natural and the natural as normative without requiring such strict construction. For one thing, the individual's genome may contain "contradictory" instructions, so technology may assist nature in one sense by overcoming it in another. Or some harmful instructions may have their source in the mutation of ancestral genes, including mutations caused by such "unnatural" insults as radiation from a nuclear power plant. Moreover, the specific configuration of genes in the individual patient result, in part, from the myriad of social decisions that shaped that individual's pedigree. Accordingly, the construction of what is natural in the genome may involve many of the same moral and logical issues that arise in the decision about whether to regard the natural as normative in the first place.

On a looser or more flexible construction of the genetic code, the physician can abet salutary tendencies or strains within the genome against less salutary ones; the physician can engage in selective genetic engineering and still be regarded as working with, or assisting, nature. But even in this more flexible view, the genome is not simply the raw material with which the physician has to work to produce desired results. The physician must be guided by, and work to reinforce, the protective or healing tendencies discerned in it. The physician's interventions have to maintain a consistency or harmony with the original genome if they are to preserve the role of the physician and the identity of the patient.

It is important to note that on this more flexible interpretation, the first view of medicine and nature does not preclude either germ line therapy or enhancement, as long as the changes wrought by those interventions can be seen as strengthening what is already present or implicit in the individual's genome. Of course, given the loose, metaphoric character of this standard, it is difficult to tell how demanding it would be. For proponents of the opposing view, however, the human genome must be reckoned with, not respected. It imposes practical limits, not moral constraints.

The Distinction between Born and Made

In the literature on assisted reproductive technology, the idea of nature as a norm has been vigorously invoked and challenged.[29] As those technologies progressed, critics of appeals to nature appear to have prevailed.

Although there have been some spirited rearguard actions, few commentators now regard the creation of a child by artificial insemination or in vitro fertilization as unnatural in any sense that would make it morally objectionable or problematic.[30] The most forceful recent critiques of assisted reproductive technology have come from feminists and other writers who fear that these technologies will commodify children and subordinate women.[31] Feminist critiques rarely invoke nature except to debunk the supposition that females are somehow more nature's creatures than are men. Nevertheless, critiques of the so-called industrialization of reproduction have important affinities with theological concerns about the displacement of natural objects and processes.[32]

The distinction and tension between the notions of *producing* and *procreating* children arose long before the advent of genetic engineering. Indeed, as William Ruddick observes, both notions have shaped our traditional thinking about natural, or species-typical, reproduction. Ruddick suggests that folk wisdom regards parents as gardeners, deliberately making a product from the material that nature provides them. Folk wisdom also regards them as guardians, deputized to nurture and protect an independent being. Ruddick suggests that both notions, or analogies, are needed to capture the parental role, which involves the production of a being that becomes the moral equal of its producers, and which places special obligations on the parents by virtue of their productive efforts.[33]

One might suggest that in Ruddick's terms the delicate balance between the two aspects of reproduction is upset by genetic technology, so that the productive aspect overwhelms the procreative. There are at least two ways in which genetic engineering might threaten the balance. The first is by conferring an unprecedented degree of control and selectivity on "gardeners," who no longer need to rely on the vagaries of genetic recombination. They can pick the genes, or at least some of the genes, that they want, and thereby increase their control over the final product. The child is not only produced but manufactured; he or she is not merely a product but an artifact. It might be argued, though, that this threat is greatly exaggerated, reflecting a naive and oversimplified view of the contribution of genes to valued traits. Genetic engineering will always leave a great deal to chance and the environment. Perhaps it will confer the illusion of total control, but that illusion will eventually yield when the limitations of the technology become manifest.

Even if genetic engineering did not confer an exceptional degree of control, there is another way in which it might upset the balance between the productive and the procreative aspects of parenting. Genetic technology, one may fear, could supplant the gardeners' stock—that is, the raw material—and thereby destroy the continuity between the gardeners' product and its predecessors. Heirloom tomatoes may be exceptionally tasty, yet what makes them heirlooms is not their taste but their lineage—that they derive from an uninterrupted succession of vines, bred for centuries.[34] These varieties link the modern consumer with medieval horticulture. The introduction of laboratory-created genes into human beings would, it may be feared, disrupt a natural progression—even one that is assisted and guided by human beings—and mark the end of a natural history.[35] By severing its link with nature, genetic engineering would deny or diminish a child's moral status.[36]

Interestingly, adoption does not raise anything like this kind of concern. While there is no biological continuity between adoptive parents and children in the usual sense, adopted children are the product of a long natural history to which the parents equally belong. By analogy, gardeners merely plant seeds in different soil. Similarly, most forms of assisted reproduction do not raise this specter of ending or departing from a natural history, since these technologies merely engage artificial means to extend a natural lineage. It is not even a threat posed by cloning, which preserves the fruit of past recombination.

The concern that children be born rather than made may reflect the reasonable insistence that children should be ends in themselves, not merely instruments to achieve ends prescribed for them. This important moral principle, however, does not rule out genetic engineering as such, but only that which parents employ in search of a "perfect" baby or one that meets certain specifications. It would be just as wrong for parents, in order to fulfill their own ambitions, to insist on a course of athletic training for a child. The objection lies not in the technology but the brazen purpose to which it is put.

To see this, consider a hypothetical example. Suppose that parents filled in a child's genome by randomly selecting from a pool of manufactured genes. The child would be completely fabricated in the sense of being made not born. Yet the random method would severely limit parental control and thus preserve a substantial element of contingency or chance, thereby assuaging objections that genetic technologies may undermine the contingency that is part of the basis of commitment or love. Such a random method, however, would, no less than deliberate selection, attenuate the connection between the new being and nature—for instance, the child's genetic forebears. It is not clear that this loss of continuity entails a loss of moral status.

Why should the insertion of genes into a human organism, moreover, transform it into an artifact when the insertion of an artificial limb, hip, or even heart does not? No one thinks that by putting a Dacron valve in a patient's heart, a surgeon somehow transforms that individual from a product of nature into a machine. The crucial issue might not lie in the use of a particular technology but in the reason or purpose of its use, and whether this is consistent with treating a person with dignity and respect. In this case, genetic technology would not differ from any other—though we have to build up the concepts, intuitions, and arguments needed to distinguish legitimate from illegitimate uses of this, as any, important new technology.

The Theological Literature: Humans as Cocreators

Many of the scholars who have explored the relationship of the genome and nature have been theologians. Catholic theology, particularly that represented in and after the Second Vatican Council, presents one obvious starting point at which to examine the idea that there is a natural order that limits human activity, especially with respect to reproduction. Vatican II made no mention of genetic engineering other than to reiterate the view that "sons of the Church may not undertake methods of regulating which are found blameworthy by the teaching authority of the Church in its unfolding of the divine law."[37] Catholic theologians, including Karl Rahner, one of the leading theologians of the twentieth century, and Bernard Haring, a leader of the reform movement in Catholic moral theology, both of whom contributed to Vatican II, have vigorously debated the prospects and permissibility of human genetic engineering. The debate in Catholic theology addresses many of the major philosophical and moral issues that surround the question of the givenness of the genome and its relation to human nature.

According to Rahner, human freedom consists in our accepting the human genome from nature or God as given, for otherwise we surrender essential aspects of our freedom to those (including the state) who would regulate genetic technology. Rahner has written that "genetic technology is the embodiment of the fear of oneself, the fear of accepting one's self as the unknown quantity it is." He extended the argument to all of nature or creation: "The world can never be 'worked over' to such an extent that man is eventually dealing only with material *he* has chosen and created."[38] For Rahner as for many environmentalists concerned with the protection of the so-called wilderness or other biological remnants of a disappearing past, the sheer givenness of nature—what biologists like Stephen Jay Gould may refer to as its contingency—is what makes it valuable and morally itself.

Rahner argued, then, that to protect what is given and therefore part of our human nature, we "must cultivate a sober and critical resistance to the fascination of novel possibilities."[39] On the other hand, as Ted Peters has argued, Rahner did not rule out all genetic manipulation and remained open to the technological future. According to Peters, Rahner recognized that human history is an "active alteration of this material world itself," and that human nature "is open and undetermined."[40]

Bernard Haring took this openness to the future further. He agreed that human beings are bound by a respect for nature, a recognition of the "gratuity of all creation," as a free gift by God, without which "our exploitation of the world becomes depletion and alienation." Haring argued, however, that humans are cocreators with God; he acknowledged that humanity had to its advantage greatly altered the natural world. He maintained that our ability to improve and perfect nature should in principle extend to the genome. Yet Haring cautioned that we must bear in mind not our own instrumental goals but the vision of God's purposes for humankind: "The divine mandate to subdue the earth and to fill it includes man's mission to transform life according to his finest vision of humankind's future." Haring employed the notion of stewardship—also prominent in environmental ethics—to argue that humanity may "freely interfere with and manipulate the function of his *bios* (biological life) and psyche insofar as this does not degrade him or diminish his or his fellowmen's dignity and freedom."[41]

A cursory look at Catholic writing in medical ethics suggests that it supports Haring's position. For example, Benedict Ashley and Kevin O'Rourke, both at St. Louis University, wrote in *Health Care Ethics* that God, in giving us intelligence, regards us as "co-workers and encourages [us] to exercise real originality."[42] Even Charles Curran, who takes a generally conservative position, has said, "The genius of modern man and woman is the ability toward self-creation and self-direction."[43] Curran, however, like other Catholic theologians, would limit genetic interventions at first to somatic therapy (which virtually no one opposes), and allow it for germ line therapy only to relieve "defects" as these are rather narrowly understood; he would rule out "improvements" that suggest individuals are valued instrumentally rather than as ends in themselves. It is not clear whether striking differences in the concept of humans as cocreators within Catholic theology have practical implications for the kinds of interventions deemed acceptable.

The relevant literature in Protestant theology is vast and represents a wide variety of views. Books with titles such as *Fabricated Man* and *Brave New People* emphasize the risk that genetic engineering will rob humanity of its freedom by substituting human purpose (an instrumental ethic) for divine purpose (creation) or no purpose (evolution).[44] James A. Nash, executive director of the Center for Theology and Public Policy, explicitly connects discussions of ecological integrity in environmental ethics to allow genetic interventions for the sake of perfecting or redeeming creation, not for reshaping it to human purposes. He asks, "Is the whole of nature to be defined by human purposes and subject to human improvements?"[45]

Like Ian Barbour and Deter Hessel, Nash takes a cautious approach, also reflected in various documents issued by the World Council of Churches, that counsels against germ line therapy except in very special cases where the therapeutic as distinct from eugenic purpose is absolutely clear.[46] Nash makes the additional point that some genetic interventions, although important in preventing a disease in certain individuals, are really inconsequential *sub specie aeternitatis*. He reminds us that "the miracles of genetic engineering are trivial in comparison with the surrounding magnitude of evolutionary and ecological miracles, which deserve preservation." To preserve these latter miracles, in the environment and ourselves, we ought to restrain ourselves, or as Nash puts it, we "ought not to exercise all the limited powers that we do have."[47]

Much of the theological writing, Catholic and Protestant, that examines moral issues in genetic engineering adopts the view, as stated forcefully by geneticist Robert Sinsheimer, that as we become creators of life, we run the risk of losing reverence for it.[48] That this consequence does not or need not follow, however, has been the thesis of Cole-Turner of the Memphis Theological Seminary. He concedes that genetic manipulation may enable us to "alter our own human nature."[49] That the technology may carry us too far by no means shows that we should not use it to improve the conditions of life.

Cole-Turner forcefully argues in theological terms against genetic exceptionalism. His critique is often scathing: "To think of genetic material as the exclusive realm of divine grace and creativity is to reduce God to the level of restriction enzymes, viruses, and sexual reproduction. Treating DNA as matter . . . is not in itself sacrilegious."[50] Cole-Turner writes in a Protestant tradition that contends that God's redemptive initiative extends to the natural world—in other words, that humanity may redeem nature by technology as it redeems itself through faith and good works. (Interestingly, Al Gore writes knowledgeably about these issues in the chapter "Environmentalism of the Spirit" in his *Earth in the Balance*.)[51] Cole-Turner recognizes that the arguments made for or against the application of genetic engineering to the human genome may also apply, mutatis mutandis, to other species. He observes that "genetic engineering is being used to confer resistance to disease on agricultural plants, and to reduce their fertilizer needs. We may regard this as redemptive in that it enhances the usefulness of these plants while diminishing the environmental damage that has been part of their cultivation."[52]

Jewish theology has, in general, been hospitable to genetic engineering. While Saint Thomas Aquinas brought the Aristotelian concept of nature into Christianity, Jewish theology has had no such commitment to the idea of defining form. Perhaps for this reason, Jewish commentators have not stated categorical objections to human genetic manipulation of any kind. They have welcomed the prospect of germ line genetic therapy for well-characterized diseases, such as Tay-Sachs. A central figure in the Conservative Jewish tradition, Elliot N. Dorff, writes, "When used in this therapeutic way, genetic engineering is an unmitigated blessing."[53] This view is shared by representatives of other branches of Judaism (see, for instance, Fred Rosner [Orthodox] and Walter Jacob [Reform]).[54] Dorff adds that "since sickness is degrading, it would be our *duty* to cure the disease at its root if we could, so that future generations will not be affected."[55]

At the same time, some Jewish theologians are concerned about the difficulty of setting limits on genetic intervention when it goes beyond such a narrow therapeutic role. Dorff, among other Jewish theologians, fully recognizes that it will be difficult to tell what to count as an acceptable intervention and what to count as enhancement. He asks, "How do we determine when we are using genetic engineering appropriately to aid God in ongoing, divine acts of cure and creation and when, on the other hand, are we usurping the proper prerogatives of God to determine the nature of creation?"[56] Jewish theologians who have written on this question have taken opposing positions. In "Judaism and Gene Design," Orthodox rabbi Azriel Rosenfeld argues, "Our sages recognize, and perhaps even encourage, the use of prenatal (or better, preconceptual) influences to improve one's offspring."[57] Other rabbis—David Golinkin is an example—disagree, pointing out that Nazi and other attempts at eugenics amply demonstrate the difficulty of finding criteria for knowing what a good trait is.[58]

Genetic Engineering in the Natural Environment

There are striking parallels in the invocation of nature by proponents of environmental protection and opponents of genetic engineering. Both appeals are characterized by arguments that move between the prudential value of nature and a variety of noninstrumental values. The early conservationists sought to preserve nature because of the threat its destruction posed to human well-being, that is, to our capacity to feed and shelter ourselves. While arguments of this form are, of course, still made, often with cogency (for example, in the debate over global warming), they are no longer the sole, or even the main, basis for restraint. Rather, environmentalists have presented several other kinds of arguments for preserving nature that do not rely on the adverse effects of destroying it. Nature may be useful, but more important, it is majestic, beautiful, and sacred, either because of its randomness and spontaneity or its intricate design and balance. Destroying nature, for example, by causing the extinction of species, may be imprudent, but it is also, and not necessarily for that reason, presumptuous, arrogant, and vulgar.

Similarly, the early critics of recombinant DNA research focused on its potential harms, arguing for restraint as a matter of prudence. These fears still have credibility, but they have been joined by the more principled concern that in engaging in the unrestricted engineering of the (human) genome, we will contaminate something precious or sacred, and that our attempts to do so display presumption, arrogance, and vulgarity.

Conceptions of nature and the natural at work in controversies over genetic engineering in food and the environment closely resemble those that motivate controversies concerning manipulation of the human genome. In all of these contexts, critics often draw a distinction between the natural and the artificial; they associate the artificial with the instrumental, the commercial, and the commodified; and they draw conclusions concerning the inappropriateness and often the risk of genetic technologies.[59] If policy choices could turn simply on risk assessment—if the contentions were consequentialist at bottom—then arguments over genetic engineering would not differ from those that pertain to any medical or environmental technology.

Popular concerns over genetic engineering in agriculture often rest on notions of nature or the natural, as do animadversions on human germ line alteration. Titles of popular articles on agricultural biotechnology appeal to the same metaphors—Frankenstein, playing God—as similar essays about engineering the human genome. Thus, a *New York Times Sunday Magazine* cover article carried the title "Playing God in the Garden," and a *Newsweek* essay covered the topic as "Frankenstein Foods?"[60] The Prince of Wales, in a famous tirade against biotechnology, invoked the idea that genetic technologies are not harmonious with nature. "I have always believed that agriculture should proceed in harmony with nature, recognizing that there are natural limits to our ambitions," Prince Charles wrote, adding, "We need to rediscover a reverence for the natural world, irrespective of its usefulness to ourselves, to become more aware of the relationship between God, man and creation."[61]

In the United States, populist critics of biotechnology appeal roughly to the same idea that nature has an essence or form that we disturb when we alter genomes. This statement by Andrew Kimbrell and Jeremy Rifkin is representative:

Is there any meaning in the morphology of animals or plants, both externally and internally? Should we alter nature or mutate, perhaps permanently, the forms or shapes of the biotic community so that they better conform to our agricultural or industrial needs? . . . What are the ethical implications of the likely proposal to engineer plant or animal genetic material into humans? Finally, who is to decide these issues: Congress, Scientists, Corporations, Theologians, The Public? Federal agencies?[62]

These remarks capture what may be the most fundamental popular concern about genetic engineering in agriculture—namely, that it is less natural than conventional breeding. As one critic commented, "It is now possible to insert genetic material from species, families and even kingdoms which could not previously be sources of genetic material for a particular species, and even to insert custom-designed genes that do not exist in nature. As a result we can create what can be regarded as synthetic life forms, something which could not be done by conventional breeding."[63] That conventional breeding was limited, however, does not imply that there are limits that humanity must respect. As one expert cautioned, "The living world can now be viewed as a vast organic Lego kit inviting combination, hybridization, and continual rebuilding. Life is manipulability.[64]

Philosophers and others who are concerned with the nature of nature often take as a starting point Aristotle's concept of *telos*, that is, the functional essence or form that identifies each plant or animal according to its kind.[65] After Aquinas had appropriated Aristotelianism for Christianity, as Bernard Rollin points out, "*telos* as function became *telos* as Divine purpose, thereby indelibly tainting the concept with a supernatural flavour that potentiated its rejection by mechanistic, reductionist science."[66] Sciences that repudiate a "reductionist" method—certain "holistic" or "synthetic" branches of ecology, for example—may cling to an Aristotelian notion of structure and function, for instance, as defining species and ecosystems. For these so-called holistic sciences of the natural world, genetic engineering poses a tough conceptual challenge. Rollin explains, "For we may now see *telos* neither as externally fixed, as did Aristotle, nor as a stop action snapshot of a permanently dynamic process, as did Darwin, but rather as something infinitely malleable by human hands."[67]

British philosopher Alan Holland has explained that the distrust of genetic engineering represents what he calls a "metaphysical fear" that "centers on concerns over the implications of this technology for conceptions of identity, integrity and origin which are foundational to our world view and to our ability to classify individual beings." As the practice of animal cloning makes clear, breakthroughs in genetic technology are likely to arise in agriculture and then be applied to human beings. As Holland concluded: "Animal biotechnology is fully implicated. For a combination of the view that 'organisms are merely the vehicles for genes' with the realization that species boundaries are fully permeable, brings it home that we should ponder long over our treatment of non-human animals lest we should come to treat our fellow humans likewise."[68]

Biotechnology and the Tree of Life

Of the two meanings of the term nature that Mill identifies, only one is relevant to science—that is, the concept of nature as everything in the universe. In this sense, humanity and all it does is natural since it fits within the causal fabric of the world. The second sense of the term nature refers to all that exists independently of human action or intention. This conception of nature, while meaningless as a scientific notion, nevertheless carries a great deal of force in arguments having to do with what we ought or ought not to do. Its force may depend, however, on how one judges the moral worth of nature—for instance, whether one condemns nature as a gruesome war of each against all or reveres it as what God has made. These views, of course, are compatible; for example, in Calvinism, God is the reverse of beneficent. The Calvinist God who chooses that most human beings suffer eternal damnation could easily have created the nature we see.

To say that something occurs as a consequence of natural causes, for example, is to absolve humans of responsibility for it. An act of nature or an act of God is one that humanity had no ability to avert. In dealing with great tragedies and taking up heavy burdens, people console themselves with the thought that their plight is God's will or that it couldn't be helped. This fatalism forgoes the anger that would otherwise become anguish. There is no one to blame.

While it is entirely reasonable to rely on the concept of nature to refer to what cannot be helped, it is quite another thing to use it to refer to what should not be changed. To place nature beyond human blame or responsibility is simply to recognize the limits of our knowledge and powers. To suppose that nature has itself a moral order or purpose we should respect, in contrast, is for us to impose limits on those powers.

The problem with engineering the human genome is not so much that it will alienate or separate us from our human nature—from what is given or contingent—but that it will increasingly make us responsible for it. The nice thing about the nature we inherit—even if it is full of defects such as the propensity for disease—is that it was no one's responsibility. The more control we have, the more the genome becomes a matter of intention and choice. It falls within the reach of human freedom precisely because it comes within the causal order our science and technology may command.

In a way, there is nothing new here. Since the medieval period, people have been liberating themselves—for better or worse—from their history. A half millennium ago, one did as one's parents did. One stayed put. One accepted the religion, beliefs, language, and so forth that came with one's heritage. Five hundred years later, individuals choose religions, careers, communities, and so on. They may soon be able to choose—to some extent—the genetic characteristics of their children as well. Not only does the individual not have a nature; the individual may no longer have a history.

In Eden, nature was wholly beneficial; it cared for human beings as it did for the lilies of the field. One consequence of our eating from the Tree of Knowledge is that nature became hostile; it lost its moral order.

The temptation has been to use knowledge to return the environment to its beneficent state—in other words, to build a second nature that serves us as well as Eden did. This goal remained beyond human reach as long as we had eaten only from the Tree of Knowledge. One can hardly ponder the possibilities and the punishments that may await us as we nibble from the Tree of Life.

Notes

The author gratefully acknowledges the support of a grant from the program for Ethical, Legal, and Social Implications of the Human Genome Project of the National Institutes of Health. The views expressed are those of the author and not of any funding agency. David Wasserman contributed suggestions, criticisms, and guidance at every step in this essay, which makes him in effect coauthor.

1. Eric S. Lander, "In Wake of the Genetic Revolution, Questions about Its Meaning," *New York Times*, September 12, 2000, F5.

2. Paul Ramsey, *Fabricated Man: The Ethics of Genetic Control* (New Haven, CT: Yale University Press, 1970), 105.

3. Sean M. Fagan, *Does Morality Change?* (Dublin, Ireland: Gill and Macmillan, 1997), 27.

4. "Only Connect," *Economist*, July 1–7, 2000, 8–11.

5. Nicholas Wade, "Genome Analysis Shows Humans Survive on Low Number of Genes," *New York Times*, February 11, 2001, A1.

6. Mildred K. Cho, David Magnus, Arthur L. Caplan, Glen McGee, and the Ethics of Genomics Group, "Ethical Considerations in Synthesizing a Minimal Genome," *Science* 286, no. 5447 (December 10, 2000): 2087–2090.

7. For further discussion, see Robert Cook-Deegan, *The Gene Wars: Science, Politics, and the Human Genome* (New York: W. W. Norton, 1996); Tristram H. Engelhardt, "Germline Genetic Engineering and Moral Diversity: Moral Controversies in a Post-Christian World," *Social Philosophy and Policy* 13, no. 2 (Summer 1996): 47–62; and Joseph Fletcher, *Humanhood: Essays in Biomedical Ethics* (Buffalo, NY: Prometheus Books, 1979).

8. Jon Turney, *Frankenstein's Footsteps: Science, Genetics, and Popular Culture* (New Haven, CT: Yale University Press, 1998).

9. Cited in Marcia Barinaga, "Asilomar Revisited: Lessons for Today?" *Science* 287 (2000), 1584.

10. Thomas H. Murray, "Genetic Exceptionalism and 'Future Diaries': Is Genetic Information Different from Other Medical Information?" in *Genetic Secrets: Protecting Privacy and Confidentiality in the Genetic Era*, ed. Mark A. Rothstein (New Haven, CT: Yale University Press, 1997), 61.

11. Glenn McGee, "Ethical Issues in Genetics in the Next 100 Years" (lecture, UNESCO Asian Bioethics Conference, Kobe, Japan, November 6, 1997), <*http://www.biol.tsukuba.ac.jp/~macer/asiae/biae245.html*> (Accessed January 20, 2004) 248; and "Generic Exceptionalism," *Harvard Journal of Law and Technology* 11 (Summer 1998): 565–568. See also Glenn McGee, *The Perfect Baby: A Pragmatic Approach to Genetics* (Lanham, MD: Rowman and Littlefield 1997).

12. Dorothy Nelkin and M. S. Lindee, *The DNA Mystique: The Gene as a Cultural Icon* (New York: W. H. Freeman, 1995), 2.

13. See Thomas H. Murray and Mark A. Rothstein, eds., *The Human Genome Project and the Future of Health Care (Medical Ethics Series)* (Bloomington: Indiana University Press, 1996).

14. Ronald Cole-Turner, *The New Genesis: Theology and the Genetic Revolution* (Louisville, KY: Westminster John Knox Press, 1993), 8.

15. See Gretchen Dailey, ed., *Nature's Services: Societal Dependence on Natural Ecosystems* (Washington, DC: Island Press, 1997); and Donella H. Meadows, Dennis L. Meadows, and Jorgen Randers, *Beyond the Limits: Confronting Global Collapse, Envisioning a Sustainable Future* (Post Mills, VT: Chelsea Green Publishing, 1992).

16. On responsibility, see John Passmore, *Man's Responsibility for Nature* (New York: Scribner's, 1974). On respect, see Paul Taylor, *Respect for Nature* (Princeton, NJ: Princeton University Press, 1986). On stewardship, see Robin Attfield, *The Ethics of Environmental Concern* (New York: Columbia University Press, 1983). On love, see Stephen R. Kellert and Edward O. Wilson, eds., *The Biophilia Hypothesis* (Washington, DC: Island Press, 1993; and D. W. Ehrenfeld, "The Conservation of Non-resources," *American Scientist* 64 (1986): 648–656. On rights, see Christopher Stone, *Should Trees Have Standing? Toward Legal Rights for Natural Objects* (Los Altos, CA: Kaufmann, 1972). On reverence, see Clarence Glacken, *Traces on the Rhodian Shore: Nature and Culture in Western Thought from Ancient Times to the End of the Eighteenth Century* (Berkeley: University of California Press, 1967).

17. William Cronon, "The Trouble with Wilderness; or, Getting Back to the Wrong Nature," in *Uncommon Ground: Rethinking the Human Place in Nature*, ed. William Cronon (New York: W. W. Norton, 1996), 69–90.

18. Carolyn Merchant, *The Death of Nature: Women, Ecology, and the Scientific Revolution* (London: Wildwood House, 1982); and Bill McKibben, *The End of Nature* (New York: Random House, 1989).

19. John Stuart Mill, "On Nature," in *Three Essays on Religion* (1874; repr., New York: Greenwood Press, 1969), 28–29.

20. Ibid., 28–29.

21. Ibid., 16.

22. Ibid., 19–20.

23. Leon Kass, *Triumph or Tragedy: The Moral Meaning of Genetic Technology* (March 18, 1999), http://www.rand.org/publications/mr/mr1139/mr1139. appf.pdf. (Accessed January 20, 2004).

24. See Eric Juengst, "Should We Treat the Human Germ Line as a Global Human Resource?" in *Germ Line Intervention and Our Responsibilities to Future Generations*, ed. Emmanuel Agius and Salvino Busuttil (Boston: Kluwer Academic, 1998), 85–102.

25. See Agenta Sutton, "The New Genetics and Traditional Hippocratic Medicine," in *Man-Made Man: The Genome Project The Faustian Dream Come True?* ed. Peter Doherty and Agneta Sutton (Dublin, Ireland: Four Courts Press, 1997), 58–70.

26. Leon Kass, *Toward a More Natural Science* (New York: Free Press, 1985); and Daniel Callahan, *Setting Limits: Medical Goals in an Aging Society* (New York: Simon and Schuster, 1987); and *What Kind of Life? The Limits of Medical Progress* (New York: Simon and Schuster, 1990).

27. See Callahan, *Setting Limits*, and *What Kind of Life?*

28. On enhancement, see Erik Parens, ed., *Enhancing Human Traits: Ethical and Social Implications* (Washington, DC: Georgetown University Press, 1998); Erik Parens "The Goodness of Fragility: On the Prospect of Genetic Technologies Aimed at the Enhancement of Human Capacities," *Kennedy Institute of Ethics Journal 5*, no. 2 (1995): 141–153; Erik Parens "Is Better Always Good? The Enhancement Project," *Hastings Center Report 28*, no. 1 (January–February 1998): S1–S17; and McGee, "Ethical Issues in Genetics." On aging, see Arthur Caplan, "Is Aging a Disease?" in *If I Were a Rich Man Could I Buy a Pancreas? And Other Essays on the Ethics of Health Care* (Bloomington: Indiana University Press, 1992).

29. See John Harris, *Wonderwoman and Superman: The Ethics of Human Biotechnology* (Oxford: Oxford University Press, 1992); and *Clones, Genes, and Immortality: Ethics and the Genetic Revolution* (Oxford: Oxford University Press, 1998).

30. For one such "rearguard action," see Leon Kass, "The Wisdom of Repugnance," *The New Republic* (June 2, 1997), http://www.catholiceducation.org/medicalethics/md0006.htm. (Accessed January 20, 2004).

31. See Gina Corea, *The Mother Machine: Reproductive Technologies from Artificial Insemination to Artificial Wombs* (New York: Harper, 1985); and David Wasserman and Robert Wachbroit, "The Technology, Law, and Ethics of In Vitro Fertilization, Gamete Donation, and Surrogate Motherhood," *Clinics in Laboratory Medicine 12*, no. 3 (September 1992): 429–448.

32. See Jonathan Glover, *What Sort of People Should There Be?* (New York: Random House, 1977).

33. William Ruddick, "Parenthood: Three Concepts and a Principle," in *Morals, Marriage, and Parenthood: An Introduction to Family Ethics*, ed. Laurence D. Houlgate (Belmont, CA: Wadsworth, 1999), 242–251.

34. See Gerhold K. Becker, *Changing Nature's Course: The Ethical Challenge of Biotechnology* (Hong Kong: Hong Kong University Press, 1996); and David Goodman and Michael Redclift, *Refashioning Nature: Food, Ecology, and Culture* (London: Routledge, 1991).

35. See Michael J. Reiss and Roger Straughan, *Improving Nature? The Science and Ethics of Genetic Engineering* (New York: Cambridge University Press, 1996).

36. See Andrew Kimbrell, *The Human Body Shop: The Engineering and Marketing of Life* (Washington, DC: Regnery Publishing, 1998).

37. Second Vatican Council, "Gaudium et Spes," in *Renewing the Earth: Catholic Documents on Peace, Justice, and Liberation*, ed. David O'Brien and Thomas Shannon (New York: Image Books, 1997), 229.

38. Karl Rahner, "The Problem of Genetic Manipulation," in *Theological Investigations* (New York: Seabury Press, 1975), 9: 244, 245.

39. Ibid., 250.

40. Ted Peters, *Playing God? Genetic Discrimination and Human Freedom* (New York: Routledge, 1997), 143.

41. Bernard Haring, *The Ethics of Manipulation* (New York: Seabury Press, 1975), 70, 161.

42. Benedict Ashley and Kevin O'Rourke, *Health Care Ethics: A Theological Analysis* (St. Louis, MO: Catholic Health Association, 1982), 306.

43. Charles C. Curran, *Moral Theology: A Continuing Quest* (Notre Dame, IN: University of Notre Dame Press, 1982), 112.

44. Ramsey, *Fabricated Man*; and Gareth D. Jones, *Brave New People: Ethical Issues at the Commencement of Life* (Leicester, UK: Inter Varsity Press, 1984).

45. James A. Nash, *Loving Nature: Ecological Integrity and Christian Responsibility* (Nashville, TN: Abington Press, 1991), 61.

46. See Ian Barbour, *Ethics in an Age of Technology* (San Francisco: Harper, 1991); Deter T. Hessel, "Now That Animals Can Be Genetically Engineered: Biotechnology in Theological-Ethical Perspective," *Theology and Public Policy* (Summer 1993); and World Council of Churches, "Manipulating Life: Ethical Issues in Genetic Engineering" (Geneva: World Council of Churches, 1982); and "Biotechnology: Challenge to the Churches" (Geneva: World Council of Churches, 1989).

47. Nash, *Loving Nature*, 63.

48. Robert L. Sinsheimer, "The Prospect of Designed Genetic Change," in *Ethics, Reproduction, and Genetic Control*, ed. Ruth F. Chadwick (New York: Routledge, 1987).

49. Ronald Cole-Turner, *The New Genesis: Theology and The Genetic Revolution* (Louisville, KY: John Knox Press, 1993), 13.

50. Ibid., 13.

51. Al Gore, *Earth in the Balance* (Boston: Houghton Mifflin, 1992).

52. Cole-Turner, *The New Genesis*, 96.

53. Elliot N. Dorff, *Matters of Life and Death: A Jewish Approach to Medical Ethics* (Philadelphia: Jewish Publication Society, 1998), 161.

54. Fred Rosner, "Genetic Engineering and Judaism," in *Jewish Bioethics*, ed. Fred Rosner and J. D. Bleich (New York: Sanhedrin Press, 1979); and Walter Jacob, "Jewish Involvement in Genetic Engineering," in *Questions and Reform Jewish Answers: New American Reform Responsa*, ed. Walter Jacob (New York: Central Conference of American Rabbis, 1992).

55. Dorff, *Matters of Life and Death*, 164.

56. Ibid., 162. See also Paul Root Wolpe, "If I Am Only My Genes, What Am I? Genetic Essentialism and a Jewish Response," *Kennedy Institute of Ethics Journal* 3 (September 7, 1997): 213–230.

57. Azriel Rosenfeld, "Judaism and Gene Design," *Tradition* 13, no. 2 (Fall 1972): 71–80.

58. David Golinkin, "Responsa: Does Jewish Law Permit Genetic Engineering on Humans?" *Moment* (August 1994): 28, 29, 67.

59. For commentary, see Paul B. Thompson, *Food Biotechnology in Ethical Perspective* (London: Chapman and Hall Blackie Academic and Professional, 1997); R. Straughn, "Ethical Aspects of Crop Biotechnology," in *Issues in Agricultural Bioethics*, ed. T. B. Mepham, G. A. Tucker, and J. Wiseman (Nottingham, UK: University of Nottingham Press, 1995), 163–176; and David Suzuki and Peter Knudtson, *Genethics: The Clash between the New Genetics and Human Values* (Cambridge, MA: Harvard University Press, 1989).

60. Michael Pollan, "Playing God in the Garden," *New York Times Sunday Magazine*, October 25, 1998 44, 13 pages; Kenneth Klee, "Frankenstein Foods?" *Newsweek*, September 13, 1999, 33–36.

61. Prince Charles, reported in "Prince warns of 'playing God,'" BBC Wednesday, 17 May 2000 http://news.bbc.co.uk/1/hi/uk/751925.stm (Accessed January 24, 2004).

62. Andrew Kimbrell and Jeremy Rifkin, "Biotechnology: A Proposal for Regulatory Reform," *Notre Dame Journal of Law, Ethics, and Public Policy* 3 (1987): 126.

63. Michael Hansen, *How Gene-Splicing Is Radically Different from Conventional Agriculture* (January 27, 2000), http://www.orapnicconsumers.org/ge/hansenGEexpl.cfm. (Accessed January 20, 2004).

64. Edward Yoxen, *The Gene Business: Who Should Control Biotechnology?* (New York: Harper Collins, 1984), 2.

65. Aristotle, *Physics* 2.

66. Bernard E. Rollin, "On Telos and Genetic Engineering," in *Animal Biotechnology and Ethics*, ed. Alan Holland and Andrew Johnson (London: Chapman and Hall, 1998), 157. See also Bernard Rollin, *The Frankenstein Syndrome:*

Ethical and Social Issues in the Genetic Engineering of Animals (New York: Cambridge University Press, 1995).

67. Rollin, "On Telos and Genetic Engineering," 157.
68. Alan Holland, "Species Are Dead: Long Live Genes!" in *Animal Biotechnology and Ethics*, ed. Alan Holland and Andrew Johnson (London: Chapman and Hall, 1998), 239.

Selected Bibliography

Appleyard, Bryan. *Brave New Worlds: Staying Human in the Genetic Future.* New York: Viking Press, 1998.

Brock, Dan. "Enhancements of Human Function: Some Distinctions for Policymakers." In *Enhancing Human Traits: Ethical and Social Implications*, edited by Erik Parens, 48–69. Washington, DC: Georgetown University Press, 1998.

Byk, Christian. "A Map to a New Treasure Island: The Human Genome and the Concept of Common Heritage." *Journal of Medicine and Philosophy* 23, no. 3 (June 1998): 234–246.

Callahan, Daniel. "Manipulating Human Life: Is There No End To It?" In *Medicine Unbound: The Human Body and the Limits of Medical Intervention*, edited by Robert H. Blank and Andrea L. Bonnicksen, 118–131. New York: Columbia University Press, 1994.

Clark, Stephen R. L. "Natural Integrity and Biotechnology." In *Human Lives: Critical Essays on Consequentialist Bioethics*, edited by David S. Oderberg and Jacqueline A. Laing, 58–76. New York: St. Martin's Press, 1997.

Dobson, Andrew. "Biocentrism and Genetic Engineering." *Environmental Values* 4, no. 3 (August 1995): 227–239.

Dobson, Andrew. "Genetic Engineering and Environmental Ethics." *Cambridge Quarterly of Healthcare Ethics* 6, no. 2 (Spring 1997): 205–221.

Evernden, Neil. *The Social Creation of Nature.* Baltimore: Johns Hopkins University Press, 1992.

Holland, Alan, and Andrew Johnson, eds. *Animal Biotechnology and Ethics.* London: Chapman and Hall, 1998.

Juengst, Eric T. "Can Enhancement Be Distinguished from Prevention in Genetic Medicine?" *Journal of Medicine and Philosophy* 22, no. 2 (April 1997): 125–142.

Juengst, Eric T. "What Does 'Enhancement' Mean?" In *Enhancing Human Traits: Ethical and Social Implications*, edited by Erik Parens, 29–47. Washington, DC: Georgetown University Press, 1998.

Kass, Leon R., and James Q. Wilson. *The Ethics of Human Cloning.* Washington, DC: AEI Press, 1998.

Kevles, Daniel J., and Leroy Hood. "Reflections." In *The Code of Codes: Scientific and Social Issues in the Human Genome Project*, edited by Daniel J.

Kevles and Leroy Hood, 300–328. Cambridge, MA: Harvard University Press, 1992.

Kilner, John F., Rebecca D. Pentz, and Frank E. Young, eds. *Genetic Ethics: Do the Ends Justify the Genes?* Grand Rapids, MI: Eerdmans Publishing, 1997.

Kitcher, Philip. *The Lives to Come: The Genetic Revolution and Human Possibilities.* Touchstone Books, 1997.

Lappe, Marc, and Britt Bailey. *Against the Grain: The Genetic Gamble with Our Food.* Monroe, ME: Common Courage Press, 1998.

Lyon, Jeff, and Peter Gorner. *Altered Fates: Gene Therapy and the Retooling of Human Life.* New York: W. W. Norton, 1996.

McGee, Glenn, ed. *Pragmatic Bioethics*, 2nd ed. Cambridge, MA: MIT Press, 2003.

National Council of Churches in Christ. *Genetic Science for Human Benefit.* New York: National Council of Churches, 1996.

O'Donovan, Oliver. *Begotten or Made?* Oxford: Clarendon Press, 1984.

O'Neill, Onora, and William Ruddick. *Having Children: Philosophical and Legal Reflections on Parenthood.* New York: Oxford University Press, 1979.

Peters, Ted. "Genome Project Forces New Look at Ethics, Law." *Forum for Applied Research and Public Policy* 8, no. 3 (Fall 1993): 5–13.

Peters, Ted. "Theological Questions Raised by the Human Genome Initiative." *Midwest Medical Ethics* 8, no. 1 (Summer 1992): 12–17.

Pope John Paul II. Speech, Pontifical Academy of Sciences, October 28, 1994; reported with text in *L'Osservatore Romano* 45, November 9, 1994, 3.

Ramsey, Paul. "Moral and Religious Implications of Genetic Control." In *Genetics and the Future of Man,* edited by John D. Roslansky. New York: Appleton-Century-Crofts, 1996.

Reichenbach, Bruce R., and V. Elving Anderson. "Stewardship and the Human Genome." In *On Behalf of God: A Christian Ethic for Biology,* 171–214. Grand Rapids, MI: Eerdmans Publishing, 1995.

Resnik, David B. "The Morality of Human Gene Patents." *Kennedy Institute of Ethics Journal* 7, no. 1 (1997): 43–61.

Resnik, David B., Holly B. Steinkraus, and Pamela J. Langer. *Human Germ Line Gene Therapy: Scientific, Moral, and Political Issues.* Austin, TX: R. G. Landes, 1999.

Rothstein, Mark A., ed. *Genetic Secrets: Protecting Privacy and Confidentiality in the Genetic Era.* New Haven, CT: Yale University Press, 1997.

Shannon, Thomas A. "Ethical Issues in Genetic Engineering: A Survey." *Midwest Medical Ethics* 8, no. 1 (Summer 1992): 26–29.

Shannon, Thomas A. "Genetics, Ethics, and Theology: The Roman Catholic Discussion." In *Genetics: Issues of Social Justice,* edited by Ted Peters, 144–179. Cleveland, OH: Pilgrim Press, 1998.

Shannon, Thomas A. *Made in Whose Image: Genetic Engineering and Christian Ethics*. New York: Humanities Press, 2000.

Shinn, Roger L. "Genetics, Ethics, and Theology: The Ecumenical Discussion." In *Genetics: Issues of Social Justice*, edited by Ted Peters, 122–143. Cleveland, OH: Pilgrim Press, 1998.

Tudge, Colin. *Engineer in the Garden*. New York: Hill and Wang, 1993.

Wikler, Daniel. "Can We Learn from Eugenics?" *Journal of Medical Ethics* 25, no. 2 (April 1999): 183–194.

Williams, Raymond. "Ideas of Nature." In *Problems in Materialism and Culture: Selected Essays*, 67–85. London: Verso, 1980.

4

Life Sciences: Discontents and Consolations

Paul Rabinow

There is little doubt that the March 24, 2000, issue of *Science* titled "The Drosophila Genome" marks a threshold in scientific achievement. This threshold, it is true, is only one in a much longer series of such achievements, many of them of recent vintage. In turn, these impressive techno-scientific achievements pose a host of other questions ranging from the metaphysical to the political.

Today, there is widespread consensus that one of the central, if not the central, developments and consequently concerns in the Western world is that scientists are now capable of purposively changing the nature of living beings. They have achieved this power through what was originally called genetic engineering, although today it is more commonly referred to as genetic manipulation. The fear exists that molecular biologists and others in the cutting-edge life sciences as well as those who finance them (states, corporations, philanthropies) have entered into the ambit of self-production. This state of affairs has been characterized with the attendant gravitas by an apparently endless procession of *prophètes de malheur* as alternatively Faustian, Promethean, Frankensteinian, or most amusingly of all among this hodgepodge of metaphoric excess and confusion, godlike.[1]

But the diagnosis of a crossing of a threshold with the introduction of the techniques of genetic manipulation, while no doubt perceptive and pertinent, must be complemented by further considerations. These considerations turn on the following claims, which I can only assert here (but for which I have attempted to provide detailed demonstrations elsewhere). An individual's self-production is a diacritic of modernity as both epoch and ethos.[2] Following from Michel Foucault's definition of "man" in his 1966 *Les Mots et Les Choses* on the intersection of labor, language, and life, we can establish a historical series in the process of self-production. Labor was the first modern domain where what were proclaimed to be an unsettling, unprecedented, and epochal set of changes were taking place. The thesis that "man makes himself" through his labor was argued for philosophically by the young G. W. F. Hegel and then given world historical importance in the writings of Karl Marx. The modernization of labor—with its positive and negative effects on *anthropos*—was followed by that of language. The theme of a human being's self-formation through discourse is developed most clearly in the structuralism of Claude Lévi-Strauss, Jacques Lacan, and Roland Barthes, but also Roman Jakobson and many others. Hannah Arendt's claims that it is only through public discourse that humans become fully human continues the tradition.[3] So, just as "society" and "discourse" have been modernized through science and planning, now it is the turn of life.[4]

Drosophila Lessons: Function Not Substance

The humble fruit fly has been the twentieth century's organism of choice for studying genetics, the basis of life. Its centrality has endured from its early fame at Columbia University, where it was chosen as a model organism in part because its reproductive habits fit the academic calendar, up to the present, when a hybrid consortium of public university labs (especially Berkeley) and the controversial biotechnology company Celera Genomics chose Drosophila as a demonstration project for their genome mapping strategies. Celera did so in part to prove to its competitors (especially the U.S. government–funded university/philanthropy consortium mapping the human genome) the power of its approach. The Drosophila map was also presented as a gift to science (free CD-ROMs are available), a token of this early twenty-first-century triumph of utter technological bravura.

It may be only a slight exaggeration to say that more has been learned in the last four years about Drosophila genetics than had been painstakingly accumulated in the previous seventy-five. Eventually, as Max Weber pointed out, what is known today will also seem "historical." The historicizing process has already begun with the juxtaposition by the press of photographs of mustachioed and suited Drosophila scientists posed at their glass-jar-encumbered lab benches and the consortium team leaders in late twentieth-century casual attire, coiffed with headphones linking them to teams of computer geeks annotating the cascade of data flowing from Celera's array of imposing sequencing machinery. In sum, "The Drosophila Genome" issue of *Science* contains much matter to ponder for geneticists and nongeneticists alike.[5] And of course, it won't be long before *Science* publishes its special issue on "The Human Genome."

One of the elder statesmen of genetics, the wise and witty Sydney Brenner, in a trenchant summary piece preceding the Drosophila genome map aptly titled "The End of the Beginning," brilliantly frames the significance of the current conjuncture in genetics. Brenner, himself the leader of the project to map the worm, *C. elegans*, opens his *Science* article by observing that "in classical experimental genetics, we could not assert the existence of a wild-type gene until a mutant version with an altered function had been isolated" [a series: one gene, one function, one phenotypic difference]. "But," he continues, "if one asked how many genes were required to make a bacteriophage or a bacterium or a fly or a mouse, no answer could be given."[6] Classical geneticists could never have produced "The Drosophila Genome" special issue because although they had developed techniques to isolate and map genes (in fact, decades before anyone knew what genes were biochemically), classical genetics had no concept equivalent to what is today called a genome. Consequently, and not surprisingly, there were neither the experimental systems nor the technologies yet invented that might have provided an answer to a question that had not been posed: What is a genome? The full impact of this conceptual shift in our understanding of living beings has perhaps not yet achieved an adequate place in public understanding given all the attention that the media have lavished on the gene for this, that, and the other thing, as well as such hot-button issues, seemingly rife with epochal significance, such as patenting life, cloning humans, and genetically modified foods. In fact, the gene for this, that, and the other thing probably should have been seen as one of the last triumphs of what Brenner calls "classical genetics" (remember, it used to be called modern genetics) rather than serving as the herald of the dawning of the new genomics. Consequently, it is eminently worth underscoring Brenner's point that locating genes is not the same thing as mapping genomes. All involved in the latter enterprise are clear that mapping genomes is only one step in understanding them.

Just as genes and genomics are not the same thing, so too, genes and DNA are not the same thing. Indeed, DNA plays the intermediary role between genes and genomes in the story we are telling. The major shift that has eventuated in the invention, discovery, and mapping of genomes during the later 1990s arguably began with the shift from genes to DNA. Following the great discoveries of the 1950s and 1960s in which the fundamentals of the double helix and genetic code were painstakingly made, the 1970s and 1980s saw the invention of a series of technologies devoted to manipulating DNA (regardless of its function); the most important were DNA sequencing, cloning DNA in bacteria, and the polymerase chain reaction (referred to as in vitro cloning), a technique that enabled the rapid, efficient, and inexpensive production of large quantities of specific DNA sequences. With the invention of the polymerase chain reaction at Cetus Corporation, a scarcity of DNA available for experimentation turned into a bounty of DNA available for experimentation.[7] The 1970s and 1980s were also the decades during which the material conditions for the production of truth in molecular biology, biochemistry, and genetics were undergoing, not coincidentally, equally significant changes. These were the decades of the emergence of the biotechnology industry—the end of an elite, artisan craft culture in molecular biology and its rapid replacement with a distinctive type of heavily machine-mediated, costly mode of quasi-industrial production, replete with a much larger and more functionally diverse labor force including computer technicians, lawyers, CEOs, and advertising agencies. Joining the crowded world of DNA was another new player, bioethicists. While companies such as Genentech, Cetus, and Biogen were shaping the field, the university world was itself moving significantly closer to this new industrial mode of operation. By 1989, it was daring but plausible for the U.S. National Institutes of Health and Department of Energy (involved in radiation research since the dropping of the atomic bombs on Japan) to announce a human genome initiative, designed to map (and eventually sequence) the human genome—defined ambiguously as the total complement of DNA in a human cell—and thereby to bring health and prosperity—eventually—to many.[8] Coincidentally, 1989 was the year of the fall of the Berlin wall.

Today, fifteen years later, a series of genomes have been mapped through massively funded, international, industry-government-university-philanthropy consortia. Many consequences and questions follow from this achievement. Among them, there needs to be a rethinking of what a gene is, because scientifically speaking genes are not what they used to be. Brenner ruefully remarks: "Old geneticists knew what they were talking about when they used the term 'gene,' but it seems to have been corrupted by modern genomics to mean any piece of expressed sequence." Instead of the misleading and anachronistic term gene, Brenner proposes to substitute the phrase "genetic locus" to indicate "either an open reading frame or a site to map mutations." An open reading frame is "a DNA sequence that potentially can be translated into protein." Brenner continues, "As proteins are the workhorses of organisms, an approach from the sequences that tells you in a mechanical fashion what the amino acids are in each protein is infinitely more economical than purifying and analyzing the vast number of proteins. The genes can then be cloned and studied, often through mutation."[9] It should come as no surprise to learn that proteomics companies are appearing, and calls for inventories of proteins are increasingly mentioned as vital.

Once the genomes are mapped and sequenced, and once the basic proteomic cataloging work is accomplished, the functional biology will only just have begun. Brenner observes that these maps are static. None of the information in them as it is currently collected tells us when genes are switched on and off, and for how long. Such information, Brenner notes, is "absolutely essential . . . because in complex organisms, evolution does not proceed by enlarging the protein inventory but by modulating the expression of genes."[10]

Thus, our understanding of the genome stands clearly in a period of transition from so-called classical genetics to modern genomics and proteomics, from expecting a thing to deciphering a function. Further, all that rested on that classical expectation stands in need of reassessment, even the assumed genetic gulf separating Drosophila from Homo sapiens; hence the questions facing this volume. While there is perhaps room for metaphysicians and ethicists to worry about the larger consequences of such surprises, an equally serious concern is with the state of the science that brought about this transformation and that promises more.

Discontents

In 1930, Sigmund Freud, already in a somber, pessimistic mood about the state of the world, one reinforced shortly thereafter by the victories of the National Socialists, published *Civilization and Its Discontents*. Perhaps defiantly, Freud conspicuously continued the scientifically detached stance he had fashioned in *The Future of an Illusion*. This stance, with its resigned distance and its self-control, was both the price to be paid and the constraint required, or so it seemed to Freud, to pursue successfully the project of demystifying humankind's deepest illusions. By means of this ascetic exercise, Freud believed he could, or had already, achieved essential insights that others, mired in illusion, lacked. That lack (Freud was lucid about this point) provided its own benefits in the world—benefits that those pursuing science would have to forgo as the price of insight. Basically, for Freud, what had to be abandoned was hope, or at least, childlike or naive hope.

It would seem to follow that abandoning this type of hope was a necessary, if not definitive, step toward maturity or perhaps wisdom. But is there such a thing as scientific maturity or wisdom? Much turns on the term *Wissenschaft*, science. And what it offered. And to whom. For several reasons that appear pertinent to the question modern science poses to our understanding of human nature and well-being, I take Freud's claims and the position he claimed them from as a starting point to explore these issues. The hope is that such an effort might help us to better understand—and renew—the historical complexities of Wissenschaft as well as the commitment to making it a central component of a human life.

One of Freud's central claims was that humankind, for most of its history, had unknowingly projected its ideals onto its gods. Recent advances in civilization, however, had complicated this millennial process; not only were some of these delusionary processes now understood (thanks to the scientific advances Freud himself was spearheading) but additionally, and this was more complicated yet, humankind was close to turning its ideals into realities: "Man has, as it were, become a kind of prosthetic God." This double turning of increased self-awareness and increased power constituted the diacritic of the present. What Freud held to be certain was: first, that the process would continue indefinitely into the future, and second, that "present-day man does not feel happy in his Godlike character."[11] And humans, according to Freud, desire to be happy. Consequently, discontent was another diacritic of humans' plight, especially as science advanced and its achievements yielded instrumental capacities.

Freud's diagnosis of the present, in 1930, was therefore gloomy. While scientific and technical advances were unquestionably accumulating, the contemporary mix of scientifically achieved self-understanding (of the self and civilization) and technical advance was, however, not yet coordinated. Humankind was pursuing its illusions with more power than ever before. Freud's effort was to question the project of coordination or at least to temper the expectations it engendered. Of course, Freud himself was deeply committed to a scientific project of his own.

Wounded Pride

In 1916, a younger Freud had written a small article for a Hungarian journal titled "A Difficulty in the Path of Psycho-Analysis." The piece, which appeared early in 1917, was intended for an "educated but uninstructed audience" (an interesting distinction when you think about it). Freud remained content with the article's basic points and repeated them (albeit phrased a little differently) in his subsequent *Introductory Lectures in Psychoanalysis*.[12] The difficulty alluded to in the title of Freud's essay was not humanity itself but rather its pride. It is worth remarking that the question of who exactly this humanity or humankind is (Europe's educated classes perhaps?), is not explored in the essay. Freud's core argument is that throughout history, scientific advance had run counter to humanity's megalomania, its self-importance. Thus, it was consistent to assume that any truly significant scientific advance concerning a human being's relation to the cosmos, nature, other humans, or itself would be resisted, for longer or shorter periods of time.[13] Freud's core position is that as science discovered and demonstrated what was true, humankind ultimately had no rational alternative but to adapt its own self-understanding to scientific discoveries. In this article as elsewhere, Freud presents himself as a scientist, even a great scientist; by so doing, his self-presentation constitutes an audacious challenge to his readers to accept his theories and no doubt offers some comfort to himself. After all, the article was written to explain why Freud's theories were not being generally accepted.

Furthermore, in his defiant faith in the inevitable triumph of science over the blind forces of irrational resistance to its discoveries, Freud can be understood not merely as a scientist but an *Aufklärer*, a man of the Enlightenment. The distinction rests on the observation that there is nothing within the disciplinary confines of this or that science to direct the historical fate of its discoveries. An Aufklärer is someone who pursues increased understanding of a rational sort wherever it leads, believing that it will lead somewhere beneficial. Enlightenment affect (belief, hope, desire) is a surplus, a supplement, to scientific achievement. An Aufklärer follows Immanuel Kant's dictum, *"Sapere Audere!"*— "dare to know!"[14] As Kant argued, enlightenment is simultaneously a scientific, moral, and political undertaking. Such a project constitutes a commitment to a kind of truth and a way of life linked to an understanding of the good. Enlightenment, one might say, is a culture, an ethos, or a form of life. It is a form of life that can never be complete. It is a form of life that is both arrogant and humble. It is arrogant insofar as it acts for humanity with a confidence that it is right; it is humble in that enlightenment is an infinite project whose achievement lies in the future.

As such, an ethos of enlightenment is a way of life that requires a certain understanding of maturity—that is to say, a view of the past, the future, and the present that links them together in a hopeful manner, but one whose proof can only lie in the future of humanity, not in any individual life. The question is whether there is a corresponding ethos within a scientific attitude. I will raise the issue of maturity and its relation to science, enlightenment, and history recurrently in this chapter. The reason for this repetition is that there are different and contrastive understandings of each of the terms. Those differences depend in part on an evaluation of the history of science and enlightenment—and of the present moment.

To return to Freud, he proposes "to describe how the universal narcissism of men, their self-love, has up to the present suffered three severe blows from the researches of science"[15]—in other words, how the belief in a fixed and knowable human essence that accorded it a superior rank in the hierarchy of beings came under attack from various sides.

• The *cosmological* blow. Humans believed that their abode, the earth, was the stationary center of the universe. This perception fit well with an individual's "inclination to regard himself as lord of the world."[16] The first blow to humankind's lordly status was dealt when humanity learned that the earth was not the center of the universe but only a tiny fragment of a cosmic system of scarcely imaginable vastness. The destruction of this narcissistic illusion came to general acceptance in the sixteenth century with Nicolaus Copernicus, although Freud is at pains to underscore that the discovery had been made millennia before.

• The *biological* blow. "In the course of the development of civilization man acquired a dominating position over his fellow-creatures in the animal kingdom. Not content with this supremacy, however, he began to place a gulf between his nature and theirs. He denied the possession of reason to them and to himself he attributed an immortal soul, and made claims to a divine descent that permitted him to break the bonds of community between himself and the animal kingdom." Charles Darwin put an end to this presumption. "Man is not a being different from animals or superior to them; he himself is of animal descent, being more closely related to some species and more distantly to others."[17] Although this point has been hard for civilized adults to accept, Freud insists that children and primitives readily accept, even assume, a closeness with animals.

• The *psychological* blow is, in Freud's self-serving opinion, probably the most wounding. Humans have been humbled externally, but now must accept that they are not sovereign within their own minds. Philosophers had previously understood this point, but its scientific demonstration has been fiercely resisted. Humans, it seems, must also accept that they are thinking about sex all the time, and only Freud has explained why.

Regardless of how one evaluates Freud's overall thesis, the main thing that he does not explain, or even address, is under what *historical* conditions scientific truth becomes socially acceptable. Greek scientists knew the earth traveled around the sun, children felt a kinship with animals, and philosophers knew we know not what we think. Yet somehow, eventually, even grown-up Europeans saw, and would see, the light of day. In this faith, despite all his pessimism about civilization and its discontents, Freud remains an Enlightenment thinker. Not only does he dare to know—the highest commandment—but he assumes that ultimately the truth will, as it were, come to light. That light, sooner or later, will shine forth and humanity will awaken. The question certainly remains open as to whether Freud's faith is not his ultimate defense mechanism or a sign of his maturity, a maturity running ahead of and presaging where the rest of humankind is heading.

Science as a Vocation: Truth versus Meaning

In 1917, perhaps on the very day of the Bolshevik seizure of power in Russia, Weber delivered a lecture titled "Science as a Vocation" (*"Wissenschaft als Beruf"*) to a crowded hall of German university students in Munich.[18] It stands as one of the great—unsurpassed in my view—twentieth-century statements of the ethics and ethos of science and scientists. It may well be considered one of the first twentieth-century statements, especially if one agrees with my old humanist German professors at the University of Chicago who felt that Western civilization had come to an end by 1917. The lecture fits within the general framework that Weber had elsewhere set for himself of characterizing the "life orders" (*Lebensführung*) under modern capitalism. Although Weber does not phrase it this way, the central theme of the lecture might well be: What is maturity, within modernity, for those who dedicate their life to seeking knowledge and understanding? In the triad of science, enlightenment, and history, Weber privileges history and science. He presents a challenging diagnosis of the historical moment and the ethical demands it poses for those who desire to remain loyal to science. Loyal, that is, without illusions. Weber chillingly refers to the Enlightenment as "the laughing heir" of capitalism—an heir that by 1917, had long lost its "rosy blush."[19] For Weber, we lived enmeshed in processes of modernity rather than enlightenment.

Weber divided his lecture, in classical didactic fashion, into three parts: (1) the material conditions of science, (2) the inner ethic of science, and (3) the cultural—or value—significance of science in modernity. Although this set of distinctions is totally out of fashion today, I believe it remains a powerful mode of orientation for those who study science and practice Wissenschaft.

Material Conditions

Weber cast his discussion of the material conditions of science as a comparison between the work conditions and career trajectory of graduate students in Germany and the United States. German students, after a lengthy apprenticeship and the publication of a book, received permission to begin offering lectures, for which they were compensated only by the fees of those students who attended their lectures. While providing limited monetary resources, this system left the student a good deal of freedom of thought and time to conduct research. In the United States, an academic career began with a regular faculty position; hence, the young person joined a bureaucratic system and was assured of being paid, often, Weber observes dryly, the equivalent wages of a semiskilled laborer. Only football coaches were well paid in U.S. universities, Weber noted. In return for this money and position, the young scientist was required to do a great deal of teaching, although ultimately a person's career would be judged on one's research. Whatever else it might be, for Weber, Wissenschaft required labor and institutional resources.

With a certain regret he sought to contain, Weber observed that the old humanist university in Germany was on its last legs:

In very important respects German university life is being Americanized, as is German life in general. The large institutes of medicine or natural science are "state capitalist" enterprises, which can not be managed without considerable funds. [As in all such enterprises, there is a separation] of the worker from his means of production. The worker, that is, the assistant, is dependent upon the implements the state puts at his disposal; hence he is just as dependent . . . as is the employee in a factory upon the management . . . [A]s with all capitalist, and at the same time bureaucratized enterprises, there are indubitable advantages in all this.[20]

And Disadvantages

Not only was science operating under capitalist and bureaucratic constraints, but it further labored, like the Vatican, under conditions of consensus formation that rarely rewarded exceptional people. Weber paints a stern, stinging, and remarkably contemporary portrait of the role played by chance, arbitrariness, and consensus formation in academic life: "It would be unfair to hold the personal inferiority of faculty members or educational ministries responsible for the fact that so many mediocrities play an eminent role at the universities. The predominance of mediocrity is rather due to the laws of human co-operation." Consequently, he admonished his audience, a young person contemplating a scientific or scholarly future must ask herself, "Do you in all conscience believe that you can stand seeing mediocrity after mediocrity, year after year, climb beyond you, without becoming embittered and without coming to grief?"[21] Although, Weber remarked, enthusiastic young people always answer that their "calling" for science will see them through, Weber cautions that few actually make it without succumbing to ressentiment or resignation.

Finally, not all were allowed to play the game of science. Although Weber does not mention gender, even though his wife was an ardent socialist-feminist, he does add that if the would-be scientist was "a Jew, of course one says *lasciate ogni speranza* ['abandon all hope']."[22] This equation of the gates of Wissenschaft with the gates of hell is, on reflection, a rather bizarre one. It should serve as a reminder to those who pine for the good old days when science was pure. By this I do not mean that the recent couplings of science and industry are unproblematic, only that historically their separation contributed to a certain castelike recruitment within Germany and beyond.

Internal Situation: Inward Calling for Science

Weber opens the section in his lecture on the "inward calling for science" by continuing to specify the conditions under which science operates. The essential feature of contemporary science is that it has entered an irreversible "phase of specialization previously unknown, and that this will forever remain the case."[23] Science is not wisdom; science is specialized knowledge. A number of important consequences follow from this situation. First, "scientific work is chained to the course of progress."[24] Any scientist knows that by definition, and in part due to their own efforts, their work is fated to be outdated. Every scientific achievement opens new questions. One might say that a successful scientist can only hope that one's work will be productively and fruitfully outmoded rather than merely forgotten. Second, the knowledge worker must live with the realization that not only are specialized advances the only ones possible but that even small accretions require massive dedication to produce. Dedication or enthusiasm alone, however, is not sufficient to produce good science. Nor does hard work guarantee success. As Weber puts it, "Ideas occur to us when they please, not when it pleases us."[25] The calling for science thus must include a sense of passionate commitment combined with methodical labor and a kind of almost mystical passivity or openness. The scientific self must be resolutely willful and patient, yet permeable—androgynous, if you will.

Here, Weber opens a parenthesis that is one of the most celebrated in his entire work. What exactly, he asks, does scientific progress provide to the individual, society, and civilization? Weber's answer amounts to the stark conclusion that not only does science alone produce neither enlightenment nor meaning but furthermore, under the conditions of modernity, science stands in a fraught, perhaps mortal, tension with both enlightenment and meaning.

For Weber, scientific work forms part of a larger "process of intellectualization" that has been developing for thousands of years. What does this mean?

Does it mean that we, today, for instance, have a greater knowledge of life under which we exist than an American Indian or a Hottentot? Hardly. Unless he is a physicist, one who rides on the streetcar has no idea how the car happened to get into motion. And he does not need to know. [He can depend on others.] The savage knows incomparably more about his tools. The savage knows what he does in order to get his daily food and which institutions serve him in this pursuit. The increasing intellectualization and rationalization do *not*, therefore, indicate an increased and general knowledge of the conditions under which one lives. It means something else, namely, the knowledge or belief that if one but wished one could learn it at any time. Hence, it means that principally there are no mysterious incalculable forces that come into play, but rather that one can in principle, master all things by calculation. This means that the world is disenchanted. One need no longer have recourse to magical means in order to master or implore the spirits . . . technical means and calculations perform the service.[26]

Now, regarding these processes of disenchantment, which have continued to exist in Occidental culture for millennia, Weber asks, "Do they have any meanings that go beyond the purely practical and technical" including the meaning of human life as it is lived.[27] His answer is a resounding "no." Strictly speaking, within the constraints of the question of the inward calling for science, there can be no answer because it is not a question that science can answer scientifically. If we recall that when Weber refers to Wissenschaft, he means all forms of disciplined knowledge, we are unlikely to be let off the hook by bringing William Shakespeare to the physicians or ethics committees to the molecular biologists. For that move risks instrumentalizing the cultural sciences (*Geisteswissenschaften*) rather than humanizing the life sciences.

What Is the Value of Science?

"To raise this question," responds Weber, "is to ask for the vocation of science within the total life of humanity."[28] The value of science is quite specific: to invent concepts and conduct rational experiments. These concepts, however, no longer provide a window onto eternal verities or essences, and the experiments no longer reveal God's truth. Furthermore, they tell us nothing about the meaning of the cosmos, nature, or the psyche. Weber heaps scorn on those who think otherwise. "And today?" he scoffs, "Who—aside from certain big children who are indeed found in the natural sciences—still believes that the findings of astronomy, biology, physics, or chemistry could teach us anything about the *meaning* of the world?" Or, "After Nietzsche's devastating criticism of the 'last men' who invented happiness, I leave aside altogether the naïve optimism in which science—that is, the technique of mastering life which rests upon science—has been celebrated as the way to happiness. Who believes in this?—aside from a few big children in university chairs or editorial offices."[29] Or, "Natural science gives us an answer to the question of what we must do if we wish to master life technically. It leaves quite aside, or assumes for its purposes, whether we should or do wish to master life technically and whether it makes ultimate sense to do so."[30] Weber shares with Freud the view that science and its associated growth of instrumental capacities was not the path to happiness. He differs from Freud in refusing to believe that scientific truths yielded meaning. For Weber, science alone could not yield meaning, especially about the human condition. The only possible path toward that goal was experience-yielding *phronesis*. Weber deeply desires to follow this path, but despairs that he is making any progress in doing so.

For Weber, science contributes methods of thinking, the tools and the training for disciplined thought. It contributes to gaining clarity. That is all. Hence for Weber, science contributes to an ethics, a critical ethos of "self-clarification and a sense of responsibility." This sense of responsibility turns on a specific conception of truth. Such an ethics is a form of critique, in the Kantian sense of establishing where the limits of thought lie. It is also critical in the sense that it displays a suitable scorn for those who cannot accept what Wissenschaft can and cannot provide. That science "does not give an answer to . . . questions [of meaning] is indubitable." On that claim Weber broached no gainsaying. Yet that insight constituted not the end but rather only the beginning of the problem of science, ethics, and modernity. "The only question that remains," Weber continued, "is the sense in which science gives 'no' answer, and whether or not science might yet be of some use to one who puts the question correctly."[31] In the conclusion, we will return to Weber's far-reaching, still-unanswered, and entirely contemporary query.

Today, however, it seems clear that Weber's view of history and science (Wissenschaft) requires modification. Specifically, it is too monotone and too substantialist. At times, Weber remains a neo-Kantian seemingly forcing science into a priori categories. At other times, there are grounds for reading him as holding a view of rationalization as the master term of Western history (although in other places he resists this hypostatization). Both tendencies go against the grain of other parts of Weber's thought, where one could argue that categories such as science are ideal types and hence stem from value orientations. And thus are historical and contingent. Wherever one comes down in these debates, Weber's question and concern about the status and challenge of the life orders within modernity, it seems to me, remains a compelling one, even if his answers seem dated.

Enlightenment Betrayed, 1917–1989

The twentieth century, amply endowed with megalomaniac projects, was the scene of further wounds to humankind's naïveté and its narcissism. The ever-reasonable, prudent, and cautiously hopeful Jürgen Habermas observes that "historical skepticism about reason belongs more to the nineteenth century, and it was not until the twentieth century that intellectuals engaged in the gravest betrayals."[32] Although Habermas is presumably referring to intellectuals such as Martin Heidegger (and his obscene allegiance to the Nazis) and Georg Lukács (and his horrific indentureship to Joseph Stalin), his point relates to natural scientists as well. The twentieth century was a time of the establishment of the most intimate and systematic connections between knowledge and the military (or forces of destruction more generally): from the horrific effects of poison gas (and other gifts of the chemical industries), through the atomic bomb (and other gifts of physics and engineering), through the Nazi nightmare of racial purification (and other gifts of anthropology and the biosciences), through the indigestible fact that close to three-quarters of the spending on scientific research during the cold war was devoted to military ends. The industries and sciences of Thanatos had a glorious century. We should never forget that what is now nostalgically seen as the golden age of science—the one before capitalism supposedly despoiled the life sciences—was really the age of the cold war.

Today, it seems implausible to maintain any longer that accumulating knowledge per se automatically leads to beneficial results, or given its fragmentation, that knowledge furthers our general self-understanding. Nor—and this is where Weber helps us avoid the fatuous denunciatory cant so widespread at present—can we unambiguously maintain that the opposite is the case.

It is striking that in 1958 when Hannah Arendt published *The Human Condition*, the science she chose as exemplary was physics. In the same year, C. P. Snow in *The Two Cultures* had done the same thing. Four years later in the book's second edition, however, Snow replaced physics with molecular biology. He was prescient. The immense achievements of molecular biology and biochemistry during the 1960s and 1970s—the discovery of the fundamental principles and mechanisms of the genetic code and its operation—will surely stand as a monumental threshold in the history of science. Nevertheless, with the invention of recombinant DNA technology and the ascendancy of a new type of industry—the biotechnology industry—another blow was dealt to those who wanted to believe that the production of truth about life must remain pure of worldly taint. It has been shown over the last few decades that there can be no life sciences without substantial amounts of money. During the cold war, this money came from nation-states. Although there is still a substantial contribution to the life sciences from the State, there is an even greater flow of funds from the huge multinational pharmaceutical industries and the fleet-footed and highly mobile purveyors of venture capital. Please note that I am not claiming that this situation is intrinsically either horrific or terrific; I have no regrets for the passing of the cold war, or for much of what nationalistic science produced in the twentieth century. I have no doubt that the goals and the means of the capitalist enterprise and character will inflect, perhaps radically, what used to be known as the scientific ethic. My goal is to note a watershed change and to urge us to reflect on it.

Although hype and cant have dominated the coverage of the emergence of genome mapping, what we *have* learned from the first decade or so is neither the secrets of the holy grail of life, nor the meaning of the code of codes, nor that genetics inevitably brings with it a new eugenics.[33] Rather, we have learned that all living beings—at the level of the genetic code—are materially the same, and that the very techniques that were developed to make this profound discovery enable, even oblige, further intervention into that materiality. François Jacob, the French Nobel Prize winner, frames these two points in simple, elegant prose. First, Jacob notes that "all living beings, from the most humble to the most complex, are related. The relationship is closer than we ever thought."[34] Second, he adds that "genetic engineering brought about a total change in the biological landscape as well as in the means of investigating it. Where it had been possible only to observe the surface of phenomena, it now became feasible to intervene in the heart of things."[35] Of course, Jacob's tropes—"landscape" and "the heart of things"—are archaic. As he is an old European, to use a phrase from Habermas, we can be tolerant of Jacob's failing figurations; however, as Jacob is an old and wise European, we should be attentive to what he sees. But we should also be alert to the fact that our practices may well be outrunning our core metaphors.[36] In that case, inventiveness in the cultural sciences would have to be placed extremely high on an agenda of value orientations.

Consolations

Let us return to *Civilization and Its Discontents*. Freud concluded his book in a clinical manner, simultaneously incisive and hesitant: "The fateful question for the human species" is whether civilization can master "the human instinct of aggression and self-destruction." But any answer to this question is unfortunately directly linked to the problem: "Men have gained control over the forces of nature to such an extent that with their help they would have no difficulty in exterminating one another to the last man. They know this, and hence comes a large part of their current unrest, their unhappiness and their mood of anxiety."[37] And indeed, the several decades succeeding the writing of these sentences in 1930 would be a time of unparalleled slaughter and brutality in world history.

Although Freud had offered his audience a predominantly pessimistic diagnosis, his tone should not, he says, be read as cautioning any specific value judgments. "My impartiality," he adds, "is made all the easier to me by my knowing very little about these things." Nevertheless, what Freud does know "for certain . . . is that man's judgments of value follow directly his wishes for happiness—that, accordingly, they are an attempt to support his illusions with arguments. . . . I can offer them no consolation: for at bottom that is what they are all demanding—the wildest revolutionaries no less passionately than the most virtuous believers."[38] Freud was surely correct in foreseeing a prosperous, if discontented, future for the hardworking would-be gods devoted to crafting prostheses.

Freud's use of "consolation" (*Trost*) is striking and unexpected. It is unexpected because clearly it is not what would-be prosthetic gods are seeking, and hence the lack of an offering is not something they would even notice. Consequently, the gift of consolation appears to be precisely what Freud can offer to himself and those who would join him in his heroic Wissenschaft. To those, that is, who would bear their fate of unbrotherliness and incessant progress like a man, as Weber said. For these German men, the key affect to be achieved is double: uprightness in facing up to the limits of science as well as the deceptions of the world, and equally the hope of consolation. But the consolation is bitter medicine for these thinkers still living in the shadow of the death of God and its related demystification of an unchanging human nature. Their position is ever so close to nihilism. They both are living in a world in which Friedrich Nietzsche's assertion that humans would rather value something than nothing at all still holds sway: an active nihilism is better than a reactive one. Freud's and Weber's pathos and bathos turn on that hauntedness.

Consolation, however, need not be so bitter, and in English it falls on the sweeter end of a spectrum of physiognomy. *Consolation* is semantically layered. In English, the transitive verb *to console* means to "alleviate the grief, sense of loss or trouble." The Merriam-Webster dictionary claims that the verb is modern, appearing first in 1693.[39] Its core meaning is "support" as the verb is a transformation of the noun *console* first used in 1664 to refer to "an architectural member projecting from a wall to form a bracket for ornamentation." Although Freud disdained support for those seeking a firm stand for their ornamentation, he was offering the hope of some alleviation of the sense of loss or trouble for those seeking an orientation in life, or more precisely a life of science—science understood as enlightenment. Freud's enlightenment was reserved only for the few able to bear it; it was certainly no longer a wave of beneficial historical progress carrying along the many in its wake.

Equally, if differently, Weber was concerned with consolation. Or at least we can legitimately read Weber's affectively complex conclusions into the semantic space of consolation. "The only question that remains," Weber contends, "is the sense in which science gives 'no' answer, and whether or not science might yet be of some use to one who puts the question correctly."[40] That use would surely not be as a means of achieving technical mastery of the world or as a support for ornamentation. It is in this context that a further meaning of the verb is relevant. In English, the verb *to console* has an older layer of meaning. That meaning is found in the noun *consolation*, first used in the fourteenth century, to indicate "a contest held for those who have lost early in a tournament." Weber held that the "intellectual aristocracy" of the mind had been eliminated from the hotly contested and amply rewarded championship fights over meaning, history, science, and humanity—by modernity.

Recently, for many, as least for a short period of time, after the Enlightenment and modernity came postmodernity. Postmodernity has now passed, and many are presently obsessed with globalization. Let those who will, play these championship games of metanarratives; there is always an attentive and enthusiastic audience for these matches. Contemporary consolation is to be found elsewhere. It seems fair to say that Sydney Brenner is a mature scientist. His proposal to stop talking about substantive and essentialized entities that used to be called genes, and instead take up the challenge as to how to reappropriate the slot (topos) as "either an open reading frame or a site to map mutations," taking place in time as well as in a complex, multileveled environment that we have yet to forge the tools to explore, provides a very exciting prospect. It is a prospect for those practicing the life sciences as well as those conducting inquiries that link life and diverse sciences, a prospect of a vast domain opening up for scientific exploration as well as discontents and consolations yet to be known or felt. "Open reading frames" and "sites to map mutations" can be read first metaphorically and then metonymically as well by those of us in the other Wissenschaften as an encouragement to the pleasures of further inquiry. By forging a new relationship to emergent objects of knowledge, and means of knowing, we once again come across an older imperative that must today be understood differently, savored in its complex bittersweetness: "dare to know."

Notes

1. The immense complexity of what God supposedly was capable of doing and what humans could know of God's plans and actions is analyzed by Hans Blumenberg in section 2 "Theological Absolution and Human Self Assertions" in *The Legitimacy of the Modern Age* (Cambridge, MA: MIT Press, 1985). On the concept of *prophète de malheur*, see Francois Chateauraynaud and Didier Torny *Les Sombres Precurseurs, Une sociologie pragmatique de l'alerte du risque* (Paris: Editions de l'Ecole Des Hautes Etudes En Sciences Sociales, 1999), 379.

2. On this distinction, see Michel Foucault, "What Is Enlightenment?" in *The Foucault Reader*, ed. Paul Rabinow (New York: Pantheon Books, 1984), 32–50.

3. Hannah Arendt, *The Human Condition* (Chicago: University of Chicago Press, 1998).

4. Although one can establish this series (labor, life, language) as a historical progression, such a move would be misleading if it did not take into account that this is first and foremost an analytic frame, stemming from a value orientation as Max Weber has taught us. It is only within such an analytic frame that these domains can be so sharply and neatly delimited. Thus, for example, it is self-evident that considerations of labor invariably contained considerations on language and life, and so on. If one were to introduce the nondiscursive dimensions of these practices into the narrative, then the story would become more complicated and yet more interesting. For instance, social planning and its associated social technologies aimed at increasing the docility and efficiency of labor, yielded massive effects on human health and disease, demography, and so forth, as well as on what we now call the environment. Therefore, in addition to a primary diagnosis of the contemporary conjuncture, the further analytic work to be done is to see how subsidiary couplings (language/labor, labor/life, language/life) are refigured within it. How, we should inquire, do the historically forged and figured domains of labor and language change when they are brought into an encompassing frame of life understood as molecular?

5. "The Drosophila Genome," *Science* 287 (March 24, 2000). Although there is an excellent history of Drosophila genetics, Robert E. Kohler, *Lords of the Flies:* Drosophila *Genetics and the Experimental Life* (Chicago: University of Chicago Press, 1994), it is not mentioned in the entire issue of *Science*.

6. Sydney Brenner, "The End of the Beginning," *Science* 287 (March 24, 2000): 2173.

7. Kary Mullis's inspiration in thinking of the polymerase chain reaction was to move from the gene to DNA. See Paul Rabinow, *Making PCR: A Story of Biotechnology* (Chicago: University of Chicago Press, 1996).

8. Of the many books on this topic, see Robert Cook-Degan, *Gene Wars: Science, Politics and the Human Genome* (New York: W. W. Norton, 1994).

9. Brenner, "The End," 2174.

10. Ibid.

11. Sigmund Freud, *Civilization and Its Discontents*, trans. and ed. James Strachey (New York: W. W. Norton, 1961), 44–45.

12. Sigmund Freud, "A Difficulty in the Path of Psycho-Analysis," in *The Standard Edition of the Complete Psychological Works of Sigmund Freud*, trans. James Strachey (London: Hogarth Press, 1986), 17:137–144. The "three blows to human narcissism' are also described at the end of lecture 18 of Freud's *Introductory Lectures* (1916–17), in *The Complete Psychological Works*, 3:284–285.

13. Freud does not discuss resistance to claims put forward by scientists in which opinion turned out to be correct, or cases in which science could not provide adequate answers.

14. Immanuel Kant, "What Is Enlightenment?" in *Kant Selections*, ed. Lewis White Beck (New York: Macmillan, 1988), 462–467.

15. Freud, "A Difficulty," 139.

16. Ibid., 140.

17. Ibid., 140, 141.

18. Max Weber, "Science as a Vocation," in *From Max Weber: Essays in Sociology*, ed. H. H. Gerth and C. Wright Mills (New York: Free Press, 1946), 129–156.

19. Max Weber, *The Protestant Ethic and the Spirit of Capitalism* (New York: Routledge, 1992), 182.

20. Weber, "Science as a Vocation," 131.

21. Ibid., 132, 134.

22. Ibid., 134.

23. Ibid., 137.

24. Ibid., 136.

25. Ibid., 139.

26. Ibid.

27. Ibid., 140.

28. Ibid., 142.

29. Ibid., 143, 144.

30. Ibid., 143. See, by way of comparison: "Victorious capitalism, since it rests on mechanical foundations, needs [religious asceticism's] support no longer. The rosy blush of its laughing heir, the Enlightenment, seems also to be irretrievably fading, and the idea of duty in one's calling prowls about in our lives like the ghost of dead religious beliefs. Where the fulfillment of the calling cannot directly be related to the highest spiritual and cultural values, or when, on the other hand, it need not be felt simply as economic compulsion, the individual generally abandons the attempt to justify it at all. In the field of its highest development, in the United States, the pursuit of wealth, stripped of its religious and ethical meaning, tends to become associated with purely mundane passions, which often actually give it the character of sport. No one knows who will live in this cage in the future, or whether at the end of this tremendous development entirely new prophets will arise, or there will be a great rebirth of old ideas and ideals, or, if neither, mechanized petrifaction, embellished with a sort of convulsive self-importance. For the last stage of this cultural development, it might well be truly said: 'Specialists without spirit, sensualists without heart; this nullity imagines that it has attained a level of civilization never before achieved'" (Weber, *Protestant Ethic*, 181–182).

31. Weber, "Science as a Vocation," 143.

32. Jürgen Habermas, "Two Hundred Years' Hindsight," in *Perpetual Peace: Essays on Kant's Cosmopolitan Ideal*, ed. James Bohman and Matthias Lutz-Bachmann (Cambridge, MA: MIT Press, 1997), 124.

33. ¹**Cant** \'kant\ *n* **1**: monotonous talk filled with platitudes **2**: hypocritically pious language **3**: the special vocabulary peculiar to the members of an underworld group: ARGOT **4**: whining speech, such as that used by beggars **5**: the special terminology understood among the members of a profession, discipline, or class but obscure to the general population: JARGON ²**cant** *vi* [Anglo-Norman *cant*, song, singing, fr. *canter*, to sing, fr. L *cantare*] **1**: To speak tediously or sententiously: MORALIZE **2**: To speak in argot or jargon **3**: to speak in a whining, pleading tone.

34. François Jacob, *Of Flies, Mice, and Men*, trans. Giselle Weiss (Cambridge, MA: Harvard University Press, 1998), 96. Originally published as *La Souris, la mouche et l'homme* (Paris: Editions Odile Jacob, 1997).

35. "The first surprise resulted from comparing developmental genes in a range of organisms. Or rather, from attempting to find out whether genes similar to those known to act as master switches in the fly exist elsewhere. . . . For example, there seemed to be little chance of finding the famous Hom genes (the genes that in *Drosophila* establish the anteroposterior axis of the body) in organisms other than insects, because their embryonic development is so different. But geneticists looked around anyway, just to make sure. And wonder of wonders! They found them everywhere. First in the frog. Then in the mouse. Then in humans, the leech, the nematode, in amphioxus and hydra. In short, in every animal examined, a group of genes was found that presented a structure that was similar to that of

fly Hom genes. Everywhere these genes seemed to play the same role: that of defining the relative position of the cells along the anteroposterior axis of the animal. . . . That the genes that build the human body could be the same as those that direct the making of the body of a fly—now there was something unthinkable! Unthinkable, that is, that the same genetic framework might underlie processes as dissimilar as those involved in the development of these two organisms!" (ibid., 92–93).

36. On the role of core metaphors, see Hans Blumenberg, *Die Lesbarkeit der Welt* (Frankfurt am Main: Suhrkamp Verlag, 1981).

37. Freud, *Civilization*, 112.

38. Ibid., 111.

39. The *Oxford English Dictionary* tells a more complicated story. The first mention is in French in the twelfth century. Its first usage then moves into Middle English. Its usage in modern English is in the seventeenth century with Shakespeare and Milton.

40. Weber, *Protestant Ethic*, 182–183.

41. Brenner, "The End," 2174.

5

Genetic Engineering and Eugenics: The Uses of History

Diane B. Paul

The prospect of human genetic engineering is inextricably entangled with fears about eugenics. One reason for the intensity of the concern is that genetic engineering techniques seem to overcome traditional limitations on efforts to shape the course of human evolution. Past efforts to do so essentially involved the application to humans of principles of plant and animal breeding.[1] Practices such as segregation and sterilization of "defectives," immigration restriction, the Nazi murder of mental patients and *Lebensborn* program, Fitter Families and Better Babies contests, advocacy of "free love," proposals for family allowances, dissemination of birth control information and devices, and sperm banking were all directed, in whole or part, at affecting who would become parents of the next generation based on often dubious assumptions about the causal connection between visible traits and underlying heredity. Even when phenotypes were a good indication of genotypes, "positive eugenics" (which aims to increase the frequency of favorable traits in a population) depended on the uncertain cooperation of the subjects, and was limited in its effects by the process of sexual reproduction, which means that individuals transmit only half their genes. With respect to "negative eugenics" (which aims to decrease the frequency of undesirable traits), the reliance on phenotypes meant that policies could only reach those who were obviously affected, leaving mostly untouched the large reservoir of invisible carriers. From this heterozygous reserve, a new affected population would be created each generation. For all these (and other) reasons, what geneticist John Maynard Smith has termed "selectionist eugenics" is both slow and inefficient.

Genetic engineering, on the other hand, allows the isolation of specific genes and their alteration in specific ways, and is therefore potentially much more precise in its effects. And at least in theory, it makes possible entirely new kinds of improvement. Even in the 1960s, before the development of recombinant DNA technology, some enthusiasts for human genetic engineering predicted that it would one day be possible to create new traits, not simply, as with traditional breeding schemes, to increase the proportion of the most desirable existing genotypes.[2] Because it seems to promise (or threaten) a much more effective means to choose the kind of children we want—including the potential to actually transform human beings—the issue of eugenics is understandably at the forefront of discussions of human genetic engineering.

The kind of eugenics that proponents hope and critics fear will result, however, has little in common with the policies and practices typically invoked in these discussions. In warning of the eugenic potential of the new technologies, critics tend to identify eugenics with compulsory sterilization and other brutal exercises of state power. Yet today, almost no one believes that the state will force parents to genetically engineer their progeny. Indeed, what critics primarily fear is "backdoor" eugenics—the collective impact of practices voluntarily chosen by consumers (especially in the context of a largely unregulated fertility industry), rather than those mandated by governments.[3] "This is the eugenics that happens when the state is specifically excluded from reproductive decisions. It is the eugenics of the free market, and results inevitably from a combination of the current quasireligious faith in the absolute virtues of unfettered markets and the rapid growth of genetic knowledge. The whole point is that we are about to be deluged with offers of choice," writes science journalist Bryan Appleyard.[4] The same point is succinctly expressed by antibiotechnology activist Jeremy Rifkin: "The old eugenics was steeped in political ideology and motivated by fear and hate. The new eugenics is being spurred by market forces and consumer desire."[5]

Thus, if we are to look to history for lessons, the most relevant precursors would not seem to be state-sponsored policies of negative selection, such as compulsory sterilization. Their proponents aimed to cull the weak as a means to counter the degeneration resulting from profligate breeding by undesirables. In general, their goal was to maintain the status quo. As Peter Morton notes, since English eugenicists "were more impelled by the fear of social degeneration than by any genuine hope of improvement, the most common mood was one of despondency appropriate to those who believe themselves to be fighting a rearguard action."[6] But current debates are not about preventing "race suicide" by culling the unfit, and the mood of enthusiasts for human genetic engineering is buoyant, not gloomy. These optimists celebrate the prospect of radical improvement in human capabilities.

Today, some applaud the (ostensible) opportunity to transform human nature, while others view the same prospect with horror. From disparate political perspectives, a conservative member of the President's Council on Bioethics Francis Fukuyama, the left-of-center ecologist Bill McKibben, and the German philosopher and social critic Jürgen Habermas have all recently identified this prospect as the most disturbing feature of the new genetic technologies.[7] These critics are responding to exuberant predictions of a transformed humanity by biologists such as Lee Silver and philosophers such as Gregory Stock, Gregory Pence, and Peter Sloterdijk who believe we can and should remake ourselves.[8] Silver and Sloterdijk, among others, even look with equanimity on a future in which the genetically improved segment of humanity has split into a separate species.

The hopes and the fears surrounding the potential of today's technologies to transform humanity, and the arguments both in favor of and in opposition to their use, do have parallels in the past—but not where we typically look. The biological transformation of humanity has been celebrated by many thinkers; Morton notes that eugenics figured in most utopian literature after 1870, although few of the authors went beyond classical schemes for state involvement in choosing parents for the next generation.[9] More ambitious, and closer in spirit to today's enthusiasts for genetic engineering, were the scientific socialists of the 1920s and 1930s. Indeed, many current arguments in favor of remaking humanity were expressed (with much greater wit) by the Marxist geneticist J. B. S. Haldane. His 1923 *Daedalus*, and the critiques it inspired, certainly have more in common with the prophecies, ambitions, and concerns surrounding human genetic engineering than with those implicated in compulsory sterilization and other forms of negative eugenics. *Daedalus* introduces not just the Promethean imagery but virtually every theme—including the prediction that reproduction in a laboratory will replace motherhood, the futility of opposing the march of technology, the celebration of moral pioneers, and the disdain for moral objections to the project of redesigning humanity—that has emerged in the raft of recent books and essays applauding new genetic possibilities.[10] In fact, with its scathing critique of what would come to be called the "wisdom of repugnance" argument against tampering with our nature, *Daedalus* could serve as a manifesto for today's utopian geneticists. But as it is not part of the traditional narrative of eugenics, few modern utopians or their critics are likely to know it.

The standard narrative also coheres uneasily with the moral most critics want to draw from the history of eugenics. Focused as it is on brutal measures of state control, the obvious implication of that narrative is that a principal wrong of eugenics was its use of coercion. The correlative lesson is the need to be wary of any interference with reproductive decision making. That libertarian message is happily embraced by enthusiasts for all forms of human genetic engineering. But many critics wish to regulate or even prohibit the use of these technologies (or particular uses of these technologies). Thus, the history is in tension with their larger agenda.

Let me offer a brief road map to what follows: first, this chapter sketches an alternative history of plans to biologically transform humanity. This history incorporates utopian elements and takes into account that not all such plans were coercive. The chapter then analyzes the uses of history in current debates. It delineates the interests that both enthusiasts and critics have in constructing a narrative that features coercive practices, and briefly explores how the critics resolve, or at least manage, the resulting tensions.

Biological Utopians: First Generation

Eugenics, in its modern form, was a stepchild of Charles Darwin's theory of evolution by natural selection. In Darwin's view and his contemporaries' reading of his theory, selection led to the constant improvement of plants and animals. But with respect to the human species, nature's intentions had been thwarted. In modern, civilized societies, selection had apparently ground to a halt. As a consequence of medical, sanitary, and charitable measures, the weak in mind and body were no longer being effectively culled from the human stock. At the same time, the least capable were producing the largest families. Thus, the best were being swamped by the worst. If mental and moral traits were inborn, and civilization becoming increasingly complex, the future was ominous.

The effects of artificial civilization would therefore have to be countered by artificial selection. This process could take the form of negative measures intended to prevent or at least discourage mental defectives and other undesirables from breeding, or positive measures intended to encourage breeding by those superior in intellect, talent, and character. Among negative measures, segregation or sterilization of the unfit were considered most effective since they did not require the cooperation of the subjects. As Watson Davis noted, "It is almost impossible to make human beings improve their breed."[11] But the dissemination of birth control information and devices was a negative measure that did depend on cooperation. The eugenic rationale was that middle-class women already had access to contraception, whereas poor women (assumed to be hereditarily inferior) were unable to limit their births. Eugenicists assumed that the poor would do so, for their own social, economic, and health reasons, if they could. It was only necessary to provide them the means.

But a negative approach could only achieve so much. While preventing further deterioration, negative measures could not create what Charlotte Perkins Gilman in her 1899 *Women and Economics* called "the ever nobler forms of life toward which social evolution tends."[12] Eugenicists with more ambitious goals, then, generally favored a positive approach. Among them was Francis Galton. Although we know from the surviving fragment of his eugenic utopia *Kantsaywhere* that Galton imagined a future society in which, à la Plato, the state controlled breeding, segregating inferior specimens in labor colonies, his published works emphasized positive measures. As Galton wrote, "The possibility of improving the race of a nation depends on the power of increasing the productivity of the best stock. This is far more important than that of repressing the productivity of the worst."[13]

In Galton's perspective, humans were enormously varied in their inborn capacities and dispositions. By breeding from the good-tempered, brave, intelligent, and muscular, we could not only stem degeneration but create a new breed. For that to happen, eugenics would have to become a new religion, and such active efforts as providing dowries for

gifted young women and attractive houses at low rents to "exceptionally promising young couples" made to encourage "the best to marry the
best" and procreate.[14] Were appropriate measures taken, the average
standard would be raised to the level necessary for the operations of a
modern society and, through the intermarriage of those with the same
rare and similar talents, a whole new race, superior to us in physical,
mental, moral, and temperamental qualities, would ultimately develop.
"Men and women of the present day," Galton predicted, "are, to those
we might hope to bring into existence, what the pariah dogs of the streets
of an Eastern town are to our own highly-bred varieties."[15]

Unlike the politically conservative Galton, Alfred Russel Wallace considered himself a socialist. Denouncing eugenics as officious meddling
by a "scientific priestcraft," he initially counted on selection, working on
groups, to transform human nature.[16] Reasoning that tribes and nations
with the most intelligent, foresighted, and altruistic individuals would
prevail in intergroup struggles, humans would ultimately become so
perfect in their mental and moral faculties that the earth would be converted from a place of misery to a new Eden. In 1864, a year before
Galton published "Hereditary Talent and Character," Wallace wrote that
while the human physique will probably not change, human mentality
"may continue to advance and improve until the world is again inhab-
ited by a single homogeneous race, no individual of which will be inferior to the noblest specimens of existing humanity." He went on to
describe the resulting paradise:

Each one will then work out his own happiness in relation to that of his fellows;
perfect freedom of action will be maintained, since the well balanced moral faculties will never permit any one to transgress on the equal freedom of others;
restrictive laws will not be wanted, for each man will be guided by the best of
laws; a thorough appreciation of the rights, and a perfect sympathy with the feelings, of all about him; compulsory government will have died away as unnecessary (for every man will know how to govern himself).[17]

A few years later, Wallace concluded that natural selection did not
after all operate on humans, whose evolution must therefore be guided
by a higher power. But he never abandoned his vision of a transformed,
biologically rooted human nature. He instead promoted a different
mechanism to bring this about: an equalization of resources (including
the abolition of inheritance) that would unleash the power of sexual

selection. Inspired by Edward Bellamy's utopian socialist novel *Looking Backward*, Wallace (along with many social radicals on both sides of the Atlantic) concluded that, if wealth were equalized, women would choose mates not for their money but for their mental and moral qualities. According to Wallace: "The idle and the selfish [men] would be almost universally rejected. The diseased or the weak in intellect would also usually remain unmarried; while those who possessed any tendency to insanity or to hereditary disease, or who possessed any congenital deformity would in hardly any case find partners, because it would be considered an offence against society to be the means of perpetuating such diseases or imperfections."[18] As a result, the race would spontaneously improve and, ultimately, we would all become noble creatures.[19]

Wallace was forced to leave school at the age of fourteen to earn his own way in the world. He found rampant capitalism appalling. Scientifically, he was a "neo-Darwinian" who rejected the Lamarckian principle of inheritance of acquired characteristics. The contrast in social background and worldview with the classical liberal Herbert Spencer, who championed laissez-faire individualism and was a leader of the "neo-Lamarckians" in Britain, could hardly have been greater. But Wallace noted that the general argument of his 1864 essay was inspired by a reading of Spencer's works, especially his *Social Statics*. Indeed, Wallace's admiration for Spencer was so deep that he named his first son after the philosopher. That act becomes more intelligible when one considers the similarity in their visions.

In Spencer's view, unfettered economic competition would act as a spur to improvement. Competition functioned to make creatures work harder, thus exercising their organs and faculties. The mental powers, skills, and traits of character fostered by this struggle would be transmitted to future generations, resulting in constant material and moral progress. Ultimately (and inevitably), the evolutionary process would produce a perfect society, characterized by stability, harmony, peace, altruism, and cooperation. Spencer's description of the features of this utopia is remarkably similar to the one that Wallace assumed would result from the equalizing of economic conditions: land would be held in common, women would have the same rights as men, and government would become superfluous and ultimately disappear.

Biological Utopians: Second Generation

All these schemes—artificial selection, sexual selection, Lamarckian adaptation—required time. By the 1920s, some scientists were becoming impatient. Spurred by both scientific developments and the Bolshevik revolution, they began to speculate about the possibility of speeding up the process of improving the human race. The first off the mark was Haldane, whose *Daedalus, or Science and the Future* and its 1927 sequel, "The Last Judgment," inspired many others to imagine how science might transform nature, including human nature, both for better, as in J. D. Bernal's *The World, the Flesh, and the Devil*, and worse, as in Bertrand Russell's *Icarus, or the Future of Science*, and Aldous Huxley's *Brave New World*.[20]

Haldane's slim book ostensibly incorporates excerpts from an undergraduate student essay on the influence of biology on history written 150 years hence. Through this device, Haldane disparages the eugenics movement as crude in its methods, and frustratingly slow, but predicts that its aims will be achieved in a different way.[21] Mass production of individuals with exceptional qualities will occur through directed mutation and especially ectogenesis (in vitro fertilization), which will largely replace motherhood as a source of babies. The separation of sexual love from reproduction will allow for a vastly more thoroughgoing selection. That is fortunate since civilization would otherwise have gone to the dogs. "The small proportion of men and women who are selected as ancestors for the next generation are so undoubtedly superior to the average that the advance in each generation in any single respect, from the increased output of first-class music to the decreased conviction for theft, is very startling," the student writes, and goes on to add: "Had it not been for ectogenesis there is little doubt that civilization would have collapsed within a measurable time owing to the greater fertility of the less desirable members of the population in almost all countries."[22]

Many, of course, will find this vision offensive. Thus, the student notes that in some countries there was strong opposition, "intensified by the Papal Bull 'Nunquam prius audito,' and the similar fatwa of the Khalif, both of which appeared in 1960." But ultimately, our values adapted to the science (as they always do), and ectogenesis became universal.[23] In an early and apparently forgotten response to what would come to be called the "wisdom of repugnance" argument, Haldane observes that every invention initially strikes us as abhorrent. "The chemical or physical inventor is always a Prometheus. There is no great invention, from fire to flying, which has not been hailed as an insult to some god. But if every physical and chemical invention is a blasphemy, every biological invention is a perversion. There is hardly one which, on first being brought to the notice of an observer from any nation which had not previously heard of their existence, would not appear to him as indecent and unnatural." But in time, these same inventions come to seem completely natural; what began as a perversion, ends "as a ritual supported by unquestioned beliefs and prejudices."[24]

Mark Adams notes that "The Last Judgment" extends the account to the far future. Whereas *Daedalus* only looks ahead 150 years, "The Last Judgment" imagines that life on earth has been destroyed—the result of humans' inability to envision the future. However, through ten thousand years of controlled evolution, a small group is bred with the physical and psychological characteristics required for colonization of Venus (which had to be made habitable through the eradication of all its own life-forms). The new race of Venusian humans in turn sped up selection to the point where Venus could colonize other, more distant planets and eventually other galaxies—a vision that inspired Olaf Stapledon to write the influential *Last and First Men*.[25]

Daedalus created a sensation, selling almost fifteen thousand copies in the United Kingdom in its first year, and eliciting diverse responses.[26] Perhaps the most prominent critic was philosopher/mathematician Russell, whose *Icarus* appeared in the same series. (Icarus had been taught to fly by his father, Daedalus, and was killed when he flew too near the sun.) The chief point of Russell's short book was "that science will be used to promote the power of dominant groups, rather than to make men happy."[27] When it came specifically to eugenics, Russell argued that reproductive decisions would ultimately be made by officials to serve their own interests. Thus, governments would first acquire the right to sterilize individuals and use this power "to diminish imbecility, a most desirable object."[28] But over time, the program would likely be expanded to include rebels of all kinds (with opposition to the state taken as proof of imbecility) and school failures (resulting in a probable increase in the general intelligence and a decline in intelligence that was extraordinary).

Russell also notes that eugenicists in any case have more ambitious aims—not just eliminating the undesirable types but increasing the desired ones. This is the more serious worry, for in the end, individuals will be bred for characteristics that appeal to officialdom rather than to the geneticists themselves. When scientists imagine that one exceptional man might sire a legion of children by many mothers, they commit the fallacy of imagining that the program "would be administered as men of science would wish, by men similar in outlook to those who have advocated it," and Russell remarks that women who advocated female suffrage similarly envisaged that "the woman voter of the future would resemble the ardent feminist who won her the vote; and socialist leaders imagine that a socialist State would be administered by idealistic reformers like themselves." But these are all delusions, since any reform, once achieved, is administered by ordinary people. Hence, if eugenics ever reached the stage where "it could increase desired types, it would not be the types desired by present-day eugenists that would be increased, but rather the types desired by the average official," and these would likely be "a subservient population, convenient to rulers but incapable of initiative."[29] Russell later elaborated this critique in his longer 1931 book, *The Scientific Outlook*, a key source for Huxley's 1932 profoundly pessimistic *Brave New World*, which links Haldane's ectogenesis to a system of mass production.[30] Interestingly, many years later Haldane himself echoed these points, warning in *New Paths in Genetics* that what counts as a desirable trait is shaped by the environment and "so far eugenical propaganda has been written almost entirely from the point of view of the well-to-do class," and in the section on "Difficulties of Positive Eugenics" in *Everything Has a History*, that "if we try to control our own evolution, we may choose the wrong path."[31]

For the geneticist H. J. Muller, who (then) greatly admired Haldane, ectogenesis represented an ideal solution to the problem of improving the human race, but he was not willing to wait for the procedure to become practical. Like Galton, Muller considered the need for improvement dire, given that life was becoming ever more complicated, requiring "an intelligence ever higher, a cooperation ever more whole-souled, thoroughgoing, and better organized."[32] (Muller was even more concerned with cooperativeness than intelligence since he agreed with Russell's claim that an increase in knowledge without a corresponding increase in social motivation would spell disaster.) Fortunately, the Bolshevik triumph provided a favorable opportunity to intervene. In *Out of the Night: A Biologist's View of the Future*, Muller explained that improvement could be accomplished through the mass insemination of women with the sperm of men superior in intellect and fellow feeling. (Although first published in 1935, the book was written in 1925.) Such a program of mass selection would rapidly raise the level of the population. Right now, if we only had the will, it would be possible to so "order our reproduction that a considerable part of the very next generation might average, in its hereditary physical and mental constitution, half-way between the average of the present population and that of our greatest living men of mind, body, or 'spirit' (as we choose). At the same time, it can be reckoned, the number of men and women of great though not supreme ability would thereby be increased several hundred fold." But this is only the immediate result. Eventually, pace Galton and Wallace, evolution "will reach down into the secret places of the great universe of its own nature and, by the aid of its ever-growing intelligence and cooperation, shape itself into an increasingly sublime creation."[33]

An even more extreme transformist vision was articulated by the Marxist crystallographer Bernal. Bernal took the practice of ectogenesis for granted, and assumed it would result in a greatly increased life span and intelligence. Those individuals with especially powerful intellects would be plugged into an elaborate network of other superior beings. Consciousness itself would likely "vanish in a humanity that has become completely etherealized, losing the close-knit organism, becoming masses of atoms in space communicating by radiation, and ultimately perhaps resolving itself entirely into light."[34] This world-mind would then be in a position to manipulate (and experiment on) other lesser beings. Bernal equably considers the possibility that the human race will split in two, with a higher race that consists of scientists, who will also eventually become rulers with "the means of directing the masses in harmless occupations and of maintaining a perfect docility under the appearance of perfect freedom."[35]

It might be noted that the idea of a world divided into rulers who constitute a biological elite and the ruled who constitute a biological underclass stretches back to Plato's *Republic*, whose guardian class would be constantly purified through selection, and the elite restricted from breeding with civilians.[36] It has since been a recurring theme in utopian (and dystopian) fiction.[37] In *The Time Machine*, H. G. Wells describes a future age in which humanity has split into two species, the refined but decadent Eloi and the brutalized Morlocks.[38] This motif seems to be again in vogue. For example, in *Regeln für den Menschenpark*, the German philosopher Peter Sloterdijk anticipates a division of humanity into genetic engineers and the genetically engineered (zookeepers and animals in the "human zoo"). Although Sloterdijk has been compared with Adolf Hitler, his vision is actually much closer in spirit to that of Plato or Bernal. That is also true of Princeton molecular biologist Lee Silver, whose *Remaking Eden* is a kind of free market analogue to *The World, the Flesh, and the Devil*. Silver asks: "Why not seize the power?" Noting that we now control children in all kinds of ways, he suggests that using genetic engineering to this purpose is no different in principle from sending them to computer camp or an expensive college or providing all kinds of other advantages that we now find acceptable.[39] Bluntly conceding that the result will be to increase inequality, he predicts that in the distant future the species will break into two, the "genrich" and the "normals." Although the former "can trace their ancestry back directly to *homo sapiens*, they are as different from humans as humans are from the primitive worms with tiny brains that first crawled along the earth's surface."[40]

That Haldane, Bernal, and Muller (at the time he wrote *Out of the Night*), were all Marxists should perhaps not be surprising. While avoiding attribute-rich characterizations of human nature, Marxists assume that there are needs and capacities that flow from our natural condition, but also that in exercising these capacities, we transform ourselves. According to the young Hegelians (including Karl Marx), we make ourselves, and not just metaphorically. In transforming nature, we also transform our capacities and sensibilities. That vision is strikingly expressed by Leon Trotsky in *Literature and Revolution*. After reshaping the physical world, Trotsky writes,

Man at last will begin to harmonize himself in earnest. . . . The human species, the coagulated *homo sapiens*, will once more enter into a state of radical transformation, and, in his own hands, will become an object of the most complicated methods of artificial selection and psycho-physical training. This is entirely in accord with evolution. . . . The human race will not have ceased to crawl on all fours before God, kings, and capital, in order later to submit humbly before the dark laws of heredity and a blind sexual selection![41]

(Trotsky, like many Marxists in the 1920s, greatly admired Darwin.) In a passage reminiscent of Wallace or Spencer, Trotsky predicts that "man will become immeasurably stronger, wiser, and subtler; his body will become more harmonized, his movements more rhythmic, his voice more musical. The forms of life will become dynamically dramatic. The average human type will rise to the heights of an Aristotle, a Goethe, or a Marx. And above this ridge, new peaks will rise."[42]

In the Aftermath of World War II

Following the Second World War, visions of biological transformation fell from favor. Although the orientation of Nazi eugenics was overwhelmingly negative (the major exception being the *Lebensborn* program, which encouraged both married and unmarried women of superior Aryan stock to bear children of SS officers), such visions seemed uncomfortably close to the National Socialist aim of creating a master race. Indeed, in the United States at least, there was a backlash against the hereditarian assumptions on which any kind of eugenics, positive or negative, necessarily depend.[43] It is unlikely, however, that many scientists changed their minds about the importance of genes to differences in human mentality and behavior, and within a decade, there were new calls to control human reproduction. The resurgence of interest in eugenics—still unembarrassedly called that—was fueled by a number of postwar anxieties that included advances in medical treatment and the prospect of a population explosion. Of greatest importance was the threat of long-term genetic damage resulting from increased exposure to radiation.[44]

Many geneticists in the 1950s believed that radiation-induced mutation presented a new threat to the human race. This peril was vigorously publicized by Muller, whose 1947 Nobel Prize for the discovery of the mutagenic properties of x-rays allowed him now to speak with new authority. In his 1949 presidential address to the newly founded American Society of Human Genetics, Muller argued that the human

species was deteriorating under an ever-increasing "genetic load" of deleterious mutations. In his view, this burden was attributable both to
expanded medical and military uses of radiation, especially atmospheric
nuclear testing, and therapeutic advances in medicine, which allowed
individuals who would once have died before childbearing to survive and
reproduce. New radiation-induced mutations, added to the already-high
load, would be increasingly difficult to accommodate and ultimately
would threaten our viability as a species. To counter this threat, Muller
urged a less casual attitude toward the use of ionizing radiation. He also
hoped that technological advances would make it possible to survey
genotypes and identify the most burdened individuals, who he assumed
would voluntarily refrain from reproducing. In this version of eugenics,
the enemy is no longer a group, such as Slavs or the feebleminded, but
mutation, which can and does affect everyone.[45] As Muller himself put
it, "None of us can cast stones, for we are all fellow mutants together."[46]
His plan is socially neutral. It represents what sociologist Barbara Katz
Rothman, in a different context, has called the new "microeugenics,"
which concerns the genes of individuals, in contrast to the old "macroeu-
genics," which concerned groups of people.[47]

Although Muller's warnings about the dangers of increased mutation
had an enormous impact, their implications were essentially conservative: the need to reduce exposure to radiation and for some form of
negative eugenics that would rely on individuals' sense of genetic
responsibility. But the warnings also had an impact more directly related
to human genetic engineering. Although Muller did not view the genome
as sacred, he certainly considered it a precious possession, which obligations to future generations required us to protect. For environmentalists, the idea that we had a duty to prevent the degradation of our
genome proved useful in the campaign against the overuse of chemical
mutagens, especially pesticides. The more cherished the genome, the
greater the strength of the case for protecting it against environmental
insult. The link is particularly evident in Silent Spring where Rachel
Carson, citing Muller, writes of the need to protect the "genetic heritage"
of humankind, characterized as "a possession infinitely more valuable
than individual life." According to Carson, the "genome is a sacred possession," which we must preserve.[48] Ironically, given Muller's view that
the human genome could stand considerable improvement, his writings

nourished the view, later turned against genetic engineering, that humans share a common genetic heritage, which it would be wrong to modify.

In the 1960s, discussion of positive eugenics was prompted by developments in molecular biology, which made it appear that more precise and direct genetic interventions were on the horizon. In 1965, Rollin Hotchkiss's "Portents for a Genetic Engineering" warned of various dangers and difficulties on the horizon, but also portrayed efforts to improve humanity as both inevitable and, given both our physical and mental imperfections, ultimately desirable.[49] Four years later, Cal Tech molecular biologist Robert Sinsheimer termed genetic engineering a "new eugenics." Like Hotchkiss, Sinsheimer emphasized that this eugenics would be accomplished by individuals acting voluntarily in their own interests. Although his prophecy was inspired by cutting-edge science, it harked back in spirit to Haldane and the Muller of *Out of the Night*. "The new eugenics," Sinsheimer claimed, "would permit in principle the conversion of all of the unfit to the highest genetic level. The old eugenics was limited to a numerical enhancement of the best of our existing gene pool. The horizons of the new eugenics are in principle boundless— for we should have the potential to create new genes and new qualities yet undreamed."[50]

Throughout the 1960s and 1970s, the morality of genetic engineering was heatedly debated. (Indeed, it is hard not to feel that virtually everything there is to say about the ethics of cloning and so forth was said then.) In this period, the Methodist Paul Ramsey became the leading critic of the new field of genetic engineering, and the Episcopalian Joseph Fletcher one of its foremost champions. The two theologians disputed the ethics of a wide variety of existing or potential genetic manipulations, including cloning. In arguing against positive interventions, Ramsey asserted that a Christian will find "elements in the nature of man which . . . should be withheld from human handling or trespass."[51] But in Fletcher's view, there was nothing sacrosanct about human nature. "The accusation that the new biology is trying to create a 'master race' is fair enough," he wrote, "if it means that a people with fewer defects and more control over the crippling accidents of 'nature' are better able to master life's ups and downs. Most of us would want to belong to the master race in that sense. Mastery in the sense of good health and inheritance is sanity."[52]

The morality of tampering with human nature was also debated in secular circles. Critics condemned such interventions as "playing God," a phrase popularized by Ted Howard's and Jeremy Rifkin's *Who Should Play God?* Rifkin has consistently called for the "resacralization of nature," which he considers "the great mission of the coming age."[54] As Peters notes, this ethic makes no appeal to Christian or Jewish theological principles (according to which it is the Creator and not the creation that is sacred), and Rifkin himself writes from a naturalist or vitalist position.[55] Indeed, it seems that many who condemn the notion of playing God are not theists, and what is meant by the phrase is not always clear; much ink has been spilled trying to sort out the various usages. Most often, when the phrase is not employed literally, it seems to be a short-hand way of charging scientific arrogance; that is, as a protest against the readiness of some people, who are necessarily fallible, to make decisions with potentially irreversible consequences for us all. In any case, it caught on among both religious and secular critics of genetic engineering (and biotechnology more generally), and with it, the concept of an inviolate, because sacred, human nature. Physician/bioethicist Leon Kass, author of the "wisdom of repugnance" argument, was perhaps the most prominent advocate of the view that human nature is sacrosanct. Noting that biological engineering was gathering power, he warned that it would bring new opportunities for eroding "our idea of man as something splendid or divine, as a creature with freedom and dignity. And clearly, if we come to see ourselves as meat, then meat we shall become."[56]

On June 16, 1980, in the case of *Diamond v. Chakrabarty*, the U.S. Supreme Court ruled that a genetically altered organism—in this case, an oil-digesting microbe—could qualify for patent protection as a novel "manufacture" or "composition of nature" (a decision followed in 1988 by the Patent and Trademark Office's award of a patent on a transgenic mouse that made whole animals, other than humans, patentable). In his amicus brief before the U.S. Supreme Court in the *Chakrabarty* case, the biotechnology critic and Rifkin associate Ted Howard asserted in words that could have easily come from the politically more conservative Kass: "To justify patenting living organisms, those who seek such patents must argue that life has no 'vital' or sacred property. . . . But once this is accomplished, all living material will be reduced to an arrangement of chemicals, or 'mere compositions of matter.' "[57]

Rifkin's antimaterialist argument clearly struck a responsive chord with religious groups, especially Southern Baptists.[58] The alliance he formed with Christian and Jewish leaders resulted in a statement critical of *Chakrabarty* issued by the heads of the National Council of Churches, the U.S. Catholic Conference, and the Synagogue Council of America. It called for a reexamination of patent laws on the grounds that new life-forms could not have been anticipated by those who wrote the laws, and also noted that the challenges to "the fundamental nature of human life and the dignity and worth of the individual human being" went far beyond patents. One of those threats was said to be the prospect that an "individual or group" will control life-forms for the purpose of improving people. "History has shown us that there will always be those who believe it appropriate to 'correct' our mental and physical structures by genetic means, so as to fit their vision of human-ity. This becomes more dangerous when the basic tools to do so are finally at hand. Those who would play God will be tempted as never before."[59]

The alliance, later extended to other religious groups, has proved both durable and effective. Thus, in 1983, Rifkin persuaded 58 religious leaders to sign "The Theological Letter concerning Moral Arguments against Genetic Engineering of the Human Germline Cells," which opposed human germ line engineering.[60] And in 1995, he organized the "Joint Appeal against Human and Animal Patenting," signed by 180 leaders representing over 80 religious groups. At the press conference announcing the one-paragraph statement, Rifkin declared, "By turning life into patented inventions, the government drains life of its intrinsic nature and sacred value."[61]

Beginning in the 1980s, then, the issue of justice became inextricably tangled with the issue of eugenics—now understood to be wrong because our DNA is sacrosanct. Of course, this position was challenged, and not only by enthusiasts for human genetic engineering. Thus the psychia-trist/bioethicist Willard Gaylin asserted: "I not only think that we *will* tamper with Mother Nature, I think Mother wants us to."[62] Perhaps the strongest challenge came from philosopher Jonathan Glover. In *What Kind of People Should There Be?* Glover attempted to separate different strands in the discussion about the desirability of modifying human nature through genetic engineering, arguing that there were good reasons for caution, especially the risk of irreversible disasters, but also bad ones, particularly the claim that human nature is inviolate. In Glover's view, our nature left a lot to be desired. He wrote:

Preserving the human race as it is will seem an acceptable option to all those who can watch the news on television and feel satisfied with the world. It will appeal to those who can talk to their children about the history of the twentieth century without wishing they could leave some things out. When, in the rest of this book, the case for and against various changes is considered, the fact that they *are* changes will be treated as no objection at all.[63]

Contemporary Worries and the Uses of History

As late as the 1980s, the pros and cons of human genetic engineering were generally argued on their merits. That is, critics contended variously that the enterprise was too risky, the underlying scientific assumptions were too reductionist, the consequences for biodiversity were dire, the existing social inequalities would be exacerbated, or the alternative approaches to disease would be usurped. Some maintained that tampering with the genome was wrong because God—and others said that evolution—knew best. But it was rare to oppose human genetic engineering on the grounds that it constituted eugenics, at least without further argument. Indeed, many writers took for granted that human genetic engineering either was or would lead to some kind of eugenics—the question was whether it would be the good or the bad kind. That the label, in itself, did not necessarily condemn is reflected in the fact that many enthusiasts were unembarrassed to call genetic engineering a "new eugenics." Critics therefore had to explain what they thought was wrong with a eugenics that relied on individual choice.

Today, the situation has changed. Notwithstanding recent efforts by some philosophers to spur a real discussion about what, if anything, is intrinsically wrong with eugenics, in popular and even most academic discourse, to label a practice eugenics is thereby to denounce it. There is thus little felt necessity to identify the specific offense(s). There are many possible candidates, and it is often difficult to tell which are assumed. (Since some are mutually inconsistent, the answer cannot be all.)[64] But the histories that typically accompany these discussions imply that one of the worst wrongs is coercion.

If an evil of the eugenics movement was its use of compulsion, the obvious lesson would seem to be the need for freedom from interference with reproductive decisions. The moral that people should be free to reach their own reproductive goals in whatever ways they want is frequently drawn. This use of history is clearly illustrated by the Swedish libertarian philosopher Torbjörn Tännsjö, who writes,

The important thing to learn from history is that society should not meddle with our reproductive decisions. This does not only imply that no one should be compelled to have an abortion or become sterilized. It implies too that no one should be stopped from becoming a parent in the way he or she sees fit. The use of techniques for assisted reproduction should not be regulated by political authorities (nor by doctors). The decisions about prenatal diagnosis, in vitro fertilization, egg donation, preimplanatory diagnosis, and so forth, should be placed in the hands of prospective parents. The doctors should serve the needs of those prospective parents. The politicians should allow the doctors to do so.[65]

As Jean Bethke Elshtain notes, the world of human reproductive technology has "been surrounded by the halo of 'rights.'"[66] Boosters and skeptics both invoke them. For instance, the skeptical Council on Responsible Genetics believes that "all people have the right to have been conceived, gestated, and born without genetic manipulation."[67] At the same time, such enthusiasts for the new technologies as John Robertson, Leroy Hood, and Lee Silver argue that we all have the right to seek to achieve our reproductive goals, however we define them (which usually translates to the claim that we have the right to any procedure we can afford).[68] The new and prospective technologies are said to allow not just infertile couples but also gay couples and single adults to reproduce children that share their genes—thereby fulfilling their reproductive desires.[69] The principle of respect for autonomy is seen to demarcate today's reproductive opportunities from the bad coercive eugenics of the past. For example, Gregory Pence writes that allowing parents virtually unfettered choice in relation to their future children through the insertion of artificial chromosomes to extend their life span or in utero therapy to improve their memory, is exactly the opposite of the bad, state-controlled eugenics of the past, which aimed to deny parents such choices. Pence notes that he himself would feel obliged to give his future child such advantages, adding that while he would respect others' decisions not to do the same (as though he had a choice!), he was baffled by how others could possibly think it just to prevent him from providing his future children with such enhancements. He goes on to remark that he sees "no difference between such a ban and a similar ban on parents sending their children to computer camps in the summer: both are intended to better children, both will be done most by people with money, and both are not the business of government."[70]

Perhaps these quotations (which could easily be multiplied) are sufficient to illustrate the interests that are served for genetic engineering enthusiasts in telling a tale that equates eugenics with compulsion and Nazis. There are two such interests. First, it allows the enthusiasts to sharply demarcate human genetic engineering from eugenics—to say that the appalling practices we associate with eugenics have nothing to do with the practices they wish to encourage today. Second, it is easily deployed in support of an antiregulatory agenda. The obvious moral is: "The state should stay out" of reproductive decision making.[71]

Critics, on the other hand, have an interest in stressing the continuity between the practices of genetic engineering and the eugenics of the past. The standard narratives serve to associate these technologies with people and practices that we today find odious, in effect denying any rupture with the past. Commenting on a position paper issued by the Council on Responsible Genetics, Ted Peters remarks, "The structure of this argument is that because germline modification can be associated with eugenics, and because eugenics can be associated with Nazism, it follows that we can associate proponents of germline enhancement with the Nazis and, on this ground, should reject it."[72] Certainly these histories arouse strong emotion, which is at least partly their point. So both critics and enthusiasts have (disparate) interests in constructing a history that identifies eugenics with brutal coercion.

But except in relation to sterilization and abortion, critics do not draw a libertarian lesson from the history of eugenics. For those wary of genetic engineering, the fact that its practices are voluntary does not imply that they are ipso facto *harmless*. Indeed, they find consumer-oriented eugenics in some respects especially disturbing. As noted earlier, the reasons why are not always clearly articulated. But a number of issues recur with some frequency. Without any attempt to rank or evaluate them, much less to be exhaustive, some principal areas of concern are:

• The implications for justice. Physicist Freeman Dyson's comment that "market-driven applied science will usually result in the invention of toys for the rich," nicely expresses the sentiment of many skeptics.[73] Genetic engineering will be expensive. Many in the United States have no health insurance, and in any case, standard policies do not pay for high-tech reproductive services, which will be available only to the affluent.[74] The effect will inevitably be to widen already immense social inequalities.

Some believe that the elite will become a genetic aristocracy—smart, attractive, artistic, musical, athletic, resistant to disease, and so on. Scenarios sketched by enthusiasts such as Silver and Sloterdijk have sometimes been taken up by critics, who predict that we will segregate into different castes and eventually different species. Thus, Dyson warns that in the absence of regulation human germ line engineering "could cause a splitting of humanity into hereditary castes."[75] Others believe that such scenarios rest on false assumptions about the contribution of genes to differences in human mentality and behavior. Their concern is rather that the emphasis on genes will result in a shift away from more effective medical, social, and environmental means to improve human health and well-being. (In a rather bizarre reversal of the usual distributive argument, James D. Watson argues that we owe it to disadvantaged people to develop genetic engineering technologies.[76]

• The impact on parent-child relationships. The concern here is that the parental desire to have a certain kind of child or, as Barbara Katz Rothman suggests, a particular kind of parenting experience, will reduce the child to an artifact and distort parent-child relations.[77] Critics ask what will happen when after all the effort and money expended to produce a child designed to certain specifications, the result disappoints? And they worry about the psychological impact on the children, who may feel even more constrained by parental expectations than they do now.[78]

• The impact on assumptions about human worth. Some critics object to any judgment that some genes are better than others. For example, Robyn Rowland writes that "whichever way it is organized, through legislation or 'choice,' the outcome of eugenicist attitudes means selecting humans of value and nonvalue."[79] Others fear that assumptions about what is desirable will embody the values of scientists and biotech entrepreneurs, who will become the "self-appointed arbiters of human excellence."[80] (It was primarily the prospect of a socially biased definition of desirable qualities that led a once-enthusiastic Haldane to reject a positive eugenics program.)

• The impact on attitudes about disabilities. Many critics think that these technologies foster an unhealthy preoccupation with perfection, thus fostering prejudice against people with disabilities.[81] It is often noted that this category will include all of us who live long enough, and that it is therefore in our own best interest to acknowledge its inevitability and our consequent reliance on networks of support. Thus, Ruth Hubbard and Elijah Wald comment that "all of us can expect to experience disabilities—if not now, then some time before we die, if not our own, then those of someone close to us."[82]

If these are serious problems, they would seem to call for limits on consumer choice. But abortion politics has made it difficult for those on the political left to argue in favor of limiting procreative liberty in the service of other values. In the United States, access to abortion has been defended on the grounds that women have an absolute right to control their own bodies, and given that rationale, the procedure should be permitted for any reason. To argue that some genetic grounds should not be respected, or that other reproductive choices should be barred, is implicitly to limit the scope of that principle. Politically left skeptics of genetic engineering tend to assert the necessity of being resolutely pro-choice and just as resolutely opposed to human genetic modifications.[83] But if reproductive autonomy is an absolute right, it is hard to see how this can be managed.[84]

A move commonly made to resolve this quandary is to implicitly suggest that choices about the use of genetic technologies are not truly autonomous. Thus, structural constraints and social pressures are sometimes said to vitiate the claim of "free choice" (a phrase typically encased in scare quotes or characterized as so-called choice) in reproductive decision making.[85]

There is no doubt that women's decision making is influenced by economic factors and social expectations. Genetic counseling, in practice, is sometimes directive.[86] The costs of caring for a severely disabled child are large, and the fate of the child after the parents are no longer able to provide care is a source of great anxiety even in systems with national health insurance. There do exist social norms regarding what constitutes reproductive responsibility, attractiveness, and health; social attitudes about gender, sexual orientation, and race; and views about what life is like for disabled people and their families.[87] But these considerations are more germane to the realm of prenatal diagnosis than to genetic engineering. There are no *economic* pressures to design one's offspring.

In any case, the influence of norms is inescapable. The way the discussion often goes, the implication is that a choice influenced by social expectations or trends is not free. To claim that "there is no free choice and autonomy regarding eugenic practices: the decisions are all embedded in the society surrounding the person," is to assume the possibility (and desirability) of a world in which people were *not* influenced by the views of their family, communities, and the larger society.[88] But all of our choices are embedded in a social context, which necessarily includes the attitudes and desires of other people. It will not work to implicitly define an "autonomous" decision as one somehow detached from social expectations. On this understanding, no important life decision could count as free.

For those alert to the dangers of the unbridled use of genetic engineering, the crucial point is not that autonomy in reproductive decision making is always a fiction but that autonomy need not trump every other value. Acknowledging this is a necessary first step toward a candid discussion of how best to exercise some kind of social control over technologies now being developed and used in a regulatory vacuum.

Notes

I am grateful to the participants in the Philosophy and History of Biology Workshop, Center for Philosophy of Science, University of Pittsburgh, March 2002, and especially James Tabery and Jim Lennox, who were commentators on my presentation of an early version of this chapter.

1. See John Maynard Smith, "Eugenics and Utopia," *Daedalus* 94 (1965): 487–505.

2. See Robert L. Sinsheimer, "The Prospect of Designed Genetic Change," *Engineering and Science* 13 (1969): 8–13. See also Daniel J. Kevles, *In the Name of Eugenics: Genetics and the Uses of Human Heredity* (Cambridge, MA: Harvard University Press, 1995), 267–268.

3. See Troy Duster, *Backdoor to Eugenics* (London: Routledge, 1990). The idea of backdoor eugenics first appeared in an essay by Rollin Hotchkiss, who coined the term "genetic engineering." Noting that a eugenics requiring state action was no longer acceptable, he suggested that interventions made possible by developments in molecular biology "could be practiced in private and in secret on individual genes of individual persons," and also observed: "It will be much more difficult to regulate, and legislation *against* it will seem like the same invasion of

personal rights that legislating *for* eugenic measures appears to be" (Rollin D. Hotchkiss, "Portents for a Genetic Engineering," *Journal of Heredity* 56 [1965]: 198).

4. Bryan Appleyard, *Brave New Worlds: Staying Human in the Genetic Future* (New York: Viking, 1998), 84.

5. Jeremy Rifkin, cited in ibid., 128. See also Richard Wright, "Achilles' Helix," *New Republic* (July 9 and 16, 1990): 21–31; Andrew Kimbrell, *The Human Body Shop: The Cloning, Engineering, and Marketing of Life*, 2nd ed. (Washington, DC: Regnery, 1997), 147; Mae-Wan Ho, *Genetic Engineering: Dream or Nightmare? Turning the Tide on the Brave New World of Bad Science and Big Business*, 2nd ed. (New York: Continuum, 2000), 222; Jean E. McEwen, "Public and Private Eugenics," *GeneWatch* 12 (June 1999): 1–3; and Mark Frankel, "Inheritable Genetic Modification and a Brave New World: Did Huxley Have It Wrong?" *Hastings Center Report* 33 (2003): 32–33.

6. Peter Morton, *The Vital Science: Biology and the Literary Imagination* (London: George All and Unwin, 1984), 121.

7. Francis Fukuyama, *Our Posthuman Future: Consequences of the Biotechnology Revolution* (New York: Farrar, Straus and Giroux, 2002); Bill McKibben, *Enough: Staying Human in an Engineered Age* (New York: Henry Holt, 2003); and Jürgen Habermas, *The Future of Human Nature* (Cambridge, UK: Polity Press, 2003).

8. Lee M. Silver, *Remaking Eden* (New York: Avon, 1997), and "Reprogenetics: How Reprogenetic and Genetic Technologies Will Be Combined to Provide New Opportunities for People to Reach Their Reproductive Goals," in *Engineering the Human Germline: An Exploration of the Science and Ethics of Altering the Genes We Pass on to Our Children*, ed. Gregory Stock and John Campbell (New York: Oxford University Press, 2000), 57–71; Gregory Stock, *Redesigning Humans: Our Inevitable Genetic Future* (Boston: Houghton Mifflin, 2002); Gregory Pence, *Re-creating Medicine: Ethical Issues at the Frontiers of Medicine* (Lanham, MD: Rowman and Littlefield, 2000); and Peter Sloterdijk, *Regeln für den Menschenpark: ein Antwortschreiben zu Heideggers Brief den Humanismus* (Frankfurt am Main: Suhrkamp Verlag, 1999).

9. Morton, *Vital Science*, 129.

10. J. B. S. Haldane, "Daedalus, or Science and the Future," in *Haldane's "Daedalus" Revisited*, ed. Krishna R. Dronamraju (1923; repr., Oxford: Oxford University Press, 1995).

11. Watson Davis, ed., *The Advance of Science* (Garden City, NY: Doubleday, 1934), 275.

12. Charlotte Perkins Gilman, cited in Wendy Kline, *Building a Better Race: Gender, Sexuality, and Eugenics from the Turn of the Century to the Baby Boom* (Berkeley: University of California Press, 2001), 12.

13. Francis Galton, "The Possible Improvement of the Human Breed, under the Existing Conditions of Law and Sentiment," in *Essays in Eugenics* (London: Eugenics Education Society, 1909), 24.

14. Galton, *Essays in Eugenics*, 25, 28, 32.

15. Francis Galton, "Hereditary Talent and Character," *Macmillan's Magazine* 12 (1865): 166.

16. Alfred Russel Wallace, "Interview Fragment," in *Alfred Russel Wallace: An Anthology of His Shorter Writings*, ed. Charles H. Smith (New York: Oxford University Press, 1991), 77. Orig. pub. 1912.

17. Alfred Russel Wallace, "The Origin of Human Races and the Antiquity of Man Deduced from the Theory of 'Natural Selection,'" in *Alfred Russel Wallace: An Anthology of His Shorter Writings*, ed. Charles H. Smith (New York: Oxford University Press, 1991), 26. Orig. pub. 1864.

18. Alfred Russel Wallace, "Human Selection," in *Alfred Russel Wallace: An Anthology of His Shorter Writings*, ed. Charles H. Smith (New York: Oxford University Press, 1991), 60. Orig. pub. 1890.

19. Patrick Parrinder, "Eugenics and Utopia: Sexual Selection from Galton to Morris," *Utopian Studies* 8 (1997): 1–12.

20. J. D. Bernal, *The World, the Flesh, and the Devil: An Inquiry into the Three Enemies of the Human Soul* (London: Kegan Paul, 1929); Bertrand Russell, *Icarus, or the Future of Science* (New York: E. P. Dutton, 1924); and Aldous Huxley, *Brave New World* (London: Chatto and Windus, 1932).

21. Haldane, "Daedalus," 35.

22. Ibid., 42.

23. Ibid., 41–42, 46, 49.

24. Ibid., 36–37. For an interesting analysis of the ways in which myths of monstrosity, including the ancient Greek myth of Daedalus and Minatour, have stigmatized the disabled while being used to warn against genetic engineering, see Mark Jeffreys, "Dr. Daedalus and His Minotaur: Mythic Warnings about Genetic Engineering from J. B. S. Haldane, François Jacob, and Andrew Niccol's *Gattacta*," *Journal of Medical Humanities* 22 (2001): 137–152. (The title is somewhat misleading as Haldane employed the myth to celebrate biological engineering, not condemn it.)

25. Mark B. Adams, "Last Judgment: The Visionary Biology of J. B. S. Haldane," *Journal of the History of Biology* 33 (2000): 463–468.

26. See Jon Turney, *Frankenstein's Footsteps: Science, Genetics, and Popular Culture* (New Haven, CT: Yale University Press, 1998), 102. See also Adams, "Last Judgment," 462.

27. Russell, *Icarus*, 5.

28. Ibid., 49.

29. Ibid., 51–52.

30. See Turney, *Frankenstein's Footsteps*, 102, 114.

31. J. B. S. Haldane, *New Paths in Genetics* (New York: Harper and Brothers, 1942), 36–37, and *Everything Has a History* (London: Allen and Unwin, 1951), 287. James Tabery pointed out Haldane's apparent change of heart and cited

these passages in his commentary on a version of this chapter presented at the Philosophy and History of Biology Workshop, Center for Philosophy of Science, University of Pittsburgh, March 23–24, 2002.

32. H. J. Muller, *Out of the Night: A Biologist's View of the Future* (1935; repr., New York: Vanguard Press, 1984), 37.

33. Ibid., 113, 125.

34. Bernal, *The World*, 57.

35. Ibid., 72, 89. See also Gary Werskey, *The Visible College: A Collective Biography of British Scientists and Socialists of the 1930s* (London: Free Association Books, 1988).

36. On Greek eugenics in general, see David J. Galton, "Greek Theories on Eugenics," *Journal of Medical Ethics* 24 (1998): 263–267.

37. See, for example, H. G. Wells, *The Time Machine* (1895). New York: Tom Doheaty Associates, LLC, 1992).

38. Cited in Morton, *Vital Science*, 110–112.

39. Silver, *Remaking Eden*, 227. See also Silver, "Reprogenetics," 60.

40. Silver, *Remaking Eden*, 292–293.

41. Leon Trotsky, *Literature and Revolution* (1924; repr., Ann Arbor: University of Michigan Press, 1960), 254–255.

42. Ibid., 256.

43. See Dorothy Nelkin and M. Susan Lindee, *The DNA Mystique: The Gene as a Cultural Icon* (New York: W. H. Freeman, 1995), 33–34.

44. See Diane B. Paul, "From Reproductive Responsibility to Reproductive Autonomy," in *Mutating Concepts, Evolving Disciplines: Genetics, Medicine, and Society*, ed. Lisa S. Parker and Rachel A. Ankeny (Dordrecht: Kluwer Academics, 2002). See also John Beatty, "Radiation Genetics as Atomic Age and Cold-War Eugenics", annual meeting of the History of Science Society, Denuer, Colorado, November 8–11, 2001); and Celeste Condit, *The Meanings of the Gene: Public Debates about Human Heredity* (Madison: University of Wisconsin Press, 1999), 65–81.

45. H. J. Muller, cited in Beatty, "Radiation Genetics."

46. H. J. Muller, "Our Load of Mutations," *American Journal of Human Genetics* 2 (1950): 169.

47. Barbara Katz Rothman, *The Book of Life: A Personal and Ethical Guide to Race, Normality, and the Implications of the Human Genome Project* (Boston: Beacon Press, 2001), 217.

48. Rachel Carson, *Silent Spring* (Boston: Houghton Mifflin, 1962), 208, 216.

49. Hotchkiss, "Portents for a Genetic Engineering," 197–222. See also Wright, "Achilles' Helix."

50. Sinsheimer, "The Prospect of Designed Genetic Change," 13.

51. Paul Ramsey, *Fabricated Man: The Ethics of Genetic Control* (New Haven, CT: Yale University Press, 1970), 31–32. It is interesting that Ramsey favored negative eugenics, which was then much less controversial, noting that in the Christian tradition, having children was never regarded as a selfish prerogative, and suggesting that we needed to develop an ethics of "genetic duty" (ibid., 56–59). For a more detailed discussion of the argument between Ramsey and Fletcher, see Paul, "From Reproductive Responsibility to Reproductive Autonomy."

52. Joseph Fletcher, *The Ethics of Genetic Control: Ending Reproductive Roulette* (Garden City, NY: Anchor Press/Doubleday, 1974), 13.

53. Jeremy Rifkin, *Who Should Play God?* (New York: Dell Publishing Co. 1977), See also Ted Peters, *Playing God? Genetic Determinism and Human Freedom* (New York: Routledge, 1997), 186–187, n. 27.

54. Jeremy Rifkin, *Algeny* (New York: Viking, 1983), 252.

55. Peters, *Playing God?* 117.

56. Leon Kass, "Making Babies: The New Biology and the 'Old' Morality," *Public Interest* (Winter 1972): 53. A brief aside on an interesting paradox: To worry about genetically changing human nature is necessarily to assume that it is malleable—that we have or at least someday may have the capacity to genetically alter "essential" human characteristics. Thus, as recently observed in *From Chance to Choice*, once we make this assumption, we can no longer assess genetic interventions by their conformity with our (fixed) nature. Questions about whether it is morally permissible or even required to genetically intervene to change our nature cannot be settled by appealing to human nature since "consonance with a fixed human nature cannot be the touchstone for what is just or moral if there is no such thing" (Allen Buchanan, Dan W. Brock, Norman Daniels, and Daniel Wikler, *From Chance to Choice: Genetics and Justice* [Cambridge: Cambridge University Press, 2000], 87, 93). For a similar point, made in relation to Haldane's scientific utopianism, see Yaron Ezrahi, "Haldane between Daedalus and Icarus," in *Haldane's Daedalus Revisited*, ed. Krishna R. Dronamragu (Oxford: Oxford University Press, 1995) 76.

57. Ted Howard, cited in Kimbrell, *The Human Body Shop*, 225.

58. See Peters, *Playing God?* 12–13, 117.

59. Clare Randall, Bernard Mandelbaum, and Thomas Kelly, "Letter from Three General Secretaries," in *Splicing Life: A Report on the Social and Ethical Issues of Genetic Engineering with Human Beings*, President's Commission for the Study of Ethical Problems in Medicine and Biomedical and Behavioral Research (Washington, DC: U.S. Government Printing Office, 1983), 96. See also Robert B. Kaiser, "Three Clerics Urge President and Congress to Set Up Controls on Genetic Engineers," *New York Times*, July 15, 1980, A16.

60. Jeremy Rifkin, "The Theological Letter concerning Moral Arguments against Genetic Engineering of the Human Germline Cells" (Washington, DC: Foundation on Economic Trends, 1983).

61. Cited in Richard Stone, "Religious Leaders Oppose Patenting Genes and Animals," *Science* 268:5214 (May 26, 1995): 1126; and Peters, *Playing God?* 116.

62. Willard Gaylin, "What's So Special about Being Human?" in *The Manipulation of Life*, ed. Robert Esbjornson (San Francisco: Harper and Row, 1983), 53.

63. Jonathan Glover, *What Kind of People Should There Be?* (Harmondsworth, UK: Penguin Books, 1984), 56.

64. Torbjörn Tännsjö, "Compulsory Sterilization in Sweden," *Bioethics* 12:3 (1998): 236–249.

65. Ibid., 247–248.

66. Jean Bethke Elshtain, "To Clone or Not to Clone," ed. Martha C. Nussbaum and Cass R. Sunstein, *Clones and Clones: Facts and Fantasies about Human Cloning* (New York: W. W. Norton, 1998), 187–188.

67. The Board of Directors of the Council for Responsible Genetics, "The Genetic Bill of Richts, April, 2000. <http://www.gene.watch.org/programs.bill-of-rights/bill-rights-text.html> (26 January 2004), 10.

68. See John A. Robertson, *Children of Choice: Freedom and the New Reproductive Technologies* (Princeton, NJ: Princeton University Press, 1994); Gregory Stock and John Campbell, eds., *Engineering the Human Germline: An Exploration of the Science and Ethics of Altering the Genes We Pass on to Our Children* (New York: Oxford University Press, 2000); and Silver, *Remaking Eden*, and "Reprogenetics."

69. See Silver, "Reprogenetics," 58.

70. Gregory Pence, "Maximize Parental Choice," in *Engineering the Human Germline: An Exploration of the Science and Ethics of Altering the Genes We Pass on to Our Children*, ed. Gregory Stock and John Campbell (New York: Oxford University Press, 2000), 113. See also Pence, *Re-creating Medicine*.

71. James Watson, cited in Stock and Campbell, *Engineering the Human Germline*, 90.

72. Peters, *Playing God?* 150.

73. Freeman Dyson, "*Daedalus* after Seventy Years," in *Haldane's "Daedalus" Revisited*, ed. Krishna R. Dronamraju (Oxford: Oxford University Press, 1995), 62.

74. Mark Frankel and Audrey R. Chapman, *Human Inheritable Genetic Modifications: Assessing Scientific, Ethical, Religious, and Policy Issues* (Washington, DC: American Association for the Advancement of Science, 2000), 36–37.

75. Freeman Dyson, *Techno-Eugenics E-mail Newsletter*, June 12, 2000, 4.

76. James D. Watson, cited in Stock and Campbell, *Engineering the Human Germline*, 79–80.

77. Rothman, *The Book of Life*, 204–205; See also Elshtain, "To Clone," 184–185.

78. See March Darnovsky, "Human Germline Engineering and Cloning as Women's Issues," *GeneWatch* 34, no. 1 (2001): 13–14. See also Frankel and Chapman, *Human Inheritable Genetic Modifications*, 31–32.

79. Robyn Rowland, "The Control of Human Life: Masculine Science and Genetic Engineering," in *Altered Genes II: The Future?* ed. Richard Hindmarsh, Geoffrey Lawrence and R. A. Hindmarsh (St. Leonards, NSW: Allen and Unwin, 1998), 93.

80. See Ruth Hubbard and Elijah Wald, *Exploding the Gene Myth: How Genetic Information Is Produced and Manipulated by Scientists, Physicians, Employers, Insurance Companies, Educators, and Law Enforcers* (Boston: Beacon Press, 1999), 116. See also Darnovksy, "Human Germline Engineering," 1.

81. See Anita Silvers, David Wasserman, and Mary B. Mahowald, *Disability, Difference, Discrimination: Perspectives on Justice in Bioethics and Public Policy* (Lanham, MD: Rowman and Littlefield, 1998). See also Erik Parens and Adrienne Asch, eds., *Prenatal Testing and Disability Rights* (Washington, DC: Georgetown University Press, 2000); Marsha Saxton, "Why Members of the Disability Community Oppose Prenatal Diagnosis and Selective Abortion," *GeneWatch* 14 (2001): 10–12; and Lori B. Andrews, *Future Perfect: Confronting Decisions about Genetics* (New York: Columbia University Press, 2001), 97–101. For a different viewpoint, see Buchanan, Brock, Daniels, and Wikler, *From Chance to Choice*, 266–288.

82. Hubbard and Wald, *Exploding the Gene Myth*, 31. See also Saxton, "Disability Community," 6; and Alasdair MacIntyre, *Dependent Rational Animals: Why Human Beings Need the Virtues* (Chicago: Open Court, 1999).

83. See, for example, Darnovksy, "Human Germline" Engineering," 14.

84. This argument is expanded in my forthcoming "On Drawing Lessons from the History of Eugenics," in *Reprogenetics: A Blueprint for Meaningful Moral Debate and Responsible Public Policy*, ed. Lori P. Knowles and Erik Parens (Baltimore: Johns Hopkins University Press).

85. See, for example, David King "Eugenic tendencies in modern genetics," in *Redesigning Life? The Worldwide Challenge to Genetic* Engineering, ed. Brian Tokar (New York: Zed Books, 2001) 175; and Hubbard and Wald, *Exploding the Gene Myth*, 27.

86. See S. Michie, F. Bron, M. Bobrow, and T. M. Marteau, "Nondirectiveness in Genetic Counseling: An Empirical Study," *American Journal of Human Genetics* 60.1 (January 1997): 40–47.

87. See Saxton, "Disability Community," 11.

88. Gregor Wolbring, "Eugenics, Euthenics, Euphenics," *GeneWatch* 12 (June 1999): 10.

II
Embodiment and Self-Identity

6

The Body and the Quest for Control

Jean Bethke Elshtain

In our fast-paced, fitness- and youth-oriented culture, perfecting the human body has become a messianic project. In this chapter, I bring theological anthropology to bear on this project for the purpose of critique.[1] It is not that easy, of course, to stand apart from the dominant preoccupations of one's own culture in order that one might assess its enthusiasms critically. But I take this to be an essential task, difficulties notwithstanding. The situation that we face is this: bodies are thought of increasingly as the exclusive property of an individual for one to do with as one sees fit. Bodies are also construed as malleable and "constructable." We are all enjoined, through advertising, cultural imagery on television and in films, science joined to profit in the biotech industry, popularizers of the genetic revolution, and others, to "get with the program," to hop on board and not remain stuck in superstition that urges restraint or even curtailment of genetic and biological engineering. Philosophers and cultural critics indebted to Christianity, among whom I number myself, are poised as a matter of principle and faithfulness in a tension between *contra mundum* and *amor mundi* in ways that may be fruitful or frustrating, or both. This tension begins with the recognition that uncritical identification with the currents of one's own time is easily understood because so many of those currents speak to real human needs, fears, and desires, and the goods associated with these. Therein lies a major part of the problem, at least if one follows Martin Luther's lead. Luther insisted that all our needs are bound to be distorted given human rebellion against God, beginning with that ur-disobedience that got Adam and Eve thrown out of the garden. Ever since, the human being itself is marked by a trace of this original willfulness, or so argued the great reformer. We are separated from God, the source of undistorted love. As well, given that Christian theological anthropology presumes intrinsic relationality—there is no primordially free self—sifting our cherished and essential commonalities (and commune-alities) from unthinking absorption in dominant cultural forces is bound to be a delicate matter.

As this chapter proceeds, I will take up examples of cultural acquiescence to ever-more-radical manipulations of the human body.[2] An overarching and framing thematic of contemporary U.S. culture is a flight from finitude that undermines a recognition of the complexities and the limits as well as the joys of embodiment—the givens, if you will, of human *being* itself. One spin-off is widespread approval of the destruction of the bodies of others as part of our culture's panoply of invented rights and punishments, whether in situ (the abortion regime) or as a central feature of our system of retributive justice (the death penalty).[3] Neither the abortion "right" nor capital punishment is a focus of this chapter, but insofar as each practice involves the destruction of a human body—one developing, and the other developed—these practices help to structure the overall cultural frame in the matter of the differential value we assign to some human bodies in contrast to others.

Having noted Luther's mordant view about the lingering implications of human defiance of the Creator, let's flesh matters out beginning with reminders about the nature of Christian freedom, and the fact that we are both creatures and creators. As creatures we are dependent. It follows that our creaturely freedom consists in our recognition that we are not abstractly free but free only in and through relationship. A limit lies at the very heart of our existence in freedom. Christian freedom turns on the recognition of the limits to freedom.

German theologian and anti-Nazi martyr Dietrich Bonhoeffer, in *Creation and Fall*, frets that humans as creators easily transmogrify into destroyers as they misuse freedom.[4] There is a big difference between enacting human projects as cocreators respectful of a limit because, unlike God, we are neither infinite nor omniscient and, by contrast, those projects that demand that humans embrace God-likeness for themselves, up to the point of displacing God himself. With God removed as a brake on human self-sovereignty, we see no limit to what human power might accomplish. An alternative to this project of self-overcoming is an understanding of a humbler freedom, a freedom that never aspires to the absolute. This freedom is constitutive of our natures. Theologian Robin Lovin helps us to appreciate a specifically Christian freedom that is not opposed to the natural order but acts in complex faithfulness to it.[5]

One begins by taking human beings as they are, not as those fanciful entities sometimes conjured up by philosophers in what they themselves call "science-fiction" examples.[6] To be sure, as Lovin observes, the freedom of a real, not a fanciful, human being means, among other things, that one can "project oneself imaginatively into a situation in which the constraints of present experience no longer hold."[7] One can imagine states of perfection or nigh perfection. At the same time, actual freedom is always situated; it is not an abstract position located nowhere in particular. Freedom is concrete, not free-floating. Freedom is a "basic human good. Life without freedom is not something we would choose, no matter how comfortable the material circumstances might be."[8] Our reasoning capacity is part and parcel of our freedom. But that reasoning is not a separate faculty cut off from our embodied selves; instead, it is profoundly constituted by our embodied histories and memories.

Christian freedom, in Lovin's words, consists in our ability to "avoid excessive identification with the surrounding culture, since that tends both to lower . . . moral expectations and to deprive [persons] of the witness to alternative possibilities."[9] If the horizon lowers excessively, the possibility that we might exercise our capacity for freedom is cor- relatively negated. So the denial of freedom consists, in part, in a refusal to accept the freedom that is the human inheritance of finite, limited crea- tures "whose capacities for change are also limited, and who can only bring about new situations that are also themselves particular, local, and contingent."[10] To presume more than this is also problematic, launching us into dangerous pridefulness, often, of course, in the name of great ideals like choice or justice. So our freedom is, at one and the same time, both real and limited.

With this as backdrop, let us examine several contemporary projects of self-overcoming that involve a negation of (or an attempt to negate) finitude and that rely on uncritical endorsement of dominant cultural demands.[11] Such projects, remember, are tricky to approach critically because they present themselves to us in the dominant language of our culture—choice, consent, control—and promise an escape from the vagaries of the human condition into a realm of near mastery. Consider the fact that we are in the throes of a structure of biological obsession underwritten by pictures of absolute self-possession.[12] We are bombarded daily with the promise that nearly every human ailment or condition can be overcome if we just have sufficient will and skill and refuse to listen to any entreaties from critics, who are invariably portrayed as negative and antiprogress. For those whom philosopher Charles Taylor calls the cultural boosters, our imperfect embodiment is a problem that must be overcome. For example: a premise—and promise—driving the Human Genome Project, the massive mapping of the genetic code of the entire human race, is that we might one day intervene decisively in order to guarantee better, if not perfect, human products.[13] Claims made by promoters and advocates of this project run to the ecstatic.

Take, for instance, Walter Gilbert's 1986 pronouncement that the Humane Genome Project "is the grail of human genetics . . . the ultimate answer to the commandment, 'Know thyself.' "[14] In the genome-enthusiast camp, they are already talking about designer genes. Note, in this regard, the following advertisement reported by the *New York Times* in early spring 1999—an ad that had appeared in college newspapers all over the United States: "EGG DONOR NEEDED / LARGE FINANCIAL INCENTIVE / INTELLIGENT, ATHLETIC EGG DONOR NEEDED / FOR LOVING FAMILY / YOU MUST BE AT LEAST 5'10" / HAVE A 1,400+ SAT SCORE / POSSESS NO MAJOR FAMILY MEDICAL ISSUES / $50,000 / FREE MEDICAL SCREENING / ALL EXPENSES PAID."[15] As *Commonweal* noted in an editorial occasioned by this advertisement, this brings back eerie reminders of earlier advertisements that involved trade in human flesh (the reference point being the slave trade), and suggests that "we are fast returning to a world where persons carry a price tag, and where the cash value of some persons . . . is far greater than that of others."[16]

Soberer voices, like that of scientist Doris T. Zallen, find themselves struggling to gain a hearing above the din of the rhetoric of enthusiasm. Having observed that the early promises of genetic intervention to forestall "serious health problems, such as sickle-cell anemia, cystic fibrosis, and Huntington disease," have thus far had only the meagerest success, Zallen takes up this booming genetic enterprise that promises not prevention of harm but the attainment of perfection. It is called "genetic enhancement." One starts with a healthy person and then moves to perfect. Zallen calls this the "genetic equivalent of cosmetic surgery."

The aim is to make people "taller, thinner, more athletic, or more attractive." Zallen lists potential harms, including the reinforcement of "irrational societal prejudices. For instance, what would happen to short people if genetic enhancement were available to increase one's height?" The "historical record is not encouraging," she adds, noting the earlier eugenics movement with its hideous outcomes, most frighteningly in Nazi Germany, but evident in the United States as well where policies of involuntary sterilization of persons with mental retardation and other measures went forward apace.[17]

The calmer voices remind us that the scientific community at present has only the "vaguest understanding" of the details of genetic instruction—unsurprising when one considers that each "single-celled conceptus immediately after fertilisation" involves a "100-trillion-times miniaturised information system."[18] Yet the enthusiasts who claim that the benefits of genetic manipulation are both unstoppable and entirely beneficial, downplay any and all controversies and short-circuit any and all difficulties. In this way, they undercut (or attempt to) any and all "nonexpert" criticism in a manner that "effectively precludes others coming to an independent judgment about the validity of their claims."[19] The upshot is that it is difficult to have the ethical and cultural discussion we require. Those who try to promote such are tagged with the label of technophobes or Luddites.

Despite this, there are a few critical straws in the cultural wind. In the 1997 film *Gattaca*, for example, the protagonist (played by Ethan Hawke) is born the "old-fashioned way" (a "faith-birth") to his parents, who had made love and taken their chances with what sort of offspring might eventuate. In this terrible new world, when a child is born an immediate genetic profile is done. Our protagonist, Vincent, is a beautiful, yet it turns out, genetically hapless child (based on the standards of the barren world that is to be his lot) who enters life not amid awe and hopefulness but misery and worry. His mother clutches the tiny newborn to her breast as his genetic quotient is coldly read off by the expert. "Cells tell all," the prophets of genomism intone. Because of his genetic flaws, for his was an unregulated birth, young Vincent isn't covered by insurance; he doesn't get to go to school past a certain age; and he is doomed to menial service. He is a degenerate. Or, as the scanners immediately pronounce it, an "Invalid."

Vincent contrives a way to fake out the system as he yearns to go on a one-year mission to some truly far-out planet. Only "Valids"—genetically correct human beings—are eligible for such elite tasks. So Vincent pays off a Valid for the Valid's urine, blood, saliva, and fingerprints, and begins his arduous, elaborate ruse. For this is a world in which any bodily scraping—a single eyelash, a single bit of skin sloughing—might betray you. Why would a Valid sell his bodily fluids and properties? Because the Valid is now "useless," a cripple, having been paralyzed in a car accident. Indeed, his life is so useless according to society's standards (which he, in turn, has thoroughly internalized) that, at the film's conclusion and after having stored sufficient urine and blood that Vincent can fool the system for years to come, the crippled Valid manages to ease himself into a blazing furnace to incinerate himself—life not being worth living any longer, not for one who cannot use his legs.

As for Vincent, and despite some tense moments, life is as good as it is ever going to get by the film's end: he has made love to Uma Thurman and he has faked his way (with the connivance of a sympathetic security officer) onto the mission to the really far-out planet of which he has dreamed since childhood, despite his genetically flawed condition. This is a bleak film. The only resistance Vincent can come up with is faking it. He has no language of protest and ethical distance available to him. This is just the world as he and others know it, and presumably will always know it. Thurman's intimacy with an Invalid is as close to resistance as she can get.[20] There are no alternative points of reference or resistance.

Of course, we are not in the *Gattaca* nightmare yet. But are we drawing uncomfortably close? There are those who believe so, including the mother of a Down syndrome child who wrote me after she had read one of my columns about genetic engineering in the *New Republic*. In that piece, I reflected on what our quest for bodily perfection might mean over the long run for the developmentally different. My interlocutor, whose child died of a critical illness in his third year, wrote me that she and her husband were enormously grateful to have had "the joyous privilege of parenting a child with Down syndrome. . . . Tommy's [not his real name] birth truly transformed our lives in ways that we will cherish forever. But how could we have known in advance that we indeed possessed the fortitude to parent a child with special needs? And who would have told us of the rich rewards?" She continued:

The function of prenatal tests, despite protestations to the contrary, is to provide parents the information necessary to assure that all pregnancies brought to term are "normal." I worry not only about the encouragement given to eliminating a "whole category of persons" (the point you make), but also about the prospects for respect and treatment of children who come to be brain-damaged either through unexpected birth traumas or later accidents. And what about the pressures to which parents like myself will be subject? How could you "choose" to burden society in this way?

In the name of expanding choice, we are narrowing our definition of humanity and, along the way, diminishing a felt responsibility to create welcoming environments for all children. Can we simply declare that they chose to have an "abnormal" child and now they must pay the consequences? This declaration, if it is generalized, takes us, as individuals and a society, off the hook for the purpose of social care and concern for all persons, including those with bodies and minds that are not supposedly normal. The trend I note here stitches together a cluster of views under the rubric of expanding choice, enhancing control, and extending freedom. The end result is a diminution of the sphere of the "unchosen" and an expansion of the reign of control. Rather than viewing children who are not considered normal in their development simply as a type of child who occurs from time to time among us, and who, in common with all children, makes a claim on our tenderest affections and most fundamental obligations, we see such children as beset by a "fixable" condition: there must be a cure. The cure, for the most part, is to gain sufficient knowledge (or at least to claim to have such knowledge) that one can predict the outcome of a pregnancy and move immediately to prevent a "wrongful" birth in the first place. The fact that "curing" Down syndrome means one eliminates entirely a type of human being is no barrier to this effort. People alive with Down syndrome must simply live with the knowledge that our culture's dominant view is that it would be better were no more of their "kind" to appear among us.

In a recent book, *The Future of the Disabled in Liberal Society: An Ethical Analysis*, philosopher Hans S. Reinders argues that, despite public policy efforts to ensure equal opportunity and access for all, liberal society (including our own) cannot sustain equal regard for persons with disabilities. This is especially true if the disabilities in question are "mental." The liberal presupposition that privileges choice as the primary category in public life and the apogee of human aspiration, paired with modern technologies of reproductive and genetic engineering, dictate that it would be far better if human persons who are incapable of choosing on the liberal model were not to appear among us.

So strong is the prejudice in this direction that we simply assume that hypothetical unborn children with cognitive disabilities would, if they could, choose not to be born. Reinders, a professor of ethics at the Vrije University in Amsterdam, argues that the regnant view among liberal philosophers is that human beings with mental retardation may be regarded as members of the human species, but they do not have full moral standing in the secular community. Because they lack such standing, the barriers to eliminating such persons will slowly but surely wither away. To be sure, given the religious derivation of so much of our ethical thinking, barriers to simply killing persons with disabilities remain. But such barriers, Reinders contends, are under continuous pressure from "secular morality" and are likely to be bulldozed out of the way by the potent machine of biotechnology backed up by medical authority. So it is not at all irrational for those with mental disabilities and their families to worry about the future. The proliferation of genetic testing, concludes Reinders, will most certainly have discriminatory effects because it puts everything under the domain of choice, and parents of children with "special needs" become guilty of irresponsible behavior in "choosing" to bear such children and burdening society in this way.[21]

Increasingly we as a society expect, and even insist, that parents must—for this is the direction choice takes at present—rid themselves of "wrongful life" in order to forestall "wrongful births" which will burden them and, even more important, the wider society. Women repeatedly tell stories of the pressure from their medical caregivers to abort should a sonogram show up something suspicious. The current abortion regime often embodies in practice a burden for women who are told that they alone have the power to choose whether or not to have a child and that they alone are expected to bear the consequences if they do not choose to do so. The growing conviction that children with disabilities ought never to be born and that prospective parents of such children ought always to abort undermines the felt skein of care and responsibility for all children.[22]

This is at least a reasonable worry, especially when the machinery of technology now surrounding childbirth turns every pregnancy into what was once labeled a "crisis pregnancy." HMOs are now standardizing prenatal testing and genetic screening procedures that were once called on only when couples had a history of difficulties. The point of all this is to initiate a process—should a sign even be hinted at—"of cajoling and pressuring that terminates in an abortion."[23] Jeannie Hannemann, a family life minister, "sees a culture shift taking place moving away from supporting families with special-needs children toward resenting such families as creating a 'burden' on society. [She] has heard of HMOs refusing treatment to special needs children, arguing their mental or physical problem represented a 'preexisting condition' because their parents elected not to abort them after prenatal screening indicated a problem."[24]

The heart of the matter lies in a loss of appreciation for the complex nature of human embodiment. The social imaginary—which the dominant scientific voices in the area of genetic engineering, technology, and "enhancement" shape—declares the body to be a construction, something we can invent. We are loath to grant the status of givenness to any aspect of ourselves, despite the fact that human babies are wriggling, complex, little bodies preprogrammed with all sorts of delicately calibrated reactions to the human relationships that "nature" presumes will be the matrix of child nurture. If we think of bodies concretely in this way, we are propelled to ask ourselves questions about the world little human bodies enter: is it welcoming, warm, responsive? But if we tilt in the biotech constructivist direction, one in which the body is so much raw material to be worked upon and worked over, the surroundings in which bodies are situated fades as the body gets enshrined as a kind of messianic project.

In this latter scenario, the body we currently inhabit becomes the imperfect body subject to chance and the vagaries of life, including illness and aging. This body is our foe. The future perfect body extolled in manifestos, promised by enthusiasts, embraced by many ordinary citizens is a gleaming fabrication. For soon, we are promised, we will have found a way around the fact that what our forebears took for granted—that the body must weaken and falter, and one day pass from life to death—will soon be a relic of a bygone era. The future perfect body will not be permitted to falter. Yes, the body may grow older in a strictly chronological sense, but why should we age? So we devise multiple strategies to fend off aging even as we represent aging bodies as those of teenagers with gleaming gray hair. A recent *New York Times Magazine* lead article on "The Recycled Generation" extolled the "promise of an infinite supply of replaceable body parts" via stem cell research, although that research is now "bogged down in abortion politics and corporate rivalries." One of the entrepreneurs, who stands to make millions of dollars in what the article calls the "scientific chase" for "the mother of all cells—the embryonic stem cell," bemoans the fact that the rush forward is being slowed down by a terrible problem—namely, the "knee jerk reaction" on the part of many people to "words like 'fetal' and 'embryo.' "[25]

The image that came bounding out of the piece is that genetic innovators who face opposition from religious and superstitious people, who go "completely irrational" when they hear certain words, fearlessly forge forth in the teeth of sustained opposition—thus reversing the actual situation in which critics are compelled to fight a rearguard battle against a powerful, monied, and influential set of cultural forces who, in line with the story our culture likes to tell about itself, represent progress and a better future.[26] The upshot is that rather than approaching matters of life, death, and health with humility, knowing that we cannot cure the human condition, we seek cures based on the assumption that the more we control, the better. As I completed a final revision of this chapter, word came that a human embryo had been cloned. Television commentary resounded with the promise that this will make possible, in the future, an endless supply of body parts that can be harvested to indefinitely prolong human life. Hence, even before a grown clone appears— and let us pray this does not happen—the clone is reduced to property to be harvested for the benefit of others.

The underlying presupposition is, of course, that nothing is good in itself, including embodied existence. It therefore becomes easier to be rather casual about devising and implementing strategies aimed at selective weeding out or destruction of the bodies of those considered imperfect or abnormal, or even the bodies of the "perfect" if that human entity is cloned. Questions about whether the path we are racing down might not turn old age itself into a pathology and at some point usher in a cultural "encouragement" for the "unproductive" elderly to permit themselves to be euthanized because they are extra mouths to feed and a nuisance to just about everybody are cast as part of a sci-fi dystopian mentality.

It is difficult to overstate just how widely accepted the technocratic view is and how overwhelmingly we, as a culture, are acquiescing to its premises. In a review in the *Times Literary Supplement* of four new books on the genetic revolution, the reviewer matter-of-factly opined that "we must inevitably start to choose our descendants," adding that we do this now in "permitting or preventing the birth of our own children according to their medical prognosis, thus selecting the lives to come." So long as society does not cramp our freedom of action, we will stay on the road of progress and exercise sovereign choice over birth by consigning to death those with a less-than-stellar potential for a life not "marred by an excess of pain or disability."[27] Molecular biologist Robert Sinsheimer calls for a "new eugenics," a phrase most try to avoid given its association with the biopolitical ideology of mid-twentieth-century National Socialism. As Sinsheimer writes, "The new eugenics would permit in principle the conversion of all the unfit to the highest genetic level."[28] With the widespread adoption of prenatal screening, now regarded as routine, so much so that prospective parents who decline this panoply of procedures are treated as irresponsible, we see at work the presumption that life should be wiped clean of any and all imperfection, inconvenience, and risk. Creation itself must be put right.

The *New York Times* alerted us to this fact on December 2, 1997, in an article titled "On Cloning Humans, 'Never' Turns Swiftly into 'Why Not'" by science editor Gina Kolata.[29] Kolata points out that in the immediate aftermath of Dolly the cloned sheep who stared out at us from the covers of so many newspapers and magazines, there was much consternation and rumbling.[30] But opposition dissipated quickly, she continues, with fertility centers soon conducting "experiments with human eggs that lay the groundwork for cloning. Moreover, the Federal Government is supporting new research on the cloning of monkeys, encouraging scientists to perfect techniques that could easily be transferred to humans." A presidential ethics commission may have recommended a "limited ban on cloning humans," but after all, argues Kolata, "it is an American tradition to allow people the freedom to reproduce in any way they like." This claim is simply false in terms of both the historical and the legal record. In common with any society of which we have any knowledge, past or present, U.S. society has built into its interstices a variety of limitations on so-called reproductive freedom. But the view that freedom means doing things in "any way one likes" now prevails as a cultural desideratum.[31] It is, therefore, unsurprising that the *New York Times* describes a "slow acceptance" of the idea of cloning in the scientific community that took just six months to go from shock and queasiness to acquiescence and widespread approval. The article concludes that "some experts said the real question was not whether cloning is ethical but whether it is legal." And one doctor is quoted in the piece: "The fact is that, in America, cloning may be bad but telling people how they should reproduce is worse. . . . In the end . . . America is not ruled by ethics. It is ruled by law." The implication of this view is that no ethical norm, standard, commitment, or insight can or should be brought to bear on whether to criticize, caution against, or checkmate statutory laws should they be unjust or unwise. The point is that with each new development that is presented to us in the name of a radical and benign extension of human freedom and powers, we pave additional miles on the fast track toward the eradication of any real integrity to the category of *the human.* Debate and discourse about such matters in the public square has turned into a routine in which a few religious spokespeople are brought on board to fret a bit and everything marches on.[32]

That the prospect of human cloning is fueled by narcissistic fantasies of radical sameness, that it represents fear of the different and the unpredictable, and that it speaks to a yearning for a world of guaranteed self-replication, matters not; indeed, such concerns are rarely named, save by those speaking from the point of view of theological anthropology. As the Pontifical Academy noted in a statement on human cloning issued June 25, 1997,

Human cloning belongs to the eugenics project and is thus subject to all the ethical and juridical observations that have amply condemned it. As Hans Jonas has already written, it is "both in method the most despotic and in aim the most slavish form of genetic manipulation; its objective is not an arbitrary modification of the hereditary material but precisely its equally arbitrary fixation in contrast to the dominant strategy of nature."[33]

Dreams of strong, wholesale self-possession grounded in attaining full control over human "reproductive material" lie at the heart of the eugenics project, despite the risk of damaging biogenetic uniformity, since much of the basic genetic information that goes into the creation of a child from two parents emerges as a result of sexual reproduction, something not replicable by definition when you pick one parent to clone. This latter is evidently a small price to pay.

What, then, about embarking on an experimental course that would likely result in flawed "products"?[34] It is convenient to forget that it took nearly three hundred failed attempts before Dolly the sheep was cloned successfully. As Leon Kass has noted, the image of failed human clones leads the soul to shudder. Abandoning what Kass terms "the wisdom of repugnance," we embark on a path that constitutes a violation of a very fundamental sort. Kass calls on us to pay close attention to what we find "offensive," "repulsive," or "distasteful," for such reactions often point to deeper realities. He writes that "in this age in which everything is held to be permissible so long as it is freely done, in which our given human nature no longer commands respect, in which our bodies are regarded as mere instruments of our autonomous rational wills, repugnance may be the only voice left that speaks up to defend the central core of our humanity. Shallow are the souls that have forgotten how to shudder."[35] Kass is arguing that repugnance is not the end of the matter but instead a beginning. Those philosophies that see in such reactions only the churnings of irrational emotion, misunderstand the nature of human emotions. Our emotional reactions are complex, laced through and through with thought. The point is to bring forward such reactions and submit them to thought.

Would we really want to live in a world in which the sight of anonymous corpses piled up elicited no strong revulsion, or a world in which the sight of a human being's body pierced through and through in dozens of places and riddled with pieces of metal was something we simply took for granted? The reaction to the first clearly gestures toward powerful condemnation of those responsible for creating those mountains of corpses, and anguish and pity for the tortured and murdered and their families. In the case of the heavy-metal-pierced person, we may decide it is a matter of little import and yet ask ourselves why mutilation of the body that goes much beyond the decorative is now so popular? Does this tell us anything about how we think about our bodies?[36] And so on.

Kass points out that the "technical, liberal, and meliorist approaches all ignore the deeper anthropological, social and, indeed, ontological meanings of bringing forth new life. To this more fitting and profound point of view, cloning shows itself to be a major alteration, indeed, a major violation, of our given nature as embodied, gendered and engendering beings—and of the social relations built on this natural ground." The upshot is that critical interpreters cede the ground too readily to those who want to move full steam ahead when, in fact, it should work the other way around. "The burden of moral argument," observes Kass, "must fall entirely on those who want to declare the widespread repugnances of humankind to be mere timidity or superstition."[37] Too many theologians, philosophers, and cultural critics have become reticent about defending insights drawn from the riches of the Western tradition.

As a result, Kass argues, we do the following things: we enter a world in which unethical experiments "upon the resulting child-to-be" are conducted; we deprive a cloned entity of a "distinctive identity not only because he will be in genotype and appearance identical to another human being, but, in this case, because he may also be twin to the person who is his 'father' or 'mother'—if one can still call them that"; we deliberately plan situations that we know—the empirical evidence is incontrovertible—are not optimal arenas for the rearing of children—namely, family fragments that deny relationality or shrink it; and we "enshrine and aggravate a profound and mischievous misunderstanding of the meaning of having children and of the parent-child relationship. . . . The child is given a genotype that has already lived. . . . Cloning is inherently despotic, for it seeks to make one's children . . . after one's own image . . . and their future according to one's will."[38] The many warnings embedded in the Western tradition, from its antique forms (pre-Christian) to Judaism and Christianity, seem now to lack the power to stay the hand of a "scientized" anthropocentrism that distorts the meaning of human freedom.[39]

Within the Hebrew and Christian traditions, a burden borne by human beings after the fall lies in discerning what is natural or given, presuming that what is encoded into the very nature of things affords a standard, accessible to human reason, by which we can assess critically the claims and forces at work in our cultural time and place. (This isn't the only available standard, of course, but it was long believed an important feature of a whole complex of views.) The great moral teachers, until relatively recently, believed that "nature" and "the natural" served as standards. Within Christian theological anthropology, human beings are corporeal beings—ensouled bodies—made in the image of their Creator.

According to Pope John Paul II, this account of our natures, including the ontological equality of male and female as corporeal beings, is "free from any trace whatsoever of subjectivism. It contains only the objective facts and defines the objective reality, both when it speaks of man's creation, male and female, in the image of God, and when it adds a little later the words of the first blessing: 'Be fruitful and multiply and fill the earth; subdue it and have dominion over it'" (Gen 1:28).[40] Dominion here—it is clear from the overall exegesis—is understood as a form of stewardship, not domination. John Paul's account of Genesis is presaged in Karol Wojtyla's prepapal writings. For example, in a series of spiritual exercises presented to Pope Paul VI, the papal household, and the cardinals and bishops of the Roman Curia during a Lenten retreat in March 1976, the then cardinal Karol Wojtyla argued that "one cannot understand either Sartre or Marx without having first read and pondered very deeply the first three chapters of Genesis. These are the key to understanding the world of today, both its roots and its extremely radical— and therefore dramatic—affirmations and denials." Teaching about human origins, human beginnings, in this way offers "an articulation of the way things are by virtue of the relation they have with their creator."[41] Denying that relationship, we too easily fall into subjectivism, into a world of rootless wills.

With this Bonhoeffer would agree. In his discussion of "The Natural" in the *Ethics*, Bonhoeffer observes that the natural fell out of favor in Protestant ethics and became the almost exclusive preserve of Catholic thought. He aimed to resurrect the natural, insisting that human beings still have access to the natural, but only "on the basis of the gospel."[42] In his move to redeem the concept of the natural, Bonhoeffer argues that human beings enjoy a "relative freedom" in natural life. But there are "true and . . . mistaken uses of this freedom," and these mark "the difference between the natural and the unnatural." It follows that the "destruction of the natural means destruction of life. . . . The unnatural is the enemy of life."

It violates our natures to approach life from a false "vitalism" or excessive idealism, on the one hand, or on the other, from an equally false "mechanization" and lassitude that shows "despair towards natural life" and manifests "a certain hostility to life, tiredness of life and incapacity for life." Our right to bodily life is a natural, not an invented, right and the basis of all other rights, given that Christians repudiate the view that the body is simply a prison for the immortal soul. Harming the body harms the self at its depth. "Bodilyness and human life belong inseparably together," in Bonhoeffer's words. Our bodies are ends in themselves. This has "very far-reaching consequences for the Christian appraisal of all the problems that have to do with the life of the body, housing, food, clothing, recreation, play and sex." We can use our bodies and the bodies of others well or ill.

The most striking and radical excision of the integrity and right of natural life is "arbitrary killing," the deliberate destruction of "innocent life." Here, Bonhoeffer mentions examples such as abortion, killing defenseless prisoners or wounded soldiers, and destroying lives we do not find worth living—a clear reference to Nazi euthanasia and genocidal policies toward the ill, the infirm, and all persons with handicaps.[43] As Bonhoeffer puts it, "The right to live is a matter of the essence" and not of any socially imposed or constructed values. Even "the most wretched life" is "worth living before God." Other violations of the liberty of the body include physical torture, arbitrary seizure, enslavement (American slavery is here referenced), deportations, separation of persons from home and family—the full panoply of horrors that the twentieth century, in particular, has dished up in superabundance. The fragment by Bonhoeffer on the natural is powerfully suggestive and worth pondering as an alternative to those cultural dictates that declare any appeal to nature or the natural as a standard illegitimate. It goes without saying that much more work would need to be done in order to redeem the categories of nature and the natural, but I here simply want to note that our present circumstances resist this conceptual and ethical possibility even as the need for some such standard becomes ever-more exigent. We need powerful and coherent categories and analyses that challenge cultural projects that deny finitude, promise a technocratic agenda that ushers in almost total human control over all of the natural world including those natures we call human, push toward an ideal of sameness through genetic manipulation and self-replication via cloning, and continue with the process of excision of bodies deemed unworthy to appear among us and share our world.[44] Perfection requires manipulation and elimination: there is a kind of purificationist imperative at work here as we aim to weed out the flawed, and recognize only the perfect and the fit. Wrapped up in a quest for control, immersed in the images and rhetoric of choice and self-possession, we will find it more and more difficult to ask the right sorts of questions as we will slowly but surely lose the rich languages of opposition, like that embodied in Christian theological anthropology.

Notes

1. This chapter draws on my book, *Who Are We?* as well as an essay written as a participant in a three-year study group headed by Professor William Schweiker of the University of Chicago Divinity School on "Property and Possession."

2. The United States is clearly my focus, although much, if not all, of what I say is applicable to the developed or, in John Paul II's terms, the "superdeveloped cultures of consumption" of the West.

3. Abortion on demand at any stage of pregnancy and the death penalty would be the two prime candidates here. This chapter's length is such that I will not be able to discuss these in full.

4. Dietrich Bonhoeffer, *Creation and Fall: A Theological Exposition of Genesis 1–3* (Minneapolis: Fortress Press, 1997).

5. This is not the time and the place to unpack ethical naturalism and moral realism. Suffice it to say that I am committed to the view that there is a "there there," that there are truths to be discerned about the world, and that the world isn't just so much putty in our conceptually deft hands. The world exists independent of our minds, but our minds possess the wonderful capacity to apprehend the world—up to a point, given the fallibility of reason.

6. One example would be the work of philosopher Judith Jarvis Thompson, known for her current support of physician-assisted suicide, but who first made her reputation by providing justifications for abortion by analogizing from a woman hooked up during her sleep to a violinist for whom she was then required to provide life support, to a woman in relationship to the fetus she is carrying. Thompson claimed that the woman would be within her rights to unhook the violinist, even if it meant the violinist's death; similarly, a woman is not required to carry a fetus to term. I have never understood why a reasonable person would find this argument compelling. Fetuses do not get attached covertly but emerge as a result of action in which the woman is implicated. As well, the fetus's dependence on the mother for sustenance for nine months is part of the order of nature—it simply is the way humans reproduce. There are many ways to sustain violinists in need of life support, and an adult violinist is scarcely analogous in any way to the life of a human being in situ.

7. Robin Lovin, *Niebuhr and Christian Realism* (Cambridge: Cambridge University Press, 1995), 123.

8. Ibid., 126.

9. Ibid., 94.

10. Ibid., 130.

11. This, too, is more complex than simple acquiescence. For example, where the matter of abortion is concerned, there is enormous popular support for some forms of restriction and restraint on the practice. The elite culture (the media, those with incomes over $50,000 per year, and lawyers, as the most reliable social science studies demonstrate) long ago fell in lockstep with an absolute abortion "right," including partial birth abortion, a practice that the American Medical Association itself has declared not to be a legitimate medical procedure. So on the level of opinion all is not homogeneous. But this opinion rarely translates into action of any sort. Thus, the atrophy of civic habits of the past four decades or so goes hand in hand with the triumph of projects that constitute flights from finitude.

12. Not ours alone, of course, but I will concentrate primarily on North American culture in depicting this obsession and grappling with its hold on the collective psyche.

13. Just to be clear at the outset, I do not intend to issue strictures against any and all attempts to intervene through modern forms of gene therapy in order to forestall, say, the development of devastating, inherited conditions or diseases. There is a huge difference between preventing an undeniable harm—say, a type of inherited condition that dooms a child to a short and painful life—and striving to create a blemishless, perfect human specimen. How one differentiates the one from the other is part of the burden of argument. One example of justifiable intervention would be a method of gene therapy that spares children "the devastating effects of a rare but deadly inherited disease. In the condition, Crigler-Najjar syndrome, a substance called bilirubin, a waste product from the destruction of worn-out red blood cells, builds up in the body. . . . Bilirubin accumulates, causing jaundice, a yellowing of the skin and the whites of the eyes. More important, bilirubin is toxic to the nervous system, and the children live in constant danger of brain damage. The only way they can survive is to spend 10 to 12 hours a day under special lights that break down the bilirubin. But as they reach their teens, the light therapy becomes less effective. Unless they can get a liver transplant, they may suffer brain damage or die" (Denise Grady, "At Gene Therapy's Frontier, the Amish Build a Clinic," *New York Times*, June 29, 1999, D1, D4). Because previous attempts at gene therapy have all fallen far short of expectations, none of this may work. But it would spare a small number of children tremendous suffering, and this sort of intervention is entirely defensive—it involves no eugenics ideology of any kind.

14. Walter Gilbert, cited in Roger Shattuck, *Forbidden Knowledge* (New York: Harcourt, Brace, 1996), 178.

15. As reprinted in an editorial in *Commonweal*, March 26, 1999, 5.

16. Ibid.

17. Doris T. Zallen, "We Need a Moratorium on 'Genetic Enhancement,'" *Chronicle of Higher Education*, March 27, 1998, A64.

18. James LeFanu, "Geneticists Are Not Gods," *Tablet*, December 12, 1998, 1645–1646.

19. Ibid.

20. A bit reminiscent of Julia, the young female sexual revolutionary, in George Orwell's 1984. She is, of course, defeated and comes to love Big Brother.

21. Hans S. Reinders, *The Future of the Disabled in Liberal Society: An Ethical Analysis* (Notre Dame, IN: University of Notre Dame Press, 2000).

22. Please note that I do not want in any way to diminish the difficulties involved in parenting a child with disabilities. As the mother of an adult daughter with mental retardation, I understand this very well. Instead, I am trying to capture the present temperament that dictates that such births are calamitous and ought never to occur.

23. "Search and Destroy Missions," *U.S. Catholic Conference*, January 2000, 16.

24. Jeannie Hannemann, cited in ibid.

25. Stephen S. Hall, "The Recycled Generation," *New York Times Magazine*, January 30, 2000, 32.

26. Ibid.

27. But who defines excess? This is a squishy, soft criterion that comes into play at present for such "abnormalities" as a cleft palate.

28. Robert Sinsheimer, quoted from the *Journal of Engineering and Science*, in Shattuck, *Forbidden Knowledge*, 193–194. The literature of reportage, enthusiasm, concern, and so forth is nearly out of control. A few magazine and newspaper pieces worth reading include: Jim Yardley, "Investigators Say Embryologist Knew He Erred in Egg Mix-Up," *New York Times*, April 17, 1999, A13; Martin Lupton, "Test-Tube Questions," *Tablet*, February 20, 1999, 259–260; David L. Marcus, "Mothers with Another's Eggs," *U.S. News and World Report*, April 13, 1999, 42–44; Nicholas Wade, "Panel Told of Vast Benefits of Embryo Cells," *New York Times*, December 3, 1998, A24; Anne Taylor Fleming, "Why I Can't Use Someone Else's Eggs," *Newsweek*, April 12, 1999, 12; Nicholas Wade, "Gene Study Bolsters Hope for Treating Diseases of Aging," *New York Times*, March 5, 1999, A12; and Lisa Belkin, "Splice Einstein and Sammy Glick, Add a Little Magellan," *New York Times Magazine*, August 23, 1998, 26–31, 56–61. For a chilling piece that shows the many ways in which geno-enthusiasm and commodification fuse, see Stephanie Armour, "Could Your Genes Hold You Back?" *USA Today*, May 5, 1999, B1–B2. An example of how the bizarre becomes commonplace is Gina Kolata, "Scientists Place Jellyfish Genes into Monkeys," *New York Times*, December 23, 1999, 1–20. We have normalized the preposterous and do not even ask, Why on earth would anyone do that— put jellyfish genes into monkeys?

29. The article begins on page 1 and continues on A17 of the *Times* for that day.

30. This foreboding also comes through in Bryan Appleyard, *Brave New Worlds: Staying Human in the Genetic Future* (New York: Viking, 1998).

31. I cannot here deal with the commercialization of genetics, but alas, the huge profits to be made drive much of the scientific and technological work. See, for example, Belkin, "Splice Einstein and Sammy Glick," 26–31.

32. Think, by the way, of what this would have done to Martin Luther King's protest: simply stopped it dead in its tracks. For the law of the Jim Crow South was the law of segregation. And no ethical argument can challenge the law. End of story. A comeback would be that you need to make a legal argument to change the law. But King's call for legal change was an ethical one. The reductive assertion that law and ethics must never touch is a crude form of legal positivism or command-obedience legal theory. What is right doesn't enter into the picture at all.

33. Pontifical Academy for Life, "Reflections on Cloning," *Origins* 28, no. 1 (May 21, 1998): 14–16. The popular press has been filled with cloning articles. A few include: Sheryl WuDunn, "South Korean Scientists Say They Cloned a Human Cell," *New York Times*, December 17, 1998, A12; Nicholas Wade, "Researchers Join in Effort on Cloning Repair Tissue," *New York Times*, May 5, 1999, A19; and Tim Friend, "Merger Could Clone Bio-Companies 'Creativity,'" *USA Today*, May 5, 1999, 13A. See also Lori B. Andrews, *The Clone Age: Adventures in the New World of Reproductive Technology* (New York: Henry Holt, 1999).

34. But we have a solution to that one, too, don't we? We can be certain that the creatures nobody wants, whose lives are not "worth living," can be easily dispatched to spare their suffering. Physician-assisted suicide, the track down which we are moving, is, of course, part and parcel of the general tendencies I here discuss and criticize. Although I do not focus specifically on this matter, I recommend the following two essays for the general reader: Paul R. McHugh, "The Kevorkian Epidemic," *American Scholar* (Winter 1997): 15–27; and Leon R. Kass and Nelson Lund, "Courting Death: Assisted Suicide, Doctors, and the Law," *Commentary* (December 1996): 17–29, See also the late Cardinal Bernardin's "Letter to the Supreme Court," which was appended to a friend-of-the-court brief filed by the Catholic Health Association in a U.S. Supreme Court case testing the appeals of two lower court decisions that struck down laws prohibiting assisted suicide in the states of Washington and New York; and a brief by the U.S. Catholic Conference, "Assisted Suicide Issue Moves to Supreme Court," *Origins* 26, no. 26 (December 12, 1996): 421–430.

35. Leon R. Kass, "The Wisdom of Repugnance," *New Republic*, June 2, 1997, 20.

36. There is a big discussion here yearning to breathe free, of course—namely, the connection between beauty and truth. But it is one I cannot even begin to enter into at this point. The truth is often described as splendid and beautiful—Augustine's language—and God as beautiful in and through God's simplicity. The aesthetic dimension in theology, and most certainly in ethics, is underexplored.

37. Kass, "The Wisdom of Repugnance," 20, 21.

38. Ibid., 22–24.

39. See Roger Shattuck's wonderful discussion of Faust and Frankenstein in *Forbidden Knowledge*.

40. John Paul II, *Original Unity of Man and Woman: Catechesis on the Book of Genesis* (Boston: Daughters of St. Paul, 1981), 23.

41. Karol Wojtyla, *Sign of Contradiction* (New York: Seabury, 1979), 24, 124.

42. This discussion in Dietrich Bonhoeffer's *Ethics* (New York: Macmillan Company, 1965) appears on pages 143–186, and all quoted matter is drawn from those pages inclusively.

43. This is an area that deserves more treatment than I can give it here. Fortunately, and at long last, there are texts in English on Nazi euthanasia as part of its general biopolitics. Of especial note is Michael Burleigh, *Death and Deliverance* (Cambridge: Cambridge University Press, 1994). This is a tremendously disquieting book for a contemporary U.S. reader. So much of the language of our own genetic engineering and "assisted suicide" proponents echoes National Socialist propaganda. The Nazis covered the waterfront, so to speak, justifying their programs of systematic selective elimination of the "unfit," of life unworthy of life (congenitally "diseased," handicapped, and so forth) on a number of interrelated grounds, including cost-benefit criteria, perfecting the race, and compassion. The Nazis also controlled the media on this issue (it goes without saying), producing short propaganda films and full-length features, lavishly produced and starring German matinee idols, to promote their euthanasia efforts.

44. In a longer work, the death penalty would come under critical scrutiny here as an act of such radical excision.

7

Visions and Re-visions: Life and the Accident of Birth

Richard M. Zaner

In the late 1950s, the great English sci-fi writer James Blish wrote a charming little novel suggestively titled *The Seedling Stars and Galactic Cluster*.[1] It had a simple premise, as inventive as it was remarkable for its prescience. Habitable planets for human beings had become premium, for straightforward reasons. Interstellar travel had become routine even as the population had long since burgeoned beyond Earth's and other planets' resources. Most of the planets that were discovered, however, turned out to be fiercely uninhabitable. Making them habitable required immensely complicated, expensive, and only rarely effective labor, by means of a process Blish called "terra-forming." To make a place human-friendly, in these terms, required either transforming that environment and its atmosphere, or protecting people from its hazards by special shelters, breathing apparatuses, and the like.

The science of biology, Blish also postulated, had undergone a sweeping revolution—the beginnings of which were already apparent when his novel appeared, and, as we have since become acutely aware, it is a revolution matching if not surpassing the earlier one in physics. In the novel, biological manipulations are routinely developed and designed for population projects using the most elementary reproductive life processes, including cloning and other types of genetic engineering.

Blish's tale is delightful. In his imaginative hands, the deliberate, literal redesigning of human individuals by other human individuals is an accomplished fact. Changes are brought about that need neither centuries of evolutionary change nor spontaneous mutation, only the ingenuity and sportive inventiveness of highly powerful biomedical scientists possessing "the secret of life," now avidly in pursuit of ever-new ways to design people. Much of the same aim was overtly advocated in the

1960s by Joshua Lederberg, a Nobel laureate in genetics, and in the late 1970s by two Nobel laureates, John Eccles and Macfarlane Burnett, and first became a reality for complex animal vertebrates in the 1990s' work of Ian Wilmut and his colleagues at the Roslyn Institute in Scotland.[2] What Blish only imagined has now begun to be more than a mere promissory note.

More recently, another Nobel Prize winner in genetics, Walter Gilbert, expressly, if with some hyperbole, portrays just that underlying vision as the "holy grail" of our times. The secret foundations of human life (in the multiple shapes proteins can take) seem now to have come close within sight. The unraveling, mapping, and sequencing of the human genome being accomplished in countless projects around the world, Gilbert avers, promises to "put together a sequence that represents . . . the underlying human structure . . . our common humanity." Soon, he is convinced, we'll be able "to pull a CD out of one's pocket and say, 'Here is a human being; it's me'!"[3]

The response to the ultimate questions of human life will thus be that it is either the genes or in the genes, and that it will not be found in the quaint metaphysical quests that moved Plato or Aristotle, Saint Thomas Aquinas or William of Ockham, Immanuel Kant or Martin Heidegger. Something like a full circle will then be reached, for at the time of DNA's discovery—what a 1961 *Life* magazine cover declared as the "secret of life," and what Kurt Vonnegut satirized in his classic first novel, *Cat's Cradle*—it was thought that the new genetics was indeed the holy grail of science and society.[4] The human genome is thus regarded as the secret hiding place of the self, indeed of life itself—a notion already somewhat passé perhaps as there is now talk of digitizing the entire genome onto ever-tinier chips that can be embedded in any cell, a sort of postmodern covert mole always on call and ready to be pulled out, read, and possibly cloned.

This motif is historically fascinating as well, for it is of a piece with one of the core convictions in medicine's long history, as articulated in one or both of two fundamental visions. Ancient physicians were struck by the ways in which the human body and soul could be changed by either medicines or, more likely, dietary regimens. Galen went so far as to assert the need to "clear the path for using bodily factors to elevate man beyond the possibilities of purely moral teaching."[5] Galen's concern, then, was as much to improve the human condition as it was to treat diseases—and in this regard was closer to Blish's biologists in his vision. Contrary to this, however, reports from the Human Genome Project mainly highlight the therapeutic potential of new discoveries while almost always downplaying the eugenic designs that fascinated both the ancients and much of science fiction.

His colorful portrait aside, Gilbert is hardly alone in his emphasis on the visionary theme of genetic research. Other distinguished geneticists— as mentioned above, Lederberg, Eccles, and Burnett, among others— have long articulated portions of that vision. Nevertheless, despite the hype and repeated promises of therapy that are invariably part of the frequent announcements about new genetic discoveries, anyone seriously considering these and related issues is well-advised to bear prominently in mind a "haunting memory—that most of the world still consists of things and creatures that neither scientists nor social theorists had any hand in making."[6] There is also the apparent need to be reminded of the not especially agreeable record of so many technological projects—one need not go much beyond that of nuclear power to fuel our modern age's incessant appetite for the always more and ever new, while pretty much ignoring and evading essential questions such as the disposal of the inevitable toxic wastes. And then there is the uneasiness we feel when attending carefully to the record of disasters and abuses that is so much a part of the history of biomedical research—the radiation experiments first publicly disclosed by Congressman Edward J. Markey (D-MA) in 1986, the syphilis experiments at Tuskegee, or the many questionable experiments highlighted by Henry Beecher and others.[7] How can we make sense of this? An indirection will be useful here.

Mendel's Dwarf

In Simon Mawer's engaging novel *Mendel's Dwarf*, the principal character is Benedict Lambert, who is a world-renowned geneticist, the great-great-great-nephew of Gregor Mendel, and a dwarf (achondroplasia).[8] Whether as a professional delivering a scientific lecture, a student sitting in a college class, or simply a citizen walking the streets of a city, Ben is made acutely aware of himself by those "phenotypically normal" people who invariably gawk at him, no matter where he happens to be.

At the start of the novel, Ben accepts a crescendo of applause after his much-anticipated lecture at the Masaryk University of Brno, where he was invited by the Mendel Society to celebrate the life and work of his great-great-great-uncle, Gregor. Ben is then greeted by the society's secretary, a "large and quivering mountain of concerned flesh," who says, "Gee, Ben, that's wonderful. So brave, so brave." At this, Ben thinks to himself, "Brave. That was the word of the moment. But I'd told Jean [his ladylove] often enough. In order to be brave, you've got to have a choice."9 Of course, choice about his dwarfism was what he never had. Rather, like the rest of us, he had only that "tyranny of chance" when just one of the countless spermatozoa from his father's erupting orgasm found (or was subtly and successfully attracted to) and penetrated his mother's ovum and, shedding its tail, managed to impregnate and fertilize—those magic moments of entrance, penetrance, implantation, and conception thanks to which a specific child, Ben, is conceived, borne by his mother, and later born into the world. After Ben suffers a typical round of teasing from his classmates ("Mendel, Mendel, Mendel's dwarf") the headmaster of his elementary school remarks that "it's a problem you have to live with," Ben objects silently to himself that achondroplasia is not like premature baldness, a birthmark, or a stutter, "it is me. There is no other."10

At another point, after he declares his love for Dinah—the first girl he ever kissed (or rather, "*she* kissed *me!*")—and helps her get through a genetics class—she dismisses him with a "thanks everso" and a final "it can't be." His response is harsh: "I'll say it for you: you can't love me because I'm hideous and deformed, a freak of nature, and people would stare. . . . You can say this: 'I would love you if you weren't a shrunken monster.' "11

Indeed, after a highly successful career in human genetics, Ben had been invited to be the Mendel Society's honored speaker at the Brno conference not because of his kinship with Mendel but rather because he had identified the achondroplasia gene—the very gene whose flawed working (or whose correct working with an incorrectly "spelled" gene) resulted in the dwarf, Ben. When Ben's results were first made public, the media took a shine to him, and a major newspaper reported on the discovery with the headline: "Dwarf Biologist Discovers Himself." His sister telephoned him to tell him about it, reading the text of the report to him: "Super geneticist Ben Lambert has finished his search of a life-time. Genetic engineering techniques and years of patience have finally led him to discover the gene that has ruled his own existence, for Ben, thirty-eight and a researcher at one of the world's leading genetics labo-ratories, is . . . a dwarf. Little in body but big in spirit."[12]

It is clearly awkward at best to contemplate Ben's condition from the perspective of medicine, with its traditional emphasis on restoring body functions and organic processes lost or compromised by illness or injury. In the first place, though severely compromised by being a dwarf, he isn't sick in any conventional sense operative in this tradition. Even while shunned in multiple ways by other people, he is also a genius—and in this respect, he enjoys a privileged place and the admiration of other people and colleagues, especially among those in restorative med-icine.[13] Despite that, as a dwarf he is *beyond* the limits of restorative medicine, *outside* its purview, unless he is sick in a conventional sense (flu, pneumonia, cancer, and so on). If the dwarf is outside the conven-tional and the customary, and if clinical, restorative medicine can do nothing for his condition as a dwarf, what exactly *is* he in conventional terms?

As he knows intimately, being outside the usual and the routine means that he is phenotypically *ab*normal—despite his condition having resulted from the tyranny of chance of disfiguring achondroplasia (though of course, we are all configured, if not abnormal and disfigured, by chance's tyranny). He may be "hideous and deformed, a freak of nature . . . a shrunken monster," but he is neither "sick" nor "injured." In this sense, geeks and freaks, dwarfs and hybrids, and other genetically or congenitally disabled individuals are socially constructed by pheno-typic normals as beyond repair, and thus fit mainly for carnivals and backstreet sideshows. Medicine's restorative approach to illness and injury cannot bring such freaks and hybrids back even approximately to accepted social norms. A dwarf may be puckish, an imp, or a good fellow, while another may be a rogue and a cad, but all of them are beyond the social limits due to the tyranny of chance of their births and how the others construe that.[14]

As I noted, Ben *can* be restoratively treated: if he gets the flu, renal disease, cancer, or any of the many illnesses that can afflict any human being, for the most part just like any of us normals. But when he is not conventionally ill, the reasonable and even required thing for the restorative physician to do about Ben is to stand back from him, trying (most often unsuccessfully, as Ben learns) not to judge his condition as abnormal—precisely his normal condition.

Yet if you were to ask him, Ben certainly does try, at times desperately, to be like others—if only he could do that. Faced with Ben in whatever situation, restorative physicians must surely sense his plight and, given this, would surely wish it were otherwise. The point is obvious when Ben talks with Dinah, or later with Jean. His body is seen as lacking—by others and thus by him. Hence, *he* is lacking, Ben is less than he should be, and this targets him as the object of gawks, the butt of jokes, a creature of side-glances and sly pranks, ridiculed, ignored, abandoned, bypassed, looked-over, mocked.

But Ben would have it otherwise. In fact, this becomes evident when, as an expert in embryo transfer and in vitro fertilization, he agrees to perform the procedure for Jean using his own sperm—and suffers the choices with which he is then confronted. As his training in genetics makes clear as well, however, this signal event in the novel finds him—and us, the readers—at a very different place than we might have expected. For now, even embryo transfer and in vitro fertilization is transformed when it is in the hands of a geneticist accomplished in the arcane arts of recombinant DNA techniques—and the sperm donor for the process. Now, truly awesome issues, previously only barely beneath the surface, explode onto the scene. More on this in a moment; for now, other aspects of the phenomenon need to be probed.

The "Scandal" in Medicine's "New Paradigm"

Most of us sense the frustration of being unable to do anything to change things for Ben. We sense as well the injustice in our social values that work so powerfully and severely to circumscribe his life. And there is a cutting irony: Ben is himself a renowned geneticist, the descendant of Mendel—also a geneticist—and Ben has succeeded in identifying the "dwarf gene." Indeed, using rDNA techniques, Ben is even capable of splicing the achondroplasia gene out of or into his and Jean's resulting embryo—or, as happens in the novel, of choosing to implant an affected or unaffected embryo into Jean's uterus.

Ben also knows the sharp edges of the new genetics. After delivering his speech to the Mendel Society, he meanders through the tiny village where his great-great-great-uncle had worked and reflects, "This acre of space was where it all started, where the stubborn friar lit a fuse that burned unnoticed for thirty-five years until they discovered his work in 1900 and the bomb finally exploded. The explosion is going on still. It engulfed me from the moment of my conception. Perhaps it will engulf us all eventually."[15]

Although a science of genetics could not truly get going until Mendel's work had been discovered and understood, this has now been done; reality has swiftly caught up with Blish's and Mawer's imaginative skills. The human genome has been almost completely mapped and sequenced, and, although understanding lags far behind, it too is picking up momentum. But here something quite different has appeared. Now, unlike any other time in medicine's history, the ground has shifted and what is still called medicine might soon be capable of *doing something* for Ben— something that could hitherto only barely be imagined. A fundamental limit in restorative medicine seems now more a challenge and problem to be surmounted by molecular medicine.

To be sure, there is still a kind of limit: it remains true that nothing can be done at the moment to change Ben's body into a "phenotypically normal" one. What's already happened cannot be altered—at least in his case, at least not yet. In other cases (cystic fibrosis, breast cancer, and others), the same techniques that Ben uses to discover his gene and later for his and Jean's embryos, can now be used with very different aims in mind—even, it may be, for the fully formed child or adult. That, at least, is part of the promissory note of the unraveling of the genome, the location and functional identification of each gene.

The implications of this are remarkable. Rather than being beyond the limit or norm, much of the sort of human affliction hitherto outside now seems capable of being brought inside. That is, in the end, not even Ben's warped and gnarled body is any longer thought to be beyond the pale— as within traditional restorative or curative medicine it had to be—no more than, say, is the neural regeneration of a quadriplegic's spine. Where the traditional view of medicine put in place the long-standing, still-viable endeavor of restoration, that approach and its limitations are now being challenged and potentially changed, decisively. Beneath the awesome potency that haunts the phenomenon of human cloning lies this astounding possibility, this fundamental shift in what medicine, disease, and health have long been thought to be all about.

This shift seems to be something not merely unparalleled but appalling. Thinking about just these matters, Hans-Jörg Rheinberger concludes that a "new medical paradigm: molecular medicine," already ongoing for the past century, has more fully blossomed over the past several decades and is well on its apparently unstoppable way to taking over the entire garden.[16] He insists, however, that there is a fundamental scandal at the core of this new paradigm, in the sense diagnosed by Claude Lévi-Strauss at the core of the incest taboo.[17] Rheinberger notes Jacques Derrida's observation that this taboo is right at the edges of, if not actually within, the "domain of the unthinkable," for it challenges the very thing that makes possible the distinction and opposition between "nature" and "culture." That distinction, Derrida contends, has for centuries been at the heart of philosophy and theoretical thinking generally.[18] Thus, the very possibility of philosophical conceptualization itself has come under severe threat, if not actual collapse, as that distinction itself loses its sense in the presence of this scandal.

Lévi-Strauss argues that "everything that is universal in man belongs to the order of nature and is characterized by spontaneity, and that everything bound to norms belongs to culture and is . . . relative and . . . particular." From this, he then identifies the epitome of scandal, "the incest prohibition," which, he thought, "escapes any norm that . . . distinguishes between . . . culture and nature. It leaves in the realm of the unthinkable what has made it possible."[19]

Although Derrida has far more subtle issues in view than can be explored here, he emphasizes that the taboo exists solely within a context that accepted the opposition between nature and culture. The fact is, Derrida says, the scandal is "something which no longer tolerates the nature/culture opposition he has accepted."[20] It is unthinkable in the sense that it makes possible both the distinction and the opposition between nature and culture, thereby grounding the very possibility of philosophy and knowledge.

In the same way that the incest taboo is scandalous, Rheinberger is convinced that there is also a scandal at the heart of the new medicine. We may catch a glimpse of what he has in mind if we think about a key feature of biomedical science: informed consent. If medicine's point is to help sick, compromised people who cannot help themselves—people who for that very reason are multiply disadvantaged and at their most vulnerable—how could there ever be any question at all about informing people and ensuring that nobody takes advantage of them?[21] Yet just that doctrine of informed consent has become a centerpiece of medicine and biomedicine, not only in research, but in daily clinical practice as well.

In both cases, there would be no need for either a taboo (in the case of incest) or the legal requirement for informed consent (in the case of human subjects research) if there were not a preexisting context requiring the one or the other. If vulnerable patient-subjects were not abused in some manner in the first place, the demand to obtain informed consent would be pointless—as would a taboo on incest, if no parent or sibling engaged in sexual activities with children or other siblings. Just as incest seems barely capable of being spoken or thought about, so is it scandalous that otherwise-decent people who are researchers (not simply those who were Nazis) must be subject to the rule of informed consent, as if they could not be trusted.

Rheinberger is in any event clear about what especially concerns him as scandalous (in the same sense as the incest taboo):

With the acceleration of a historical, irreversible alteration of the earth's surface and atmosphere, which is taking place within the span of an individual human's lifetime; with the realization that our mankindly, science-guided actions result, on a scale of natural history, in the mass extinction of species, in a global climatic change, and in gene technology that has the potential to change our genetic constitution, a fundamental alteration in the representation of nature is taking place, which we are still barely realizing.[22]

To be sure, discovery and diagnosis continue to occupy the limelight of human genetics research—even with its newly acquired name, genomics—with treatments and understanding lagging far behind. Nonetheless, the regularly stated, almost mantralike discourse about (and often justifications for) genetics projects, and the probable future reality of genomics, is that clinical practice will be totally transformed as new genetic knowledge leads eventually to effective treatment modalities. With that eventuality, a wholly new meaning of "health" must shortly follow: it will be more a matter of healthy genes (with the ability to make and keep them healthy) than of the absence of health or the workings of some pathological process or entity.

At this point, it is necessary to take a few cautious steps of my own into the unforgiving unthinkable.

Beginning to Think about the Unthinkable

In traditional, restorative medicine, there is nothing that can be done for Ben's condition. If he is injured or becomes ill, of course, as much can be done for him as for anyone else—taking into account that his condition may itself require one or another regimen. While changes in social attitudes and acceptance, along with support to pursue accepted goals or careers, even if not done or not done well by those who meet or know such dwarfs, can be recommended, they are plainly sufficiently rare as to prompt some cynicism.

But is this sort of encouragement medicine's business? Should physicians be involved with or even concerned about the mistreatment Ben regularly receives? Doesn't this sort of thing fall to others, such as social workers, ministers, rabbis, or therapists? In the end, why should any of us be much concerned about dwarfs like Ben? What we were born with is, after all, neither more nor less thanks to chance than is Ben's condition. Indeed, unlike most of us, Ben is a famous scientist appointed to a famous institute. What need does he have for anything from medicine or the rest of us? If he is singled out for special consideration, doesn't this simply defeat the very purpose of special consideration?

Still, even considered merely as a body, we are obliged to recognize that while currently nothing can be done for Ben and others like him, in the new genetic, molecular model, such people may no longer be so obviously off the medical agenda, and in any event their progeny most surely will be squarely on the agenda of future, frankly eugenic medical interventions—much of it done while progeny are still embryonic.

What is novel about molecular biology and genetics is that very little, perhaps nothing, will be regarded as automatically beyond the social or medical pale. Everything, in short, formally beyond the limit is now up for review, study, design, and possible if not yet probable reversal, correction, or even replacement if need be. We ought not fear being on a slippery slope; instead, we should welcome and even relish the novel vistas, prospects, and exhilarating ride—which are potent indeed.

In Mawer's novel, Dinah is deeply ambivalent toward Ben, at once attracted and repelled—not unlike many others of us when we are in the company of the likes of Ben. Ben, on the other hand, is not only extremely nice to Dinah but goes out of his way to help her get through a genetics class. Why, then, are the Bens of the world so disturbing? Dinah is beside herself when she passes the course and spontaneously kisses Ben, then promptly tries to take it back. Befuddled, on fire, Ben tells Dinah that he loves her, and she responds, "I knew you'd do this. ... [C]an't you see it's impossible?" Ben replies, "Of course it's impossible. It's the impossible that attracts me. When you're like I am, who gives a toss about the possible?"[23] He then says what she cannot bring herself to mention: that he is a dwarf.

At this point, there is something left unsaid, unspoken, perhaps unthinkable even as Ben himself tries to think and say it—or perhaps, it can be spoken only because the unspeakable one himself, Ben the dwarf, says it for her. Why, we must wonder, is it so hard for her to say what she actually thinks, and to say it directly to Ben? Isn't utter honesty called for? Why would it be difficult for any of us to say it to someone like Ben? Why do we hesitate to say it when, on the other hand, what is unsaid is, if anything, utterly decisive for what we then think about and how we act toward Ben the dwarf?

When discussing using human subjects for research in 1865, Claude Bernard did not mention, nor presumably did he intend to mention anything like informed consent. Rather, he said, that "it is our duty and our right to perform an experiment on man whenever it can save his life, cure him, or gain him some personal benefit. The principle of medical and surgical morality, therefore, consists in never performing on man an experiment which might be harmful to him to any extent, even though the results might be highly advantageous to science, i.e., to the health of others."[24]

Commenting on this passage, Jay Katz notes "that Bernard spoke about 'our duty' and 'our right'; he said nothing about research subjects' consent." And, continuing to reflect on this remarkable passage, Katz seems taken aback by the realization that one question has not been thoroughly analyzed to this day: When may investigators, actively or by acquiescence, expose human beings to harm in order to seek benefits for them, for others, or for society as a whole? If one peruses the literature with this question in mind, one soon learns that no searching general justifications for involving any human beings as subjects for research have ever been formulated. . . . Instead, in the past and even now, it has been assumed without question that the general necessity for experimenting with human beings, while requiring regulation, is so obvious that it need not be justified. . . . I do not contend that it cannot be justified. I only wish to point to the pervasive silence . . . and, more specifically, to the lack of separate justifications for novel interventions employed for the benefit of future patients and science, in contrast to those employed for patients' direct benefits.[25]

At the heart of this is "a slippery slope of engineering consent," one that leads "inexorably to Tuskegee, the Jewish Chronic Disease Hospital in Brooklyn, LSD experiments in Manhattan, DES (diethylstilbestrol) experiments in Chicago"—and many others might be added—all of which are "done in the belief that physician-scientists can be trusted to safeguard the physical integrity of their subjects."[26]

It might be said, of course, that the physician-scientists involved in these events, like those who conducted the experiments in the Nazi concentration camps, the Gulag Archipelago, Willowbrook, or others, are perverse or even evil persons. Science and medicine are value neutral; they are "intrinsically benign," it might be said.[27] Evil actions stem not from science but from individuals who are evil, or who do evil things because of the ways they use science and medicine. To suggest otherwise, Katz verges on saying, would be to court something scandalous—if not unspeakable or unthinkable, then surely repugnant, and that would be something awful, appalling even, quite as much as engaging in an act of incest.

A few things are clear. In the new genetics, nothing seems beyond the limits of newly possible interventions designed to correct, refigure, conquer, or replace—most of all before flawed genes can do their inevitable work. Reflecting on Mawer's narrative about Ben Lambert, something unspeakable emerges as somehow connected to this point: that we dare not say what we truly believe about individuals such as dwarfs—that is, until and unless something can be done to correct or ameliorate phenomena such as achondroplasia. Then, there is that "pervasive silence" that puzzles Katz.

There seems nowadays to be the possibility, at least, of a sort of license for genetic medicine to try and outdo, replace, or even transcend nature and natural evolution, to remake Ben, because being Ben is regarded as profoundly offensive—in much the same way that the "feebleminded" were regarded by Charles Darwin:

> With savages, the weak in body or mind are soon eliminated; and those that survive commonly exhibit a vigorous state of health. We civilized men, on the other hand, do our utmost to check the process of elimination; we build asylums for the imbecile, the maimed, and the sick; we institute poor-laws; and our medical men exert their utmost skill to save the life of every one to the last moment.[28]

Saving the imbecile, the severely disabled, the simpleminded, the hopelessly confused and nonproductive—even encouraging them to reproduce—can only be "highly injurious to the race of man," Darwin believed, and eventually leads to the degeneration of "man himself." The sensible thing for nature, God, or whatever set evolution in motion in the first place would have been to prevent such individuals from reproducing. Since that did not happen on its own, so to speak, Darwin and his legacy took it on themselves to do it by inspiring, if not recommending, various sterilization laws to prevent the feebleminded from reproducing. It then naturally follows, Kurt Bayertz argues, that with this striking failure of "natural selection," the ground was well prepared for the more recent proposals for deliberately controlled experiments to produce more useful citizens, precisely as Eccles, Burnett, and other geneticists and molecular biologists had proposed, using whatever means necessary.[29]

Then we must wonder about that pervasive silence by the research community. As Katz sees it, it leads to a slippery slope of engineering consent for research projects, and this in turn inexorably leads to the dreadful perversions of Tuskegee, the radiation experiments in the United States with whose outrageous aftermaths we are still living, but that took so long even to acknowledge publicly. How could any of this happen? How can any of it be understood? How could any physician in the restorative, Hippocratic tradition ever be caught up in such deliberate designs not only to ignore, abandon, and literally overlook individual human beings but to do so in the name of science and medicine?

Speaking to the Unspeakable

What does Rheinberger mean when, taking off from the incest taboo, he writes, "Just as the incest prohibition became the scandal of anthropology, so has the commandment of truth become the scandal of the sciences of natural things," including the human body? Is it that, say, with the "deliberate 'rewriting' of life" that is the basic aim of the new genetics, there is introduced what is also capable of fundamentally altering the very life that conceived of and then carried out the new genetics— such that, perhaps, the very possibility and ability of future generations to do this as well can and will be made impossible?[30] Because we *can*, are we then free to try and cancel the same sort of freedom of action of those future generations?

Or is it like the Pasteurian program a century ago, cited by Rheinberger, that rejected the entire question of theories or goals, but thought of means merely, which is precisely what is now being embraced by the handful of molecular biologists and project managers at the National Institutes of Health and the Department of Energy on establishing the Human Genome Project? Rheinberger quotes Bruno Latour to make his point: those Pasteurians, not themselves especially potent in political terms, nonetheless "followed the demand that [their own weak] forces were making, but imposed on them a way of formulating that demand to which only [they] possessed the answer, since it required [men and women] of the laboratory to understand its terms."[31]

Nothing, Rheinberger insists, "could describe the political moves of James Watson, Walter Gilbert and their combatants better than this quotation."[32] Is this then the scandal: the spectacle of this remarkable finesse of politicians by, of all things, scientists who are typically thought to be politically ineffective, but who yet secured immense funding for a scientific project riding on the back, it seems, of what Rheinberger gently calls a "misunderstanding"? He means, I gather, that genetics is not so much about diagnosis or even the curing of disease as it is about improving people (or some of them) by controlling and "exploiting" (in Eccles's view) human and animal evolution—aims that, because they do not sit well with a largely uninformed public, must be somewhat hidden behind stated aims such as treatments for diseases that are valued by that same public.

The new genetics is for all practical purposes capable right now of serious control of human reproduction; experiments with animals since the early 1980s demonstrate that the same can be done with humans. Is the scandal, then—what either should not, cannot, or will not be openly admitted—that only those with the power to control the knowledge and exploit the technology will do so, and they will never let the truth of what's happened be known—a type of potent, silent priesthood? Is the point that scientists should or must give politicians the ammunition needed for their reelection—marching out genetics under the banner of changing medical practice by finding ways to cure disease—and the money mill will open wide? And that the rest of us will not be able to know before or after the fact what went on behind closed doors?

Politics, Power, and the Loss of Norms

This may be at least partly what Rheinberger is saying with his talk about scandals. But for his case to be well argued, it seems to me, there is something else that needs an accounting. How and why is it that such widespread suspicion, with distrust spreading to everyone and everything, has come about, especially toward one of the last bastions of social prestige and authority: medicine (and the biomedical sciences)?[33] And why is there distrust, even cynicism, concerning those people who can and will actually control procreation?[34] As Barbara Ehrenreich caustically noted in her editorial for *Time* on the occasion of the first (although mistaken) announcement in 1993 that human cloning had been achieved: we should be apprehensive, not about twenty-first-century technology—which promises the kind of genetic cloning Blish forecast in his cunning novel, technology with which to "seed" the stars—but about putting such potent technologies into the hands of twentieth-century capitalists, whose money, after all, pays for such adventures.[35] If our concern is not about the scientists whose research results in the feared technologies, then it has to do with a distrust of the genetic engineers who will put the theories to work; and if not them, then toward those who provide the funding for the enterprise, or possibly those with positions in policy formulation and enactment.

Is this passion for control, for epistemic and political power, then, the real scandal? If so, then Rheinberger's point about science and the loss of truth makes a good deal of sense—the crucial point isn't what you know, but who owns the means and product of research. To be sure, this is a scandal in the sense that, if present trends continue, the very sciences that proudly parade a commitment to truth would, in their constant and upward-spiraling escalation of costs (and their search for escalating financial support), be for sale to the highest bidder and thus undo that very commitment to truth.[36] Is the scandal, then, that once on this fateful path, a course is inexorably set, like the best of slippery slopes, even if concealed by nice words?

The reminder is inevitable: the astounding Grand Inquisitor scene in Fyodor Dostoyevsky's *The Brothers Karamasov*, where, after hearing Ivan's tale of the return of Christ and the priest's objections to that, Alyosha cries out with his riveting question, Is anything then permitted? Is nothing forbidden? Can anyone then do anything they want, simply because at this or that moment they by chance happen to want it—and can pay for it?[37]

It would appear that modern medicine's impending realization of its ancient dream to improve the human condition is set deeply within something that resists being expressly spoken. Such may be the actual scandal, for must we not wonder about the wisdom of the choices that will, it seems, inevitably be made by those who will make them simply because they alone understand the technologies, or have paid for them? We must wonder, too, with Hans Jonas, about efforts to rectify and alleviate the "necessities and miseries of humanity" in the manner of Francis Bacon by technological means, at the same time so conceiving of knowledge that no room is left for what can alone provide guidance, a knowledge of "beneficence and charity."[38]

No matter how well he understood the necessity of moral guidance for that "race of inventions," Bacon's project succeeds only in creating a powerful paradox since neither theory nor practice in this usage contains or can say anything about such goals or moral governance. Neither beneficence nor charity "is itself among the fruits of theory in the modern sense," nor is "modern theory . . . self-sufficiently the source of the human quality that makes it beneficial." Indeed, Jonas argues that the fact that the results of theory are detachable and can be handed over for use to those who had no part in the theoretical process is only one aspect of the matter. Because of their expertise scientists are no more qualified than others to discern or to care for the good of humankind. Benevolence must be called in from the outside to supplement the knowledge acquired through theory: it does not flow from theory itself.[39]

Emphasizing that the prospect of genetic control "raises ethical questions of a wholly new kind" for which we are most ill prepared, Jonas later urgently suggested, "Since no less than the very nature and image of man are at issue, prudence becomes itself our first ethical duty, and hypothetical reasoning our first responsibility."[40]

H. Tristram Engelhardt, Jr. came to much the same conclusion about modern medicine. Echoing Jonas, he wrote that "man has become more technically adept than he is wise, and must now look for the wisdom to use that knowledge he possesses."[41] Recall T. S. Eliot's incisive, thundering questions: Where is the knowledge we have lost in information? And where is the wisdom we have lost in knowledge? Jonas emphasized that we are "constantly confronted with issues whose positive choice requires supreme wisdom—an impossible situation for man in general, because he does not possess that wisdom, and in particular for contemporary man, who denies the very existence of its object: viz., objective value and truth. We need wisdom most when we believe in it least."[42]

It is not so much that we are continually threatened by one or another slippery slope. Rather, I believe, being on a slippery slope is precisely the human lot, what it means to be human, at least since Darwin and in particular the disasters of the twentieth century. The dreadful has already come about, asserts R. D. Laing.[43] And I think it bears all the signs of Dostoyevsky's breathtaking "anything is permitted."

Thinking about Birth and Beyond

Even at this point, I have a sense that there is something else still lurking in the darker corners. As mentioned, at issue in the Human Genome Project is a fundamental philosophical-anthropological concern: not only how self is at all known and experienced but *whether there is self* at all, much less a person, or instead, merely genetic information encoded in or on strands of DNA/RNA nestled within any individual's body cells. Walter Gilbert's excited pronouncement, "Here is a human being; it's me'!" etched on a CD, is a challenge none of us can ignore. Does it not pose very much the same question of scandal that Rheinberger dares us to face?

To help make my way through these complex matters, I think it is helpful to dwell for a bit on several peculiar passages in the work of Alfred Schutz. One appears in his critical review of Edmund Husserl's understanding of intersubjectivity; the other in his intriguing article on Max Scheler.

After insisting that intersubjectivity is a "given" and not a "problem" to be solved, Schutz maintained that "as long as man is born of woman, intersubjectivity and the we-relationship will be the foundation for all other categories of human existence." Accordingly, he continued, everything in human life is "founded on the primal experience of the we-relationship," which, though he didn't explicitly say so, must surely be the experience of being "born of woman." Since *all* "other categories of human existence" are founded on this primal experience, our being with and among other people was for Schutz "the fundamental ontological category of human existence in the world and therefore of all philosophical anthropology."[44]

In the Scheler essay, Schutz's words are equally fascinating. He first pointed out that there is one taken-for-granted assumption that no one for a moment doubts, not even the most ornery skeptic: "We are simply born into a world of Others." Then he said: "As long as human beings are not concocted like homunculi in retorts but are born and brought up by mothers, the sphere of the 'We' will be naively presupposed."[45] Here, too, it is reasonable to surmise that what is "naively presupposed" is precisely that "primal experience" of being borne by a woman (I need to add) and born of woman, and (he added here) being raised by mothers as opposed to being "concocted . . . in retorts."

What I want to pick up on is the idea that being born of woman constitutes "the" (not merely "a") "fundamental" ontological and anthropological category of human life. It is curious to note first that few philosophers have thought it necessary or, I suppose, fruitful to focus on this phenomenon of having been born of woman. Reflections on death and dying are plentiful; those on birth, being borne and then born, or "worlded," are oddly lacking. Still, if we consider this—even if, as Schutz also said, we can get at it only indirectly, through other people[46]—still, my having been borne and born are surely as constitutive of my life as is my "going to die."

Schutz did not probe this phenomenon any more than these scant references. Still, his words have to be taken quite seriously, for in a clear and compelling way it is the primal experience of being (or having been) borne and born that constitutes the crucial other side (other than death) of the central experience of growing old together, and of our being-with-one-another—of what he terms the "tuning-in relationship" or intersubjectivity. We could not experience ourselves as growing older together, if we did not begin to be—that is, if we did not come at some always-already-ongoing time in our lives to find ourselves as having-already-been-thrust-into life: birthed and thereby worlded.

To be born as human, but more specifically as myself, is to have *received* life, to *have been given* my life—the first and fundamental sense of *gift*. And in this, it seems clear as well, lies a fundamental paradox of freedom: while a prime condition for morality (choice, responsibility, and so on), I do not choose to be free, but, as Jean-Paul Sartre saw, I am not free to choose to cease being free. Hence, an ethics that focuses on giving is seriously incomplete without a complementary reflection on the ethics of receiving; the latter may indeed be the more fundamental phenomenon.

The primal other, in short, is the mother, the one with whom each of us in the first instance grows older, in Schutz's words; and the initial and primal *place* or habitat is her body, her womb. She is the one who gifts me with myself and is progressively the one who gifts me with herself. From her we receive culture, history, world, mainly through giving the key stories by which we come to know ourselves.

I am not only, then, a being-toward-death but surely just as fundamentally a being-*from*-birth—indeed, in a sense my being is always already a being-before-birth, being already within the mother's body; this is thus the originating sense of my becoming. What and who I *am*, is what and who I in multiple ways *become*, and this is first set in motion in the essentially mysterious and accidental ways of every birth.

This returns me to Ben.

Of the Scandal, Chance, and God

As Ben reflects when he's in the passionate moment of wondering how it was that he ever came to be just this specific person, this Ben the dwarf, there simply is no way to know the why or how just one specific sperm made its way into one specific ovum, nor the countless accidental splittings, changings, connectings, shiftings, and turnabouts of both Ben and his mother as she bore him from the tiniest of the tiny into birth, and beyond, into himself. Even were there to have been an in vitro infusion of a preselected sperm—"get that one there, Shirley. . . . No, not him, *that* one . . ."—how is one to account for, how is one to make understandable, what constitutes just *that* life, *that* unique life, which then, if all goes well, becomes just that unique individual, Ben Lambert, dwarf?

Now, these reflections evoke not so much that the new genetics places this entire, awesome process at risk, as Rheinberger and many others suggest; nor do the novel genetic techniques and theories threaten my "who I am" and the variety of foundational relationships among us (father, mother, son, daughter, and so forth), as Kass insists. Rather, it is *my being at all* that is at issue, for this is now placed in a radically new light, and in this there may be a true scandal: *that* I am *at all*, *that* I have come or been brought into being (into life) neither through my own action or choice, nor through anyone's decision, while yet being born free to choose from that point on.

Nor did Ben's parents choose Ben, this unique individual. Perhaps they had wanted a baby, but *his* coming on the scene, the unique *Ben*, is wholly outside any parents' or anyone's ken, foreknowledge, or choice. Being a baby—being *this* baby—is always and essentially a surprise—to itself and its parents. But the reverse is also true, for Ben no more chose his parents than they chose him. Hence, for Ben to be what he is, to be himself, is to be an ontological surprise. He is an accident (the "accident of birth") that embodies chance in its purest form, though being himself is not only that.

What is scandalous about that? At one point in Mawer's deeply ironic novel, Ben succeeds in sequencing the genes that, incorporating a single, apparently trivial error in a single base pair in "this enigmatic, molecular world," likely eventuated in him, Ben Lambert. That so-called genetic error involves a "simple transition at nucleotide 1,138 of the *FGFR3* gene," which, in the dark recesses of his mother's womb and impregnated by a single sperm, mutated into what eventually became Ben.[47] A single mistake in the 3.3×10^9 base pairs in his genome, one mistake, one substitution of guanine for adenine, in the transmembrane domain of the protein—that part that fits through the cell membrane—and the result was Ben. Is this not a scandal: the sheer, accidental fact that of all the millions of pairings along those snaky helixical arms and spiraled columns of deoxyribonucleic acid busily replicating, churning out proteins (those building blocks of life), a single exchange, a single letter error, and there's Ben, the achondroplasic dwarf, that gnarled, disfigured "monster" who despite everything is a genius and, more, loves Jean? And Jean, the accidental outcome of the same sort of sinewy organic workings, tries mightily to love him, too, but in the end has to confess that she just cannot.

Picking up on Herbert Spiegelberg's insight, it must be noted that despite having no choice in our birth—not even that we will be born—each of us as we grow older assumes the prime responsibility for ourselves.[48] Save for that initiating happenstance, each of us is responsible for whatever may eventuate. At some also unchosen point, Ben gradually emerges from a globally undifferentiated entity at birth that we name and celebrate as "baby." From the same playing out of chance, Ben could just as easily *not* have been born, hence not *be* at all—or if born, then born without that chance mutation, and for any number of incalculable reasons themselves as accidental as that, the multiple biological processes and timings managed to eventuate in his birth. But from then on, it is his life, whatever he may subsequently do or not do about that: he, Ben, is the continuous outcome of *chance* and *choice*. Even more, beyond all that, being born as "me" with its unchosen accoutrements is, Spiegelberg is anxious for us to understand, the purest kind of "moral chance" and therefore utterly undeserved: there is no moral entitlement to what I happen to be, whatever the station of my birth, no more than what I biologically inherit is something to which I am entitled.

The phenomenon of moral chance seems quite essential to having been born of woman, mother—nor, I strongly suspect, can there be any ontological or theological accounting for that uniqueness that each of us is already at birth. As I think about Ben, it seems to me outrageous that he was, choicelessly, saddled with being *him*; it seems altogether scandalous, moreover, that he (and the rest of us) should have either advantages or disadvantages simply because of the accident of birth. But precisely the same is true for each of us, both in our biological where-withal and our initial stations in life (which family, which place, which time). Is it not outrageous that any of us is born at all, with all of what we are and who we become?

All that is a kind of prologue to something more puzzling still. This arises from the choice Ben faces when Jean, now back with her infertile husband, asks Ben to use his sperm for the in vitro fertilization she has asked him to perform. He agrees. Later, he checks the fertilized eggs, has an associate gently suck up each embryo in turn, while he himself does the polymerase chain reaction amplification. He determines that embryos two, five, six, and seven are unaffected; they show no misspelling of adenine by guanine. Yet he also determines that one, two, four, and eight show that very mutation; adenine has been replaced with guanine, and achondroplasia is irreversibly on the way.

By chance, four "normals" and four "mutations" have come about as dwarfs-to-be—if allowed to be all. What should Ben do? Note well: he *can* actually choose one or more embryos to implant; he can select which, by implanting, will be allowed to grow into a baby. Is this the way God goes about the business of human birth? Should Ben "play God"? Mawer sets the scene: "Benedict Lambert is sitting in his laboratory" with eight embryos in eight little tubes. "Four of the embryos," he reflects, "are proto-Benedicts, proto-dwarfs; the other four are, for want of a better word, normal. How should he choose? And is his choice, whatever it may be, acting or 'playing' like God?" Ben continues:

Of course, we all know that God has opted for the easy way out. He has decided on chance as the way to select one combination of genes from another. If you want to shun euphemisms, then God allows pure luck to decide whether a mutant child or a normal child shall be born. But Benedict Lambert has the possibility of beating God's proxy and overturning the tables of chance. He can choose. Wasn't choice what betrayed Adam and Eve?[49]

So, Ben is not playing God in the least; if he were to do that, he would find a way to let chance work its way, not him. But Ben can choose, and when he makes the choice, does the deed, and the baby is on its way, Jean telephones to ask him what he did: "Is it all right?" Which embryo was implanted? The conversation heats up as Ben evades and dodges, knowing full well what he has already done, and cannot now undo, and doesn't want to tell her. But Jean pleads with him, to the point where he grows angry "at the docile stupidity of her, at the pleading, whining kindness of her, at her naïveté. 'Well, you'll have to wait and see, won't you?' I said to her."[50] Then he hangs up. Was that in any sense fair? Was it just?

Spiegelberg asserts, in a certain sense addressing just this sort of issue, that there is a much "deeper sense of justice" and "injustice" than is usually discussed, something genuinely "cosmic," at the core of our lives. His point is that since "*undeserved discrimination calls for redress,*" and since "*all inequalities of birth constitute undeserved discriminations,*" he concludes that "*all inequalities of birth call for redress,*" therefore that "*inequality is a fundamental ethical demand.*"[51] If that is so, on whom does the responsibility for redress fall? But is this true for Ben? Will it eventually be true of his child, who will eventually be born from Jean's body? Is it true for Jean, too?

Does Ben's "inequality of birth" call for redress? Indeed, is it not rather the case that, while we may well feel how profoundly unjust it is that Ben was born, we cannot avoid the awesome, awful question, Was Ben's birth unjust? Even if it were, does that imply a demand for redress? If so, who redresses, and what exactly can be redressed? And finally, what exactly is unjust, cosmically or otherwise? Is it that through no fault of his own, Ben is a dwarf? At the same time, however, each of us must know that who and what we are did not come about through our own choice—and just because of that, each of us, dwarf or supposedly normal, is essentially in the same quandary as Ben might be.

Beneath the Scandal That I Am Myself

Each of us, then, is born with some initiating condition that is utterly unchosen, undeserved, and surely, an inequality of the first order. Does Spiegelberg's passionate focus work here? I think not, and *that it does not seems outrageous, a real scandal.* What happens after the brute accident of birth, that's something else, something with respect to which this or that course of life may or may not ensue, with responsibility properly meted out for these as for all other people. But for the bald, brutal fact of initial biological, familial, and in general existential wherewithal? It does not make sense to talk about redress here, and that it does not make sense is disgraceful.

On the other hand, it strikes me as clearly wrong to allege, for oneself (if born as Ben) or another (Ben's mother or pregnant Jean), that "God did it" and is responsible, and hence must be called to account for the offense. As Ben reflects, after donating his sperm,

What is natural? Nature is what nature does. Am I natural? Is superovulation followed by transvaginal ultrasound-guided oocyte retrieval natural? Is *in vitro* fertilization and the growth of multiple embryos in culture, is all that natural? Two months later . . . I watched shivering spermatozoa clustering around eggs, *my* spermatozoa clustering around *her* eggs. Consummation beneath the microscope. Is that natural?[52]

Precisely here it seems is a true scandal: as Schutz apparently appreciated, we are each of us born, and in the fact of being here at all—much less in the way and how we each are—we are initially what and who we are thanks to a plain throw of the dice, the sheerest of chance. And this, I think, openly displays the brazen hubris of Gilbert, Watson, and Eccles, and their promises of control in a world governed to the contrary by the genius of chance.

Am I Me Solely within You? Are You Solely within Me?

A way to appreciate what's so compelling about Schutz's otherwise-only-isolated suggestions is to consider them in light of that theme du jour, human cloning.

A cloned human infant is, of course, not the same as a being, in Schutz's terms, "concocted . . . in retorts," although as he apparently used this then-common term, it probably amounts to much the same thing. In any event, it is clear that a cloned human being hardly ceases to be human simply because it is cloned. As even the most hard-nosed genetic determinist knows perfectly well, moreover, in the case of cloned individuals all that's different is that they share most (one cannot overlook the fact of continuous chance mutations) of the same genome, by design and deliberate plan rather than the usual delightful way—as in the case, absent the deliberate planning, of naturally occurring identical twins (who also, of course, share the same genome).

Ian Wilmut's method, as is well known, involves the nuclear transfer of genetic material from an adult cell to an egg taken from another adult, which is then implanted into a third adult's uterus.[53] Here, it is clear, there is not only deliberation and planning, but the reproduction itself is asexual, which is the very thing that worries Kass and others. To be sure, a nonhuman uterus might conceivably be developed. It has already been demonstrated that human genes are able to be spliced into the cells of certain animals—though there are potentially serious problems with this[54]—to produce certain human proteins. Eventually, human tissues and even solid organs might well be produced. Could a full human fetus be similarly developed? It is not at all clear how or whether that question could be answered.

One thing is clear. The human fetus within a human uterus exists and has its being solely within a continuously developing context or network of intimate interactions with the mother and even other individuals, although much of this is still poorly understood. In any case, it is thanks to that developing network that what we otherwise term "fetal development" is truly "human development" in its earliest and most apparent form. I mean: to be human is to *become* human; and becoming human requires a sequential development whose primary characteristic is that each of its stages is or involves a complex context of interrelationships with a highly specific other, the mother.[55] Each of us is at the outset of our lives truly *always-already-with* mother; we are *always-already-within* the literal embrace of her body, from the earliest stirrings of semen-penetrated ovum to the full infant immediately prior to birth.

Schutz understood with remarkable, if also undeveloped, insight that the prime phenomenon here is receiving life, being gifted with myself by the mother. What he did not probe were the implications of the "primal experience"—and it is just this phenomenon that comes into question again with the advent of human cloning. He also seemed to have understood that without that ongoing biological process of pregnancy, it would be profoundly questionable whether any "outcome" could conceivably be "human." If we suppose it were possible for there to be some sort of artificial womb and placenta housed in some laboratory somewhere—a completely novel sort of intensive care unit from the earliest moments of impregnation on—and suppose further that an appropriately cloned or semen-penetrated egg could be implanted in it, we would then have to contend with the really difficult question implicit in Schutz's words. Would "homunculi in retorts" be "humans" if they did not issue from impregnation, implantation, and fertilization, and were not allowed to stay and grow in mutual relationships within that most primal of human environments, a female human being, a mother? If what I have suggested is correct, nothing but a homunculus could possibly emerge from such a retort. To be human, to repeat, is at the very least to become human, and becoming human in stages along life's way requires that temporal, sequential development within and nourished by another human body.

Thus, when Jean Bethke Elshtain asserts, in what she says is her own "nightmare scenario" (cloning human beings to serve as spare parts for, one presumes, other human beings), that "cloned entities are not fully human," she is quite evidently mistaken.[56] Her nightmare is nonsense—*unless* such an entity were conceived and carried in at least its initial journey outside the mother's womb. The uterine environment, in other words, strikes me as absolutely essential, though it is not all that is essential, for such an entity to become human.

The risk of cloning, then, is not some supposed threat that it will erase the unique individual or its network of relationships with others (mother, father, son, and so on). Rather, it is the loss of that for and in each of us, which comes to be within and by means of my relating to you and you relating to me: it is, ultimately, *we*, you and I, who are at risk. This is not true of natural identical twins, for they are both nurtured and enabled to grow toward birth within the mother's body, and, in that intimacy, come to be as and who they are—clones both of them, and none the worse for it. When born, however much alike, they are yet destined to be that self each is solely in relation both to its mother and others, but especially to its twin—who are each also a self in relation both to one another.

Concluding Reflection

The fact of the accident of birth gives a quite different sense than usual to the idea of the slippery slope, which has had such attraction over the past four decades. The horror at the bottom of the slope, it must now be clear, is that there simply is no bottom, nothing solid whatsoever, only a steady, slippery slope initiated before the accident of our individual births. It is, in a word, our human condition—to be always in search of firm or firmer footing than presently at hand, and always to be disappointed in our failure to find it. In this respect, that fabulous slope is not unlike what Albert Camus brilliantly stated in his great work *The Myth of Sisyphus*. His words allow me to bring this long reflection to some kind of conclusion.

Camus had the courage to say out loud for all to hear that any appeal whatsoever to transcendence and absolutes (the supposedly firmer footing that moves so many of us at times of radical uncertainty) can only be "absurd." Such an appeal is but one of the machinations by which control is sought; it is but a way to try and ensure that the one who asserts the transcendent or the absolute also asserts that they know better than anyone else what's good for all the others. As if there were something absolute; as if, even if there were, such an absolute would be the truth of who and what we are; as if, even were that coherent, this or that finite human being could apprehend it surely and doubtlessly; and as if, apprehending it in one grand sweep of thought innocent of every infelicity of being a specific, error-prone, historically bound individual, this were not the height of hubris.

Camus' point, or some key part of it, is that such schemes are beyond our capabilities. Such appeals to some sort of higher ledge of authority— available to no one else and from which to pronounce judgments on the rest of us—are but tacit signs of dread and doom, of the deep uncertainty and chance that constitute our condition as human. "I want to know whether, accepting a life *without appeal*, one can also agree to *work* and create *without appeal* and what is the way leading to these liberties." And this, set out as starkly as the sun-blistered sands on that striking, colorless beach in *The Stranger*, may be the sole way genuinely to reclaim our lives. "I want to liberate my universe of its phantoms and to people it solely with flesh-and-blood truths whose presence I cannot deny."[57]

Notes

1. James Blish, *The Seedling Stars and Galactic Cluster* (Hicksville, NY: Gnome Press, 1957).

2. On Joshua Lederberg, see Leon Kass, "The Wisdom of Repugnance," *The New Republic*, June 2, 1997, 17, and "New Beginnings in Life," in *The New Genetics and the Future of Man*, ed. Michael P. Hamilton (Grand Rapids, MI: William B. Erdmann's, 1972), 54. See also John C. Eccles, *The Human Mystery* (Berlin: Springer-Verlag, 1979); Macfarlane Burnett, *Endurance of Life: The Implications of Genetics for Human Life* (London: Cambridge University Press, 1978); and I. Wilmut, A. E. Schnieke, J. McWhir, A. J. Kind, and K. H. S. Campbell, "Viable Offspring Derived from Fetal and Adult Mammalian Cells," *Nature* 385 (February 27, 1997): 810–813.

3. Walter Gilbert, "A Vision of the Grail," in *The Code of Code: Scientific and Social Issues in the Human Genome Project*, ed. Daniel J. Kevles and Leroy Hood (Cambridge, MA: Harvard University Press, 1992), 95.

4. See especially John C. Eccles, *Facing Reality* (Berlin: Springer-Verlag, 1970) and his numerous references, in particular in chapters 1 and 4.

5. Oswei Tempkin, *Galenism: Rise and Decline of a Medical Philosophy* (Ithaca, NY: Cornell University Press, 1973), 85.

6. Langdon Winner, "Resistance Is Futile: The Posthuman Condition and Its Advocates," this volume.

7. In 1986, Congressman Edward J. Markey released records detailing experiments by the U.S. government between 1940 and 1971; see Subcommittee on Energy and Power, *American Nuclear Guinea Pigs: Three Decades of Radiation Experiments on U.S. Citizens*, 99R Cong., 2nd sess., 1986, 3.0727.0000643 W. On the syphilis experiments, see James H. Jones, *Bad Blood: The Tuskegee Syphilis Experiment* (New York: Free Press, 1981). On the experiments documented by Henry K. Beecher, see his *Experimentation in Man* (Springfield, IL: Charles C. Thomas, 1959), and "Ethics and Clinical Research," *New England Journal of Medicine* 74 (1966): 1354–1360. On other questionable experiments, see George J. Annas and Michael A. Grodin, eds., *The Nazi Doctors and the Nuremberg Code* (New York: Oxford University Press, 1992); Norman Howard-Jones, "Human Experimentation in Historical and Ethical Perspectives," *Social Science and Medicine* 16 (1982): 1429–1448; and William Curran, "Subject Consent Requirements in Clinical Research: An International Perspective for Industrial and Developing Countries," in *Human Experimentation and Medical Ethics*, ed. Zbifniew Bankowski and Norman Howard-Jones (Geneva: Council for International Organizations of Medical Sciences, 1982).

8. Simon Mawer, *Mendel's Dwarf* (New York: Penguin Books, 1998). Mawer himself is a microbiologist and a geneticist.

9. Ibid., 5.

10. Ibid., 21.

11. Ibid., 18.

12. Ibid., 242–243.

13. For a sense of "restorative medicine," see Richard M. Zaner, "Thinking about Medicine," in *Handbook of Phenomenology and Medicine*, ed. A. Kay Toombs (Dordrecht: Kluwer Academic, 2001), 127–144, and "Brave New World

of Genetics," in *Jahrbuch für Recht und Ethik* (Berlin: Dunchker and Humblot, 2001), 297–322.

14. Another novel well worth taking quite as seriously as Mawer's is Katherine Dunn, *Geek Love* (New York: Warner Books, 1989). Dunn lays out precisely these variations of anomaly, personality, and values among the children deliberately conceived by their parents to be freaks.

15. Mawer, *Mendel's Dwarf*, 10.

16. Hans-Jörg Rheinberger, "Beyond Nature and Culture: A Note on Medicine in the Age of Molecular Biology," *Science in Context* 8, no. 1 (Spring 1995): 254.

17. Claude Lévi-Strauss, *Les structures élémentaries de la parenté*, 2nd ed. (The Hague: Mouton, 1967), 10.

18. Jacques Derrida, "Structure, Sign, and Play in the Discourse of the Human Science," in *Writing and Difference* (Chicago: University of Chicago Press, 1980), 258.

19. Lévi-Strauss, *Les structures élémentaries*, 258.

20. Derrida, "Structure, Sign, and Play," 283.

21. See Marian Yagel McBay, "Should Routine Childhood Immunizations Serve as an Exemplar of Minimal Risk in U.S. Regulation of Research Involving Children? A Closer Look at the Minimal Risk Threshold" (PhD diss., Vanderbilt University, 2001).

22. Rheinberger, "Beyond Nature and Culture," 260.

23. Mawer, *Mendel's Dwarf*, 52.

24. Claude Bernard, cited in Jay Katz, "The Consent Principle of the Nuremberg Code: Its Significance Then and Now," in Annas and Grodin, *The Naei Doctors*, 229.

25. Katz, "The Consent Principle," 231.

26. Ibid. As Franz J. Ingelfinger, a former editor of the *New England Journal of Medicine*, once insisted: "The subject's only real protection, the public as well as the medical profession must recognize, depends on the conscience and compassion of the investigator and his peers" ("Informed [But Uneducated] Consent," *New England Journal of Medicine* 287 [August 31, 1972]: 465–466).

27. This claim is expressly made by Gerald A. Weissmann, "The Need to Know: Utilitarian and Esthetic Values of Biomedical Science," in *New Knowledge in the Biomedical Sciences: Some Moral Implications of Its Acquisition, Possession, and Use*, ed. William B. Bondeson, H. Tristram Engelhardt Jr., Stuart F. Spicker, and Joseph M. White Jr. (Dordrecht: D. Reidel Publishing, 1982), 106–110.

28. Charles Darwin, *The Descent of Man and Selection in Relation to Sex*, rev. ed. (1874; repr., Chicago: Rand McNally, 1974), 130–131.

29. Kurt Bayertz, *GenEthics: Technological Intervention in Human Reproduction as a Philosophical Problem* (Cambridge: Cambridge University Press, 1994), 42–44.

30. Rheinberger, "Beyond Nature and Culture," 259, 253.

31. Ibid., 254; see Bruno Latour, *The Pasteurization of France* (Cambridge, MA: Harvard University Press, 1988), 71.

32. Ibid., 254.

33. See Edmund D. Pellegrino, ed., *Ethics, Trust, and the Professions: Philosophical and Cultural Aspects* (Washington, DC: Georgetown University Press, 1991).

34. The distrust is open and evident in, for instance, the rejection of human cloning by Leon Kass ("The Wisdom of Repugnance").

35. Barbara Ehrenreich," The Economics of Cloning," *Time* (November 22, 1963): 86.

36. See Nicholas Rescher, "Moral Issues Relating to the Economics of New Knowledge in the Biomedical Science," in *New Knowledge in the Biomedical Sciences: Some Moral Implications of Its Acquisition, Possession, and Use*, ed. William B. Bondeson, H. Tristram Engelhardt Jr., Stuart F. Spicker, and Joseph M. White (Dordrecht: D. Reidel Publishing, 1982), 33–45.

37. Itself a stark reminder of what Edmund Husserl pointed out at the beginning of the twentieth century in his 1910 essay in the journal *Logos*, "Philosophy as Rigorous Science," published in English together with "Philosophy and the Crisis of European Man," in *Phenomenology and the Crisis of Philosophy*, trans. and intro. Quentin Lauer (New York: Harper Torchbooks, 1965). Husserl picked up the theme much later in his *The Crisis of European Sciences and Transcendental Phenomenology*, ed. Walter Biemel, trans. and intro. David Carr (Evanston, IL: Northwestern University Press, 1970).

38. Hans Jonas, *The Phenomenon of Life* (Chicago: University of Chicago Press, 1966), 189.

39. Ibid., 194–195.

40. Hans Jonas, *The Imperative of Responsibility: In Search of an Ethics for the Technological Age* (Chicago: University of Chicago Press, 1984), 141.

41. H. Tristram Engelhardt Jr., "The Philosophy of Medicine: A New Endeavor," *Texas Reports on Biology and Medicine* 31 (1973): 451–452.

42. Hans Jonas, *Philosophical Essays: From Ancient Creed to Technological Man* (Englewood Cliffs, NJ: Prentice Hall, 1974), 18.

43. R. D. Laing, *The Politics of Experience* (New York: Pantheon Press, 1967).

44. Alfred Schutz, "The Problem of Transcendental Intersubjectivity in Husserl," in *Collected Papers* (The Hague: Martinus Nijhoff, 1966), 3:82.

45. Alfred Schutz, "Scheler's Theory of Intersubjectivity and the General Thesis of the Alter Ego," in *Collected Papers* (The Hague: Martinus Nijhoff, 1962), 1:168.

46. See Alfred Schutz and Thomas Luckmann, *Structures of the Life-World* (Evanston, IL: Northwestern University Press, 1973), 46.

47. Mawer, *Mendel's Dwarf*, 197, 198.

48. See Herbert Spiegelberg, "'Accident of Birth': A Non-Utilitarian Motif in Mill's Philosophy," *Journal of the History of Ideas* 22, No. 10 (1961): 475–492. and "Ethics for Fellows in the Fate of Experience," in *Mid-Twentieth Century American Philosophy: Personal Statements*, ed. Peter Bertocci (New York: Humanities Press, 1974), 193–210.

49. Mawer, *Mendel's Dwarf*, 238.

50. Ibid., 245.

51. Herbert Spiegelberg, "A Defense of Human Equality," *Philosophical Review* 53 (1944): 113.

52. Mawer, *Mendel's Dwarf*, 214–215.

53. See I. Wilmut, A. E. Schnieke, J. McWhir, A. J. Kind, and K. H. S. Campbell, "Viable Offspring" 810–813. See also *Cloning Human Beings*: Report and Recommendation of the National Bioethics Advising Commission (Rockville, MD: The Commission, 1997), 19–23.

54. In particular, the potentially lethal consequences from alien viruses and bacteria.

55. See Richard M. Zaner, *The Context of Self* (Athens: Ohio University Press, 1981), where I used a neologism to capture this complexity: complexure.

56. Jean Bethke Elshtain, "To Clone or Not to Clone," in *Clones and Clones: Facts and Fantasies about Human Cloning*, ed. Martha C. Nussbaum and Cass R. Sunstein (New York: W. W. Norton, 1998), 182.

57. Albert Camus, *The Myth of Sisyphus, and Other Essays* (New York: Vintage, 1955), 102.

8

Aristotle and Genetic Engineering: The Uncertainty of Excellence

Harold W. Baillie

I am a mystery to myself.
—Saint Augustine

Ethics discussions have a whiff of the tragic to them; to be reflective about action is, it seems, always to be a bit too late. Like the chorus in a Greek tragedy, ethicians comment, often wisely, on the action that has just taken place. Their evaluations are a careful analysis of the events in hopes of clarifying the future. But, just as the chorus sends the audience off with the admonition to not do what this fellow did or it will turn out badly for you as well, so too ethicians admonish their readers to avoid what seems inevitable.

The discussion of genetics and our understanding of human nature has this tone to it. There is a sense of wonder when facing the capabilities of our emerging knowledge of the genome, but we are caught between an overwhelming anticipation of what that knowledge will enable us to do and a nagging dread that hidden in that future is the moment of our self-destruction. Self-destruction, brought about by the hero's own hopeful ambitions and tragic flaws, remains the key to classic tragedy, and tragedy's continued hold over us is due to nothing less than our continued ignorance about who we are and what we are doing.

We live at a time when, for example, cloning sheep and cows is a reality, and the cloning of humans will occur any day.[1] In their efforts to further both career and knowledge, scientists are pushing inexorably toward that accomplishment, and the world hangs breathlessly on every news release. At the same time, voices are raised against such cloning, from the U.S. president Bill Clinton to Ian Wilmut, the lead scientist for the team that first successfully cloned a sheep and ushered in the recognition that large mammals can indeed be cloned. Citing a variety of religious and ethical arguments, these opponents of cloning and other technologies are vigorous but seemingly ineffectual, and their ranks thin as new possible accomplishments appear on the horizon. For example, the ranks of abortion foes split over stem cell research as it became apparent that stem cells hold serious possibilities for a wide variety of treatments. The innocent personhood of the fertilized egg was suddenly not quite so sanctified when treatment for the more mature was the issue and not a woman's control over her body.

Such issues are the stuff of contemporary ethics, and the timeliness of our discussions gives rise to a sense of both urgency and an opportunity to affect the course of action. If we could only get human nature right, or lay hold of the human condition, we might—to modify Karl Marx a little—be able to change the world by describing it. But there is a nagging sense of tragic limitations to our efforts: are we the actors we would like to think we are or the chorus watching the world slip by?

Consequently, it is difficult to know what to say about genetic engineering. Events and the ambitions they generate overtake today's ethics even while today's reflections have attempted to deal only with what happened yesterday. It appears we do not even have the time for tragedy.

A Commonplace about Genetic Engineering

An example of this dynamic can be found in the discussion of genetic therapy and engineering. For some time, it has been commonplace to argue that genetic therapy is ethically acceptable, while genetic enhancement should be forbidden. Somatic genetic therapy is acceptable because, by analogy with other therapies, it focuses on treating the individual with consequences that are limited to that individual. On the other hand, germ line genetic therapy and genetic enhancement are not acceptable. Germ line genetic therapy refers to changing an inheritable but undesirable genetic trait, while genetic enhancement usually means the conscious attempt to improve an existing "normal" human genome. The effects of both are inherited, and thus they may affect future generations in ways that we cannot foresee or evaluate. Hence, there is much more at stake than treating the individual, and our ignorance of possible outcomes is the basis for a seemingly compelling "No."

Yet the argument for germ line therapy is seductive. If we can prevent future generations from suffering inheritable genetic diseases such as Huntington's Chorea, or Tay-Sachs, or even diabetes, why not? These are clear diseases; they are fatal or debilitating, and expensive to treat; they seem to be prime targets for advances in genetic medicine. This leads to an interesting slippery slope, or perhaps an invitation to the obvious: in essence, germ line therapy is eugenics, at least in the sense that we would be improving the germ line by knocking out manifestly undesirable genetic traits. If germ line therapy is acceptable, perhaps genetic enhancement should be as well. Both involve genetic engineering, the discernment of desirable genetic makeups, and a certain control over future generations. Is our understanding of disease and health so clear that we are confident in rejecting the pursuit of advantages and accepting only the avoidance of potential catastrophes?

One reading of this slippery slope is that however reasonable the argument against genetic enhancement might sound to sympathetic ears, it is inadequate, and when the case against genetic enhancement rests on this alone, it will eventually crumble. In the crunch of daily survival and immediate possibilities, arguments rooted in our obligations to the future, especially when couched in terms of a cautious ignorance, have not been observed in practice as carefully as their proponents would want; for example, concerns about the environment or the future of diverse cultures are often voiced and seldom heeded.

Metaphysics as a Prolegomenon to Genetic Enhancement

If an effective (or at least more enlightening) case against genetic engineering can be made, it will be made on grounds that have immediate bearing on those drawn to the enterprise. My purpose in this chapter is to suggest that the appropriate ground for the argument is the idea of personhood and a particular understanding of personhood.

For such an argument, certain issues must be clarified. While the notion of personhood is an ethical concern, it must also have metaphysical roots. If genetic engineering gives rise to concerns that go beyond an evaluation of the consequences of an action or the political understanding of it, then it is because such a practice would be an alteration of the metaphysical nature of the human being. Thus, if there are to be effective arguments about genetic enhancement, they must represent a metaphysical discussion about human nature.

I will argue that such a discussion is possible and is rooted in two issues: the nature of our existence as physical beings, and the effect of mortality on the urgency of creating content for our lives.

There are certain conceptions of the soul that explicitly or implicitly encourage genetic engineering while in effect begging the question of the significance of altering the body. The concept of the soul has a long and significant role in philosophical as well as theological ethics. For one, there is the Platonic, Augustinian, or Cartesian view of the soul as a separate substance that uses the body as an instrument. Given this view, certainly the condition of the body dramatically influences the quality of human life endured by the soul, and the soul's success or failure in harnessing the impulses of the body in part depends on the challenges the body presents. But it cannot be alleged that the soul requires these challenges or would be harmed by the absence of these difficulties, unless the argument is supported by a claim that the soul needs to prove itself in some fashion by overcoming these difficulties. René Descartes, for example, is explicit about the advantages of improving the body for acquiring wisdom and happiness.[2] A *res cogitans* with a healthy body will be wiser and happier simply because the absence of bodily troubles will allow the soul's natural good sense to express itself more directly and efficiently. A soul that journeys with a well-formed and harmonious body still has work to do for wisdom (most obviously for Descartes, work in learning a method and developing the discipline necessary to stick with it), but in the absence of distractions, more of the soul's energy can be focused on the end to be achieved, rather than the insufficiencies of the means.

Another important example is Jean-Jacques Rousseau's view of the human being as a free being capable of radically changing its nature through the imitation of other creatures and, ultimately, even other members of its own species.[3] If we are capable of improving ourselves through imitating others, then the perception that some other animal has an advantage of a specific type becomes a model for imitation. Thus, if working in a group, being taller, or being stronger poses an advantage, then those characteristics are desirable. If the advantage allows for imitation, then others may acquire this advantage. By watching others, I may learn to hunt or to work in a group, assuming my existing abilities allow that. For Rousseau, the history of our capacity for imitation is the source of the inequality that so characterizes and divides modern society. From such a perspective, the assertion of a particular psychological or natural structure as characteristic of a human being is an ideological claim that represents and defends a segment of the human population to the detriment of the rest. Hence, Aristotle's human essence (not to mention the virtues of the *Nicomachean Ethics*) is a representation of a gentleman (the noble and the beautiful) of Athens circa 350 B.C.E., and cannot be taken as any metaphysical claim about human nature.

With regard to questions of genetic engineering, however, freedom speaks neither for nor against the quality of the body in which it resides. Freedom is in one's response to the conditions of life, regardless of what those conditions are. This in itself may suggest the lack of a true distinction between therapy and enhancement, if my inability to work in a group is due to a physical impairment such as depression or fear. Treat my depression or fear, and with my cured psyche I may now work in a group, improving the lot of all humans by imitating other social animals. If I live in a society that gives an advantage to tall people, then if I am short, or come from a long line of short people, perhaps "correcting" the gene for shortness will be a proper response to achieve imitative self-improvement. This is much more difficult technically than learning to work in a group, but in principle the very notion of freedom as self-overcoming does not oppose the idea. All we are doing is overcoming the currently understood limitations of human nature in favor of a perceived advantage. Thus, a Rousseauian could be understood to demand genetic enhancement rather than just tolerate it.

The only way to limit this possible influence of freedom would be to condition freedom with some other concern that would address the physical makeup of the free body. For example, the general will arising from the social contract might develop a principle that for the general good, such genetic engineering would be dangerous, and thus forbid it. Or it might stipulate that a general physical equality is to be enforced through genetic engineering. One's freedom regarding genetic manipulation would then be understood as an acquiescence to this determination of the general will, and a social imperative would conclude the debate.

Consequently, neither Descartes' idea of the soul nor Rousseau's sense of freedom provides us with a ground to argue against genetic enhancement, and indeed may even encourage arguments for it. If the intuition that genetic enhancement is somehow dangerous and unethical is to be defended, it is not on the grounds of the person as a soul (at least as res cogitans) or as free (at least where freedom is taken as self-overcoming). If a claim is to be made that genetic enhancement is a good to be vigorously pursued, the very idea that the soul is free may support the contention.

Our Existence as Physical Beings

I wish to argue for a rethinking of the traditional Aristotelian view of the soul. For Aristotle, an essence (*to ti hen enai*) was what the thing is in virtue of itself.[4] This is an understanding of the experienced thing, an individual of form and matter with a *telos*, or finality, that was intrinsic to, constitutive of, and evaluative of the thing itself. The modern arguments of freedom and social constructivism have insisted that such a view of the thing is simply wrong. The structure that such a telos implies, they assert, can be better understood socially, as the historically based result of social structure or individual choices.

Against such claims, I do not wish to return to a naively metaphysical view of, in particular, human nature. But I do wish to emphasize and use some of the insights that remain enduring in Aristotle's view, and in doing so, suggest that modern disputes over such distinctions as essentialist-nonessentialist or teleological-nonteleological are not helpful. Perhaps most important is Aristotle's insistence that the subject of discussion is the *tode ti*, the concrete individual that has some sort of identity. It is this individual that we experience, not the species (or if a human individual, society or history). Aristotle preferred to settle arguments by a return to our experience of the thing, separable and this, not by turning to some theoretical criterion, even that of logical consistency.[5] He would have little truck with the Parmenidean insistence that logic speaks more loudly than experience, and it is this allegiance to the thing that separates Aristotle from some of his greatest students, notably (for modern sensibilities) G. W. F. Hegel and Marx.

This return to our experience of the individual as a *tode ti* (some-thing separable and identifiable) has several elements to it, some of which are unavoidably Aristotelian, and some of which not. The Aristotelian elements that are most unavoidable are the form and the matter of his hylomorphic psychology. This is, of course, quite traditional, but the hylomorphic psychology is worth a fresh look when it has been severed from the traditional understanding of the structured teleology of Aristotle's own position. The less-traditional Aristotelian elements are the basics of human life, which Aristotle himself, although obviously aware of, ignored in favor of his teleological ideals of human life. These basics are birth, suffering, and death (or as Aristotle insisted, that stories have a beginning, a middle, and an end; even metaphysical explanation must have a beginning, a middle, and an end). Every human being lives these events; they are not the objects of choice, they are subjects of reflection, and as such the substance of reflection.

A Hylomorphic Psychology

I would suggest that if there is to be an argument against genetic enhancement that has immediate import for us as existing persons, it is to be found in the tradition of Aristotle or Saint Thomas Aquinas—that is, in a hylomorphic psychology. There are two basic reasons for this claim, and one obvious objection. A hylomorphic psychology avoids the Scylla of the abstract comfort of freedom in the face of the material rootedness of the discussion of genetic enhancement, and the Charybdis of a materialism that issues in a genetic determinism that undercuts the very idea that there is a moral dilemma in this discussion. The obvious objection is that a hylomorphic psychology is a curiosity rooted in an outdated metaphysics, which has at best a nostalgic appeal in this postmodern age. A full response to this objection would have to take to task the predominant view of the last century, and there is no reasonable opportunity to do that here. But insofar as the points made in favor of discussing hylomorphic psychology in the context of genetic enhancement have any persuasive power, they become a suggestion of the need to question the resolutely antimetaphysical bent of contemporary philosophy. It is in human frailty rooted in materiality and the possibility of overcoming it held out by genetic engineering that we see the true advantages of a hylomorphic psychology to enhance the discussion. A hylomorphic psychology suggests that the advantages offered by genetic engineering are illusory since they at best appear to accomplish what is the function of the soul while in fact leaving that function untouched. The body is altered, but the soul is not.[6]

The basic relevant claim of a hylomorphic psychology is that, as Aristotle put it, the soul is the first *entelechia* of a body composed of organs (*organikon*).[7] The body is a natural object that possesses life: meaning, at least, it is capable of nutrition, growth, and reproduction. But the body in this sense is a composite; its material cause is the organic material, while the form is the entelecheia of that matter. Entelecheia is normally translated as actuality, the end of a motion (*kinesis*) or activity (*energeia*).[8] What matters here is its meaning. In talking about the soul, Aristotle understands the entelecheia to be a sort of transition, the completion of the body as its life, and the possibility of further activities (or energeia) of the living being. He points out that there are two relevant senses of actuality, analogous to the possession of knowledge and the exercise of it.[9] Entelecheia in this case refers to the first sense, the possession. This is because as the first end of a body, Aristotle means that the soul is the life of the body, the change that a body expresses that shows its living nature, as opposed to the inert nature of, for instance, a rock or a statue, but also to be distinguished from the particular activities that a living being might perform because it is alive.

Aristotle describes energeia in opposition to kinesis, or motion. A kinesis has its end outside itself, and it thus is interruptible. A kinesis is always incomplete; as long as the motion is present, the end has not been attained, and when the end is attained, the motion is absent. A simple example of a motion is walking to the store. As long as you are walking to the store, you are not at the store; when you are at the store, you are no longer walking to it. By contrast, an energeia contains its own end (or telos) and cannot be interrupted. It is complete whenever it occurs, and every instance it occurs. This is why the concept of energeia does the work of describing the change or process of living for Aristotle. His illustrations of this include sensing and thinking, but listening to music or even a child playing are examples as well.[10]

By defining the soul as the first *entelechia* of a body with organs, Aristotle supposes the soul to be the natural completion of the body. As he makes clear in both *de Anima* and the *Nicomachean Ethics*, the entelecheia of the body is a life of a variety of capabilities, desires, emotions, and reasoning.[11] The natural completion of the body is a process of physical and psychological growth driven by the inherent structure of the human being,[12] and for the purpose of accomplishing the activities for which the body is suited. The human being is complete as a human being, each and every instant of its existence; but this completeness is nevertheless a process by which the structure of the being is expressed, and that expression is (in the development of a happy life) made more transparent over time. This can be illustrated by looking at the differences between Thomas Hobbes and Aristotle on the subject of happiness. Hobbes rejects the reality of any entelecheia understood as making possible an energeia; so that for Hobbes life is endless motion, the pursuit of the satisfaction of desire after desire, with no particular accomplishment attributable to the satisfaction of any particular desire. For Hobbes, happiness is always temporary, satisfaction quickly overcome by new desires.[13] For Aristotle, the performance of certain capabilities is the completion of the life of the body, what the body exists to be. Happiness is the energeia of virtue, a stable, active state of completion, satisfying, pleasurable, and (for humans, to a limited extent) self-sustaining. For Hobbes, the body is always an instrument, for Aristotle, fundamentally it is not. For Aristotle, it is the presence, the actuality, of the end. In short, the concept of the entelecheia of the soul as making possible an energeia is central to the notion of a hylomorphic psychology.

But what is entelecheia when put in these terms, especially when it is applied to its obvious focus and source: human beings? One important, and counterintuitive, observation is that it is passive, or perhaps better, it is limited; it suffers the limitations of materiality. Aristotle described the soul as the completion of a body with organs. The soul, as an entelecheia, a completion, not a completer, not a doer, but an expression of the capabilities of the body itself. The passivity is an expression of what was already there, contained potentially in the body and released by the soul to be the activity, the energeia, of what was already there. The body is not the result and simple consequent of the activity of the soul; again, the soul is not a maker of the body. In a sense, the body is already there, as material cause, or as might be said today, genetics. From this perspective, the activity of the soul is constrained by the capabilities of the body and appears almost as an epiphenomenon.

Passivity and Activity

The constraints imposed by the material composition of the body are an important part of our nature. We are not gods because we have a material cause and tire in all our activities, even thinking.[14] Pleasure and pain also influence our activity, as Aristotle notes: "Our activities are sharpened, prolonged and improved by their own pleasure," and "when an activity causes pain, this pain destroys it."[15] We are constrained by the material circumstances of our lives: "Since man's nature is not self-sufficient for the activity of contemplation, [the philosopher] must also have bodily health and a supply of food and other requirements," maintains Aristotle.[16] These represent limitations on the soul that arise from the materiality of the body. Aristotle is clear that happiness requires favorable material circumstances for a happy life, among them good birth, health, satisfactory children, personal beauty, wealth, friends, political power, and a life long enough to have all of this.[17] In particular, death limits the person, and as an example, presents Aristotle with a conundrum as to whether a dead person may be considered happy and what conditions might change that evaluation. These are limits present in the person because of the material cause, and they present both obstacles and opportunities for the actualization of the person—that is, the activity that is the soul.

In addition to this passivity, the soul is also the activity of that body; it is its completion and its presence. It is the *essence* manifested in the thing; the doing of what the body both allows and is brought to. The soul brings the body to completion and makes the whole more than the sum of its parts. This completion is a discovery of the capabilities of the body, wherein the body is taken its inertness and its structured materiality (entelecheia, its actuality as a living substance) to its activity (energeia). Because it is beyond the body, because the whole person is more than the sum of its parts, the activity of the soul cannot be conclusively anticipated by the structure of its materiality. The limits of the activity—birth, struggle, death—may be anticipated, but the activity itself remains beyond any rational interpretation arising solely from the material structure itself. Rooted in a structured passivity, the activity of the soul appears as a surprise, a serendipitous discovery of the person.

This interpretation is at odds with strong criticism that Aristotle's faculty psychology, and as a result his ethics, is reflective of the Athenian social structure and hence unwittingly a social construction disguised as essentialist metaphysics. The argument of this chapter is that Aristotle's distinction between entelecheia and energeia in his conception of the soul is metaphysically deeper than is suggested by a faculty psychology, and is not wedded to the identity of virtues based on the structure of the human being as described in the *Nicomachean Ethics*. But it is not clear that the depiction of the social virtues as historical and perhaps ideological renders the metaphysical concept of the soul as the entelecheia of the body inappropriate and ethically useless; instead, this conception of the soul is useful in its establishing teleological limits rather than teleological necessities. Thus, a hylomorphic psychology need not be dismissed as merely the reification of accepted social categories and modes of interpretation. Time and again, we see the development of the life of the human body occur in ways mysterious and unexpected. It is ourselves as active beings (as energeia) we do not understand, and this is the point where genetic enhancement appears as a metaphysical issue, not simply as an ethical problem.

Human Nature: Freedom or Serendipity?

Fundamental to human life and development is an openness and responsiveness to the unexpected and serendipitous—that is, the soul as the activity of the body. This is a characteristic we find in evolutionary theory as well: random mutations are tested and selected by the challenges of the environment, and the successful mutation is the one that reproduces itself with the greatest fecundity. But what is unexpected and serendipitous occurs against a background of the expected and the routine. The difference, of course, is the claim that it is the soul that is the source and evaluator of human serendipity, while it is the environment that is such for evolution.

The point of revisiting Aristotle's hylomorphic psychology is thus not an effort to return to a discussion of the virtues as the basis for speaking of today's metaphysical or ethical problems. Criticisms of Aristotle's depiction of the human essence, its faculty psychology, its (often misunderstood) teleology, its reification of historical social roles and opportunities, may be left to stand. Rather, the issue is a reexamination of the metaphysical basis of human life and how that may cast light on the discussion of genetic engineering. Does genetic engineering touch in a profound sense what we are, and may its practice forever alter and perhaps efface human nature?

Death

The most dramatic way in which genetic engineering could alter human nature would be to slow the process of aging or do away completely with death. Our struggle with death and our desire to overcome it are illustrated throughout all forms of literature. The rewards of being a good human being are generally put in some form of eternal life, whether it be the transformation of heroes in Greek mythology, the eternal salvation of Christianity, or the release from the wheel of life in Hinduism. Another dramatic possible effect of genetic engineering would be service in the pursuit of perfection, to eliminate flaws and certain types of limitations that impede the accomplishment of a sense of the ideal. Both of these possible effects are areas of obvious linkage between cultural attitudes and medical science. As medical science is transformed by genetics, the long-standing Cartesian expectation that medicine is the most promising route for human moral, as well as physical, improvement seems well within our grasp.

The possibility of escaping death seems to be inextricably connected with the enmattered nature of human life. We die, learn, struggle, forget, and fail, all because of our physical nature. Thus, it seems that the matter of our nature is what is the matter with it.

This issue has received much attention in the history of Western philosophy; consequently, it is much too big to be adequately enjoined here. For the sake of illustration, and consistent with the approach already taken in this argument, a brief look at Aristotle's handling of the question of the limitation of being material would be appropriate. If Joseph Owens is correct, the focus and goal of the argument in Aristotle's *Meta-*

physics is the proof of the existence of an immaterial substance—that is, the unmoved mover or god.[18] Structurally, there is no doubt that the unmoved mover, or pure activity (energeia) is crucial to Aristotle's system. But is the point of the system to show the existence of god (a central concern for Aquinas), or is the importance of the existence of god not so much in the conclusion that god exists or in the work that god does in the system itself? If the former, then, like Aquinas, Aristotle will find humans existing in the shadow of God. But, if the answer is in the latter possibility, then the question of the point of the system itself becomes the primary question, and Aristotle's human is different. Metaphysically, the conceptual point of contact between humans and god regards activity (energeia). Activity is god's nature, purely actual, utterly immaterial. Humans may aspire to this (that is, happiness is the activity of virtue), but because of the simple reality of their emmattered form, they cannot achieve it.

When he describes pure energeia, the substance of god, Aristotle depicts it as thought thinking thought.[19] The basis for this is the pureness of divine activity as shown in the proof of the existence of god. Since divine existence is shown by the necessity of a prime mover, a pure activity the existence of which prevents an infinite regress of potencies actualized by another being in act that itself had an origin in potency, divine existence must be that pure activity. Such pure activity, he thinks, must be thought, following both Greek tradition (in, for example, Xenophanes and Parmenides) and his own suggestion that human thinking is the least enmattered of all human activities.

Aristotle further argues that divine thought must be about something, or else it would be more like divine sleeping and unworthy of veneration as a first cause. But if it must be about something, either a god thinks of itself or of something else; and if it thinks of something else, then it must be something that is either always the same or something that changes. But does it make any difference whether a god is thinking of that which is noble rather than of any chance thing? Would it not be absurd for such a being to be thinking of anything less than the most noble things? Clearly, then, Aristotle's god is thinking of that which is most divine and most honorable, and it is not changing, for change could only be for the worse, and this change would then be motion (kinesis).

Divine thinking must be eternally about itself, for any other subject would sully the divine purity. Thus, god's telos, contained in its activity of thinking, is clearly known because of its simplicity.

It is important for Aristotle and many others that the reality that human thought and divine thought share is this energeia. But there is no question that Aristotle's human is in fact an enmattered form, and there is no activity independent of that cause or origin (arche). While divine thinking is of itself, human thinking must have an object; we necessarily think about something that has its epistemological source in experience. Nevertheless, throughout the human thinking of an object is the activity of thinking itself, and here the descriptions of human thought and divine thought match. For example, energeia in both god and humans is life, pleasure, and self-awareness—that is, the awareness of activity or energeia as what one is doing. This similarity can lead to a perhaps too enthusiastic reading of the role of Aristotle's god as final cause and a sense that the blessed person of the *Nicomachean Ethics* somehow escapes the normal human condition; but that reading is wrong. Human thought, even in its best moments, is always enmattered, never the pure activity of divine thinking. Thus, the activity of human thought contains an end or telos that is complicated by its enmattered origins. The challenge of human thinking is found in both what it thinks about and what it does in thinking about this object of thought. Unlike divine thought, when humans think about themselves, they think about complex things they have learned about through experience, and they may respond to those complex things in many ways. There is no direct analogy between the simplicity of the activity of divine thinking and the complex activity of human thinking, nor any persuasive hope that human thought can be divine. Hence, due acknowledgment of the role of matter in human thinking, or as well, human nature, is necessary to get our understanding of human thinking right, and in so doing to get the nature of human nature complete.

Aristotle's god thinks only of itself (process) because that is what is most (Aristotle suggests) noble. But it can be objected that the absence of matter in god, and the consequent absence of death and the possibility of failure, strips god of thoughtfulness and moral life, and would do the same for us. The eventuality of our death (the most cataclysmic consequence of our enmattered nature) and, along the way, the continual possibility of failure injects conditions into our energeia (the activities of both our thinking and our life itself) and gives it content. Any attempt to remove death or failure is an attempt to deny the material cause of human life—that is, the need for and the accomplishment of development and growth. To do so through genetic engineering would be exactly what it is described as: a triumph over our nature.

Effects of Materiality: Birth, Death, Failure, and Serendipity

From the perspective of Aristotelian metaphysics, a full discussion of the role of matter in human life centers on the possibility of substantial change. We are born, and we die: that is the primary effect of our materiality. There are, of course, a variety of additional effects of materiality: the need to eat, grow, and reproduce as conditions of life itself; the opportunity to sense, imagine, and locomote as expressions of animality; and the possibility of speaking, learning, acting, and thinking as the opportunities of human life. But all these activities take place within the bookends of birth and death.

Birth makes it clear that we develop. It is a beginning, a setting off of a person, a future of possibilities.[20] But these possibilities are, for humans, human possibilities. They are the first actuality of our bodies (the entelecheia). It is at birth that our material humanness exists in the raw, so to speak, without the complications of a history. The dominant activities (energeia) are the ones basic to life: nutrition and growth.

The focus of genetic engineering is the body actualized: genetic engineering attempts to control, or at least alter, the material humanness of the person. The fallacy of genetic engineering is its claim to alter the person (the energeia built on the entelecheia of the body) by altering the body. Genetic engineering seeks to transform the body from a constant possibility of inertness into a source of direction and development for a person's life; it seeks to eliminate the need for a soul by substituting a developed genetic code for the serendipity of the soul. The person, as energeia built on the entelecheia of the body, is not defined by the structure, although it is confined by the structure. Function may be limited by form, but it is not defined by form. There is still the need for the soul as energeia.

What defines us is what we do, and we do things under the recognition of death, the recognition of the eventual triumph of the potential for inertness of our body. Death is a break in the iteration of our days; it may or may not happen now, so the recognition of our death, our finitude, becomes an issue for us. Our body (as matter) as it is, is passive; it is the true nature and source of our finitude. If there is a general desire on the part of matter for form (as Aristotle suggests), then the matter that we are seeks its actualization in the serendipity and energeia of the soul that we are.[21] The living body is the body of the activity of the soul; the soul is the living of the body that is beyond the given. The recognition of our death is the threat of being nothing beyond the inertness, the givenness, of our body. The recognition of finitude is the source of an imperative to act and do so rationally because our existence indicates itself only through such action. Thus, death is the ultimate human closure, the recognition of which is the recognition that all possibilities cannot be put off forever, and that priorities must be established and followed. It is death that forces us to face the issue of an appropriate development of content in our lives.

The threat of death forces content into our lives as the means of escaping the inertness that remains a constant possibility of the body. Hannah Arendt, for example, discusses action as the insertion of the individual into the human world.[22] Without such an insertion, the individual never exists; thus, an ultimate motive for action is the fear of never having existed. The difference is rooted in what we understand ourselves primordially to be. Arendt has the sense that there is a self, a force that motivates our speech and is revealed to others in speaking, even if we are unaware of that self ourselves. This supports the suggestion that there is a spontaneity to each life, a sense that each life is a discovery waiting to happen. This is not the assertion of a self-created self but a discovery of a self, a discovery of what was already (potentially) there, by asserting the need for it to exist.

The Possibility of Failure (We Might Be Heroes, but We Are Not Gods)

Fall 2001 was the time of one of the most thrilling World Series in the history of baseball. Games were won—and lost—in last inning, just before the last out. The reigning champions (the New York Yankees) were challenged by youth (the Arizona Diamondbacks), yet they hung on to redeem the value of age and experience, only—again at the last opportunity—to be dethroned by the slimmest of margins with the heroes thwarted after what seemed to be another improbable success. 2002 (and every next year) appeared as a challenge for the new champions, and the opportunity for revenge for everyone else.

Why do we live for such moments? The answer seems to be found in the uncertainty of the outcome, the possibility of the hoped-for success, but also the possibility of failure. It sounds a bit pessimistic, but failure is more likely than success, the mundane more likely than the extraordinary. When Arendt talks of the person as a beginning, of the insertion of the individual into public space, she allows as well for a discussion of the failure of such efforts. It has been said that life is what happens while you are making plans.[23] This is particularly true when we plan for the development of the self. Life plans are difficult phenomena in that the more explicit and rigorous they are, the more prone they are to failure or the sacrifice of one who is the subject of the plan. In large measure, this can be explained by the argument that the self is discovered, not created.

Importantly, the most serious challenge to any attempt to discover the self is the possibility of failure; I may not find what is there to be found. Since I do not know (explicitly and completely) what I am looking for, and since there may be something there for me to find, I may not find it.

From the vantage point of this observation, a significant difficulty posed by genetic engineering is brought into view. While it is generally overshadowed by the concern with death, we have an important concern with the possibility of failure. We may be put under compulsion to act by our fear of death and the possibility of never having existed, but once undertaken, our actions are dogged by our limitations. All too aware of the uncertain outcome of our intentions, we turn to whatever means available to increase the chances of success. Can we use genetic engineering to more successfully accomplish our life plans? In so doing, are we not trying to eliminate failure? Of particular interest is the possibility of living a perfect life, that is, a life completely congruent with the expectations held for that life. If failure is a large part of life, and a large part of the learning that we do in life, then the elimination of failure has serious consequences for our understanding of what it means to be human. We can applaud (and have almost always applauded) the composite who accomplishes his or her individual goals through effort and good fortune. But we seem not to feel the same way about someone who has done only what he or she could easily do. A hylomorphic psychology suggests that there is a significant difference between a life in which the composite, the whole composed of matter and form, struggles to accomplish its goal and a life in which the struggle is prevented by "perfecting" the material conditions of that life. In short, there is a difference between the person and the material cause. In a hylomorphic metaphysics, the raw material of the body is always subject to some form—the open question is the source and influence of the form. Will its source be social expectations and ideals, or the natural entelecheia of human life and the spontaneity (the energeia) that has been characteristic of human nature?

Genetic engineering affects the body as matter, not the body as form. In other words, genetic engineering is the manipulation of the body, and such manipulation works alongside and below the activities of the soul. As such, genetic engineering is the manipulation of the condition (the entelecheia) of the human person—that is, a manipulation of its limits. Matter changes up to a point without changing the substance. The point where changes in the matter change the substance is a significant issue, one that presents a discussion of the nature of the death of the individual or the evolution of the species.

It is important to remember that genetic engineering always influences the next (and possibly successive) generations. The choices that one might make regarding the genetic makeup of a future child reflect several assumptions. Perhaps the most important is the assumption about progress. To refine a future person's genetic makeup is to improve them in some way. This sense of improvement rests on a metaphysical presupposition that life moves in a (more or less) straight line; that tomorrow will be different than today, and it is open to being better or worse. We are thought to bear responsibility for the future, and for goodhearted people to shoulder that responsibility is to strive to make tomorrow better. Given such an intellectual context, the obligation to at least alleviate disease (that is, germ line therapy) seems compelling.

Yet one can question the assumption that life moves forward to a different tomorrow. There are certainly events that take place in one's life, or more comprehensively, in history, that are unrepeatable in their specificity due to the causal contribution of particular human agency. But it is still the case that those events take place within the bookmarks of birth and death, and those events are performed by agents who learned, struggled, succeeded, or failed as human beings. Those events take place within the cycle of life that grounds and contextualizes the human individual. Generation and corruption are the unavoidable metaphysical and ontological ground of human life.

When we consider the genetic manipulation of the body, a central element in our thinking will be how we think about the future. Are we making it different because it is and will be our opportunity (perhaps even our birthright) to influence how it will be different? Or are we making it different by warping the cycle so that when we look at the struggles of future generations, they will still course on the center of birth, struggle, and death, yet wobble with the added burden of self-inflicted wounds?

Personhood and the Argument against Genetic Enhancement

For my argument, I would define personhood as the entelechy of the body, Aristotle's sense of soul. Personhood thus calls for an openness to what I, or any human being, will become by the living that I do. The serendipitous ways I will respond to my biologically, socially, and temporally grounded opportunities reveal my person. When another prohibitively limits the range of my responses, on the basis of their intention or a larger social design, my personhood is diminished or even destroyed.

By contrast, John Rawls's analysis of justice as fairness suggests a different approach to this question.[24] That people become ill seems unfair. That they suffer deformities or dysfunctions due to nature seems unfair. In Rawls's famous phrase, they have lost the natural lottery, and that is not right. Given that genetic enhancement purports to mold the human genome into something more suitable to our sense of appropriateness and fairness, the problematic concern is not human nature but rather an equitable social response to unfairness. In Rawls's view, at least with regard to those issues that bear on the distribution of goods, the society has a limited obligation of justice to redress this unfairness. It is a small jump from this position to one that suggests that society has an obligation to redress the unfairness of illness and deformity, and genetic enhancement presents itself as a superb means to do this most efficiently.

This argument, however, is flawed because it ignores a larger concern with the effect that genetic enhancement has on our ability to act in our full human capacity. That nature is indeed unfair is certainly an important point, and where possible and appropriate, it is one that calls on us for redress. In part, this a justification for medical practice itself, and in particular, it has been cited as a justification for somatic and germ line therapy. But redressing inequities can level the playing field by reducing life to its least common denominators or its recognizable short-term gains. The "promise" of genetic enhancement is that we can alter and augment known and recognized human abilities. The meaning of "known and recognized" human abilities is the issue. We will (quite logically) engineer those enhancements that we understand to be beneficial to current success in society. But what we understand at any given time to be beneficial is subject to constraints established by the limits of our knowledge and the current expectations of our society. We are likely to engineer for the present we understand and not the future we do not.

But there is more to this issue than the dangers of the consequences of not knowing quite what we are doing. As Hans Jonas and others have argued, it is certainly important to wonder about and analyze the ethical implications of the very real consequences of genetic engineering on future generations.[25] But this approach is incomplete. The true impact of genetic modifications is in their ability to mask from us our own nature—that is, deny our personhood. We discover ourselves only through historical experience, the activity of the soul in completing the body (to return to Aristotle's phrasing). In that sense, we are not something made (poiesis) in which the end is generally foreseen by the artisan in commencing production. Rather, we are an activity (energeia) that opens up to an end (telos); we have within us an end discoverable only in the hard work of living what we are. If we try to make ourselves, we deny the activity of our soul by replacing it with the activity of our reason; we substitute the part for the whole.

This is the modern criticism of traditional ethics turned on modern aspirations. While it may be true that Aristotle fell victim to his culture's view of the good person—and if so, it is a serious limitation of his work—what protection do we have that we are not making the same mistake? If we choose to enhance a particular characteristic of current value, what assurance have we that we are not using our science to perpetuate our self-image?

Givenness and Serendipity

By contrast, I am arguing that we are given to ourselves, yet we do not know what has been given. Insofar as I have a future, I do not know myself. Part of that future will be the result of choices I make for reasons that I am aware of and understand. But it is also the case that my future contains surprises for me—changes in attitude, twists of fate, unintended consequences, or simple growth and maturity that I neither anticipate nor understand given my current experience and knowledge. Whatever I will be in twenty years, or twenty days for that matter, will be the result of happenings both anticipated and unanticipated. I will be more than, or less than, and in any case different than my current hopes for myself. That, of course, is what distinguishes me from my machines and my pets. The surprises my car holds for me involve how long it will work, not what kind of work it will do, while my dog holds surprises not only of longevity but also obedience. In part, what makes my pet more interesting than my car (and considerably less useful) are the surprises he holds in store for me.

My children illustrate the same point on a much more profound level. There is a role played out by my desires for my children, but there is a strange and remarkable interaction between parental design and the child's emerging life, in which both elements have their role to play, the dominant one being the child's life.

This is the point of importance for the thought of genetic enhancement. I cannot claim to know the full adequacy of my plans, nor can I claim the power to bring those plans to completion. I am a player in the drama of life and its regeneration, but only one player among many, only one limited, mistake-prone intelligence, one storm-tossed, blindly insightful emotional presence. The only antidote I have to my finitude is time, the time to let myself, my children, and my friends live themselves into what they are. If I try to choose the future of my children (or my genetic products) in the profoundly mechanistic and permanent way of altering their genetic makeup, I turn them into my limited, finite projections, stripping them of their complexity, their otherness, and their capacity to surprise. Certainly, as a parent, my goals and aspirations for my children are a part of their being and their future. But as noted above, the more power I assume for myself to engineer my children to accomplish my goals for them, the more completely I substitute the part for the whole, and in so doing alter their very being.

In the conclusion to *Frankenstein*, Mary Shelley summarizes Frankenstein's reaction to the monster as disgust at both his appearance and the malevolence of his actions. But obviously my analysis suggests that the problem is on a more profound level: the scientist's ambition to create life, rooted in the new technologies of science, blinded him to what life really is. Frankenstein assumed the monster would live the life the scientist anticipated, which is what he expected on the basis of cultural assumptions and blinkered thought, and he was unprepared for the monster's own course and own desires. Frankenstein forgot the very serendipity that is central to human life. He succeeded beyond his wildest dreams, but his dreams, however ambitious, were those limited dreams of a modern scientist, dreams of a technology of life, and thus were inadequate to the real issue. The problem was not that his techniques were crude; it was that his assumptions about personhood were deeply flawed.

This chapter began with some comments about the ability of ethics to affect basic decisions about what we, particularly those of us involved with research into genetic engineering, will do. The comments were pessimistic. To worry about the subsequent impact of genetic alteration is a real and serious concern, but a type of concern that again and again has been ignored by human risk taking and ambition. The argument of this chapter has been that the certainty and assertiveness inherent to genetic engineering is opposed to and subversive of the reality of human nature. Indeed, so compelling is the promise of the development of genetic engineering that most of this argument has been focused on identifying a way of talking about the more fragile and tentative discovering of a human being, recognizing its embodiment and yet revealing more. We are much more likely to grasp the engineered future than we are to commit ourselves to the uncertain progress of individuals buffeted by flaws, failures, and death. To do so, unfortunately, is to leach out the surprise, the beauty, and the accomplishment that is the true, yet ephemeral, fruit of human life. Since the loss of the ephemeral can be easily forgotten, the price of such a choice will not be obvious or compelling. We will simply live out the uneasy distinction of having reversed Geppetto's preference for a real son over a puppet.

Notes

1. The week I am writing this, Advanced Cell Technology has announced their (failed) attempts at cloning human embryos. The announcement of failure was made for several reasons, including the desire to be first and the desire for the research support that comes to those who are first. Apparently, it is just as good to be the first failure as it is to be the first success in today's research investment market.

2. René Descartes, *Discourse on Method*, in *The Philosophical Works of Descartes*, trans. Elizabeth S. Haldane and G.R.T. Ross (New York: Cambridge University Press, 1970), 1:119–120.

3. Jean-Jacques Rousseau, "Discourse on Inequality among Men," in *The Essential Rousseau*, trans. Lowell Bair (New York: New American Library, 1974), 146–147, 152–153.

4. Aristotle, *Metaphysics* 7.4.1029b14.

5. This is clear in Aristotle's argument that matter is not the primary sense of substance (*Metaphysics* 7.4.1029a8–30). Also for this reason, it is inappropriate to speak of natural laws in Aristotle's metaphysics; there are only natural things.

6. This is in dramatic opposition to Cartesian dualism, which takes the view that the weakness of the body causes a weakness in the mind; when the weakness of the body is removed, generally by medical care, the mind gains in wisdom: "We may find a practical philosophy by means of which . . . [we] render ourselves masters and possessors of nature. . . . This is . . . to be desired principally because it brings about the preservation of health, which is without doubt the chief blessing and the foundation of all other blessings in this life. For the mind depends so much on the temperament and disposition of the bodily organs that, if it is possible to find a means of rendering men wiser and cleverer than they have hitherto been, I believe it is in medicine that it must be sought" (Descartes, *Discourse*, 119–120).

7. Aristotle, *de Anima* 2.1.412a29.

8. Aristotle, *de Anima* 2.1.412a20–23 and *Metaphysics* 9.3.1047a30–1047b1, 1050a15–24.

9. Aristotle, *de Anima* 2.1.412a223.

10. Aristotle, *Metaphysics* 9.6.1048b28–35.

11. Aristotle, *Nicomachean Ethics* 1.8.1102a28–1103a4.

12. Or for that matter any living substance. This is presumably the source of Hans Jonas's argument regarding the role of metabolism in identifying the purposiveness of life (*The Phenomenon of Life* [Chicago: University of Chicago Press, 1982], 74–83).

13. Thomas Hobbes, *Leviathan* (New York: Penguin Books, 1985), 129–130.

14. See Aristotle, *Nicomachean Ethics* 10.4.1175a3–5.

15. Ibid., 10.5.1175b15, 1175b18.

16. Ibid., 10.8.1178b34–1179a4.

17. Ibid., 1.8.1099a31–1099b10.

18. Joseph Owens, *The Doctrine of Being in the Aristotelian Metaphysics*, 2nd ed. (Toronto: Pontifical Institute of Medieval Studies 1963).

19. Aristotle, *Metaphysics* 12.9.1074b15–1075a11.

20. See Hannah Arendt, *The Human Condition* (Chicago: University of Chicago Press, 1998).

21. Aristotle, *Physics* 1.9.192a16–19.

22. Arendt, *The Human Condition*, 176–181.

23. At least, it has been said by the secretary for the philosophy department of the University of Scranton. I do not know of a more original source.

24. John Rawls, *A Theory of Justice* (Cambridge, MA: Harvard University Press, 1971). For a development of this position in regard to genetic engineering, see Allan Buchanan, Dan W. Brock, Norman Daniels, and Daniel Wikler, *From Chance to Choice: Genetics and Justice* (New York: Cambridge University Press, 2000), 258–303.

25. See, for example, Hans Jonas, "Biological Engineering: A Preview," in *Philosophical Essays* (Chicago: University of Chicago Press, 1981), 141–167.

III

Freedom and Telos

9

Human Recency and Race: Molecular Anthropology, the Refigured Acheulean, and the UNESCO Response to Auschwitz

Robert N. Proctor

That Neanderthals are thought of in terms of a "problem" or a "question" is remarkably similar to the way in which Germans thought about Jews prior to World War II. In both instances, the objects of such treatment were cast in the role of a collective "other" whose differences have been assumed to indicate the extent of their failure to qualify for fully human status.

—C. Loring Brace, *Evolution in an Anthropological View*

When did humans become human? Did this happen five million or fifty thousand years ago? How sudden was the transition, and is this even a meaningful question? Strange as it may seem, there is radical disagreement over the timing of human evolution, understood as the coming-into-being of the language-using symbolic cultural creature of today. No one knows whether speech, consciousness, or the human aesthetic sense are fairly recent phenomena (circa fifty thousand years ago) or ten or even fifty times that old—though it seems that recency currently enjoys the upper hand.[1] For many years, it was fashionable to project "humanness" (whatever that might mean) onto any and every hominid scratched out by a paleontologist; Lucy was "our oldest ancestor," an australopithecine "woman" (versus "female"); and even older hominids were sometimes granted humanity. Today, however, it is more common to see the australopithecines as far more chimplike; humanness is often not even granted to *Homo erectus*, the earliest of our genus (itself an arbitrary designation), and there are those who do not want to see the Neanderthals or even early *Homo sapiens* as "fully human."

What is going on here? What makes us want to grant or withdraw humanity from a given or presumptive ancestor? What is the evidence one way or the other, and what larger prejudices are at stake?

Here, I would like to explore some of the separate lines of argument leading to the idea that humanness is a relatively recent phenomenon—no more than 150,000 years, and perhaps even as recent as 50,000 years, since that is when we find the first self-representation, compound tools, and other signs of human intelligence or symbolic behavior. Now, I don't want to get bogged down in definitions—and to avoid doing so, let me operationalize humanness by equating it for a moment with language and culture—recognizing also that these categories are no more secure, no less in flux, than *Menschlichkeit*: witness the recent work on "chimpanzee material culture" that casts the traditional Boasian concept in an altogether different light from how U.S. anthropologists have regarded this category.[2] Let me simply set aside some of these definitional issues for the moment, to make sure I get across the novelty implicit in recent thinking with regard to human recency.

Just to give a couple of examples: it was widely thought several decades ago that the two- and three-million-year-old hominid fossils being found in Africa had "culture" in the Boasian sense—including folkways and mores, fables and religion, and so forth. Humanness in the wake of the 1950 UNESCO *Statement on Race* was pushed back even into the middle Miocene—as when Louis Leakey and many others suggested that *Ramapithecus* circa fourteen million years ago was a hominid and tool user—both of which were taken to mean that the creature was human in some deep and inclusive sense.[3] By the mid-1970s, the hominid status of Ramapithecus had been sanctified by "millions of textbooks and *Time-Life* volumes on human evolution."[4] The equation of hominid and humanity fit with the older tradition of humans as an evolutionary *Sonderweg*: only humans use tools, tool use implies language, language implies culture, language and culture are unique to humanity, and so forth; it also had certain advantages for career-conscious fossil finders, since it was surely preferable to have found some kind of human rather than some kind of chimp. It was not until the 1960s that Allan Wilson and Vince Sarich showed that humans shared a common ancestor with chimps as recently as five to six million years ago—and not until the 1980s that this idea was widely accepted.[5] (A few maverick evolutionists as recently as the 1960s could maintain that humans and apes had not shared an ancestor since the Eocene—roughly fifty million years ago by modern counts.) It is also noteworthy that it took a racial inegalitarian (Sarich) to discover the more recent split—more on that in a moment.

Much of that consensus—equating hominid and humanity—has been broken in the past couple of decades, and here I want to explore how and why that came to pass. It has partly to do, of course, with Jane Goodall's celebration of nonhuman tool use and, to a lesser extent, the rise of "pop ethology," evolutionary psychology, and sociobiology—all of which champion the animal in humans—but there are several other key transitions that warrant an accounting. I want to focus on three of these transformations, or "crises," all of which have given force to the idea that humanness may be a relatively recent phenomenon:

1. Archaeology, and the crisis in interpretation of the oldest tools—specifically, the Oldowan and Acheulean assemblages of the Lower Paleolithic, the oldest tools to have epochal names attached and to count as evidence of hominid or human "culture." (Chimpanzee cultural traditions can be treated only ahistorically, since there is almost no "archaeological" evidence of chimpanzee tool use, though Frédéric Joulian has recently found stone anvils being used by chimps for at least two hundred years and we should, in theory, be able to find these going back millions of years.)[6] The key question here is whether Oldowan and Acheulean artifacts can be considered evidence of cultural "traditions" in any interesting sense. An argument can be made that they cannot, or at least cannot in the conventional Boasian sense, given their apparent stability and uniformity over vast stretches of time and space. Oldowan tools persist for roughly a million years in Africa (from 2.5 to 1.5 M.Y.A.), and Acheulean tools last even longer, from about 1.5 to .2 M.Y.A. The assertion has been made that one reason these tools are so stable is that their users were not transmitting knowledge of their use by means of abstract symbols (language), and that some other mechanism must account for their endurance. One possible implication is that their inventors were not yet human in some significant sense (for example, not linguistic creatures); some kind of nonlinguistic transmission might have been involved—such as imitation, the way Japanese macaques copied Imo the inventive one, who sorted grain from sand by tossing them both into the water (grain floats).[7] Independent invention is also a possibility, and could help explain the constancy of the design over time and space, if,

for instance, throwing for hunting or some other primary use were continually reconfining the shape.[8]

2. Paleontology, and the crisis deriving from the recognition of fossil hominid phyletic diversity—another innovation of the 1960s and 1970s, following spectacular south and east African hominid fossil finds (Mary Leakey's *Zinjanthropus*, Louis Leakey's *Homo habilis*, Donald Johanson's *Australopithecus* "Lucy," and so on) showing that more than one species of hominid must have coexisted at many points in the course of hominid evolution. Many paleoanthropologists today place the total number of hominid species at about twenty, in three or four separate genera (*Australopithecus*, *Paranthropus*, *Homo*, and perhaps *Ardipithecus* and others). Hominid diversity seems to have peaked about two million years ago, when three, four, five, or possibly even more separate hominid species coexisted on the planet (and all in East Africa). The present situation, in fact, where there is only one surviving species, *Homo sapiens*, seems to be an unusual state of affairs in the five-million-year span of "human" evolution. There may have been other periods with only one hominid (prior to about five million years ago, for example, when the combined number of hominid *and* chimp species may have been no greater than one), but the last thirty thousand or so years—since the extinction of the Neanderthals—is certainly unusual in having only one living representative of the hominid family. Fossil hominid diversity was not accepted without a struggle, however: there was a certain degree of ideological resistance stemming from the liberal antiracialist climate of the post-Auschwitz era, when it was dogmatically assumed that only one hominid species could exist at any given time (the "single species hypothesis"). This is interestingly tied to the reevaluation of *race* in the early post–World War II era, when a broad cultural consensus emerged that the humans living today are more or less equal in terms of cultural worth and standing in the "family of man"—culminating in UNESCO' *Statement on Race*, which branded race an "unscientific" category and "man's most dangerous myth" (Ashley Montagu's epithet).

3. Molecular anthropology, and the crisis (turning point) stemming from the recognition that all living humans have descended from a small group of Africans who lived roughly 135,000 years ago. "Modern humans" are therefore relatively recent in a *biological* sense, though nothing is

necessarily implied about *cultural* recency. This "out-of-Africa" scenario has received immense coverage in the popular press through its vivid emblem of an "African Eve," of course, but also through the clarity and simplicity of its opposition to the "multiregional" or "regional continuity" hypothesis—according to which the *Homo erectus* populations in different parts of the world didn't go extinct (as proposed by the molecularists) but gave rise to the distinct (but commingling) populations of *Homo sapiens* that eventually evolved in those regions. The opposing molecularist, sequence-based recency thesis has become the dominant view; it has done this partly through the strength of its molecular methods, but also by successfully tarring the multiregional model (inspired by Franz Weidenreich) with older polygenist traditions, which presumed deep and usually invidious racial divisions.

All three of these transformations—archaeological, paleontological, and genetic—have been important in the rising stock of human recency. Of course, the factors I have mentioned and will soon elaborate on are not the only elements at work; there are others—like the triumph of Stephen Jay Gould and Niles Eldredge's punctuated equilibrium, or efforts by paleoanthropologists like Richard Klein, who argues that the explosive growth of human innovativeness circa fifty thousand years ago—John Pfeiffer's "creative explosion" or Jared Diamond's "great leap forward"—might be traceable to some sort of "neural mutation."[9] Recency is not the same as suddenness, however, and the idea of recency has become at least as popular among anti-Gouldians as Gouldians. Indeed, it was two *anti*-Gouldian aspects of the thesis that first piqued my own interest in human recency: (1) the idea that language capacities might have developed relatively late in human evolution (albeit perhaps gradually, over a long period of time), and (2) the awkward fact that the human cultural "Big Bang" seems perilously close to the point of human racial differentiation and dispersal, raising the specter that some "races" might actually have become "human" earlier than others—a common idea among segregationalists and polygenists as late as the 1950s and 1960s.[10] Both of these are rather non-Gouldian concerns, and avoidable; both, I would say, can be rectified within an expanded theory of recency consistent with racial egalitarianism and punctuated equilibrium.

Before I turn to these crises, let me make two methodological points about opportunities for historical inquiry in this area.

The first is simply a call for historians of science and technology to entertain paleoanthropology and the Paleolithic. Paleoanthropology is a fascinating and understudied area of modern technoscience, full of adventure and ideology; but so, too, at least in this latter aspect, is the Paleolithic itself. Prehistoric tools have generally not become the objects of analysis by historians of technology, and the explanation is fairly obvious (if moronic), given that the founding mytho-myopia of our discipline (history) is that "historical" events are those that postdate the invention of writing circa 3000 B.C. The parochialism of such an approach has long been obvious to practitioners of oral history and archaeology, and to historians of material culture and so on; but the history of tools prior to text remains rather remarkably undertheorized—by historians, at least. I would therefore like to make a pitch for a "deep history of technology," closer collaborations with archaeologists and prehistorians, a serious reckoning with that 99.9 percent of hominid experience that predates what historians define as "history proper" (since the invention of script), and perhaps even an increased attention to human evolution as central to our understanding of humanness in general. The textual turn in anthropology in this sense needs to be complemented by a nontextual (or pretextual) turn; we need to problematize the disciplinary divide that has tended to isolate prehistorians from historians of technology.[11]

A second point is that we need to look for the political good in the technically bad, and vice versa, the politically bad in the technically good. The point is not that tools may be used for good or ill but rather that political evil may be creative and political goodwill stifling. Nazi tobacco research is an obvious case of the former (the fertile face of fascism).[12] The UNESCO *Statement on Race* is, I will argue, a heretofore unnoticed example of the latter, since one of my claims will be that the racial liberalism of the 1950s and 1960s was partly responsible for delaying the recognition of fossil hominid diversity by ten or twenty years. Let me turn now, though, to archaeology, moving then to paleontology, and finally to race and genetics.

Refiguring the Acheulean

In 1797 John Frere, an English country squire and former high sheriff of Suffolk, discovered a number of curious artifacts in a brick-clay pit in the parish of Hoxne. In a letter published three years later in *Archae-*

ologia, the journal of the Society of Antiquaries, Frere described the implements as "evidently weapons of war, fabricated and used by a people who had not the use of metals." The situation under which they had been found led him to believe that they must be extremely old, having been buried under ten feet of well-stratified vegetable earth and "Argill" clay. Frere concluded that this particular manner of burial, plus their association with the bones of animals no longer found in England, meant that these artifacts must date from "a very remote period indeed; even beyond that of the present world."[13]

Historians have often commented on the failure of Frere's contemporaries to recognize the antiquity of human artifacts: his paper went essentially unnoticed for more than fifty years, until the prehistoric revolution of 1859, when from diverse angles—and fairly suddenly—it was recognized that humans have a profound antiquity.[14] Paleontologists in Frere's time had already by and large abandoned Archbishop James Ussher's oft-cited estimate of six thousand years since creation (Georges-Louis Buffon in 1775 had calculated an age of seventy-five thousand years for the earth, based on experiments with cooling bodies), but the absence of human remains in geologic deposits had made it unfashionable to argue for the existence of humanity beyond the more miserly biblical chronology. Paleontological time markers were introduced in the early decades of the nineteenth century, but even Georges Cuvier, the primary architect of such markers, died in 1832 believing that there was no such thing as fossil humans.[15] It was not until the late 1850s that human antiquity was widely recognized, the key event being the acceptance by English and French geologists of the authenticity of the Acheulean "hand axes" found by Jacques Boucher de Perthes in the gravels south of St. Acheul, near Amien, northwest of Paris.[16] The discovery was interestingly coincident with the publication of Charles Darwin's *Origin of Species*, though the latter book seems actually to have had little or no immediate impact on the question of human antiquity. The leading architect of the revolution, Boucher de Perthes, was in fact a biblical catastrophist and antitransformationist who argued that humans were probably created and destroyed several times before Adam was called into being.

Acheulean tools are remarkable in several different respects—quite apart from their stunning beauty and symmetry, qualities that have earned for them recognition as the first traces of a primate (human?)

aesthetic sense (Oldowan tools, by contrast, dating back to circa 2.5 M.Y.A. look more like crudely broken rocks, though I should note that some Oldowan stonework survives long into the "Acheulean"). The oldest hand axes are about 1.5 million years old, and the youngest about one hundred thousand.[17] That brings us to one of the most remarkable features of such tools (if that is what they are): their relative uniformity over vast reaches of time and space. Acheulean hand axes are found for a span of 1.4 million years—more than fifty thousand generations—over most of the range occupied by *Homo erectus*, from the Pleistocene gravels of England (though not in Ireland, which was scoured clean by glaciers) to the open-air sites of northern Spain (Torralba and Ambrona), Algeria, and Morocco, to the famous *erectus* sites of east and southern Africa and as far east as the Urals—and occasionally beyond, as indicated by the recent finds at Nihewan and Bose Basin in southern China.[18] (Early hominids never seem to have crossed any significant body of water; that does not occur until fairly late in the evolution of *Homo sapiens*, circa forty or fifty thousand years ago, when humans voyaged into Australia. The presumption is that oceangoing rafts do not exist until that time.)

A second remarkable fact is how difficult it has been to come up with an adequate sense of how to interpret "hand axes." This is partly traceable to the lack of contemporary ethnographic evidence (Acheulean tools have not been used for one to two hundred thousand years), but also to the difficulties of understanding what life was like for creatures that may have been quite different from us. *Homo erectus* is generally assumed to have made these objects, but there are several other (albeit closely allied) candidates, including *Homo habilis*, *Homo rudolfensis*, *Homo antecessor*, *Homo heidelbergensis*, and *Homo ergaster*. The idea of the same tool type being made and used by entirely different species is not one that many cultural anthropologists are generally comfortable with—which is one reason there is room to doubt whether the Acheulean is a culture or tradition in any interesting sense. The term Acheulean itself blends paleontological and ethnic categories, nature and culture, since there are some who talk about the Acheulean as a people (strange, since it may have embraced three or four different species), and others who treat it more as a chronological or periodizing category (like Pleistocene), and still others as simply a formal tool-type designation (Acheulean hand axe). The ambiguity is reflected in how and where such artifacts are found, since they were produced for so many hundreds of millennia as to have become distributed as quasi-geologic objects. They can almost be used as index fossils, for example, to date a sediment.

Now, Paleolithic archaeology is a complex and arcane science, so let me here say a few words about the history of these artifacts and how difficult they have been to interpret. Acheulean tools have become Rorschach tests of sorts, blank slates onto which different conceptions of antiquity and humanity have been inscribed.

Frere is often credited with having been the first to recognize the antiquity of ancient stone tools, but he was by no means the first to have observed them. Stone tools of various sorts have been picked up since time immemorial—by their original makers, of course, but also by people from "historical" times, who often saw them as the work of fairies or some other natural or magical agent. (The oldest image of a Paleolithic artifact may well be the medieval French painting depicting Saint Etienne holding a typical Acheulean flint hand axe.) Georgius Agricola and Konrad Gesner in the sixteenth century had suggested that chipped-flint implements were the traces left by thunderbolts; there was also the idea that such artifacts had originally been made of iron and had converted into stone by their long continuance in the earth.[19] Stone artifacts of various sorts must have been picked up wherever people were curious—prehistory may even have been "discovered" from time to time and then forgotten—but in the absence of a well-founded belief in either human antiquity or the possibility of fossilization, prehistoric artifacts were no doubt not often recognized as such.[20] Ulisse Aldrovandi in his posthumous 1648 *Musaeum metallicum* classed stone points along with glossopetrae ("tongue stones"), or what we today would recognize as sharks' teeth; Mercatus's 1719 *Metallotheca* included stone points under the general category of ceraunia—Pliny's grouping that included belemnites. Stone points were often confused with fossils, it being not at all obvious where either of these had come from. Even some of the early utilitarian explanations strike us today as quaintly comical—for example, William Buckland's 1823 characterization of "a small flint, the edges of which had been chipped off, as if by striking a light."[21] If axes were projections of woodsmen, flints here were presumed to have something to do with the flintlock or fire lighter.

For many years after Frere's discovery, and subsequent work by Boucher de Perthes, it was argued that (what we now call) Acheulean tools were axes or hatchets—a not implausible suggestion given their symmetry, size, and cutting edge, which generally extends around the entirety of the tool.[22] In the nineteenth century, it was often suggested that these were weapons of some sort (recall Frere's account) used by primitives to defend themselves against ferocious beasts, and perhaps also to wage war against one another. Typical is Louis Figuier's 1870 *L'homme primitif*, which shows club- and ax-wielding savages from "the period of extinct animals" fending off an attacking cave bear.[23] Axes in the nineteenth-century European ethnographic imagination were often accoutrements of medieval armor, supplemented by non-Western images of dress or habit. This was consonant with older images of early man as Adam or Hercules (with club and skin) or the more or less noble savage—all of which were recycled for use in "man of the Stone Age" representations.[24] The idea of a "Stone Age man with hafted axe" was also consistent with the nineteenth-century urbanist equation, primitive = woodsman, an equation visible in countless early illustrations: Pierre Boitard's "Fossil Man" (1861), *Harper Weekly*'s "Neanderthal" (1873), Henri du Cleuzieu's "Pithecanthropus" (1887), Léon Maxime Faivre's "Deux mères" (1888), Anandee Forestier's "Modern Man, the Mammoth Slayer" (1911), and many others.

The problem with this view, as subsequent studies showed, was that none of the axes used in the Lower Paleolithic show any evidence of having ever been hafted (there are no notches, for example). This was already recognized in the nineteenth century, when Gabriel de Mortillet (1821–1898), an early French Darwinian, identified Acheulean hand axes as *coups de poing*—"blows of the fist"—the idea being that such instruments would be held in the hand to chop or dig or to butcher large animals.[25] The absence of hafting or any other kind of combined tool use prior to about fifty thousand years ago (hook with string, hoe with handle, knife with wooden grip, and so on) has been used to argue that something changed in the cognitive regimen of humans about that time— a conceptual falling-into-place that allowed some new type of inventive, recombinant capacity.[26]

Kathy Schick and Nicholas Toth in the 1990s provided experimental archaeological support for the idea that Acheulean hand axes (and Oldowan tools) could have been used to process large animal carcasses, hunted or scavenged, though that is only one of many recent theories put forward.[27] J. Desmond Clark of Berkeley has suggested their use as bark-stripping tools, to allow feeding on the cambium layer of trees; others have proposed a digging scenario, the point being to extract plant roots, water, or burrowing animals. The idea has also been put forward that hand axes were designed for myriad diverse uses, such as cutting, digging, scraping, hammering, and chopping. Hand axes in this view were the Swiss Army Knives of the Paleolithic.[28]

Evolutionary psychologists have also thrown their hats into the ring. In spring 1998, University of Reading archaeologist Steven Mithen proposed that hand axes might actually be sexual lures, bragging points made by men to attract the opposite sex, the Ferraris or Armani suits of an earlier age. The rather macho (yet thin) theory here is that females were attracted to handsome stone-ax makers, thereby causing those who made the more perfect forms to leave more offspring.[29] This could presumably help explain why many of the hand axes found in different parts of the world never seem to have been used (there is often no edge wear).[30] It might also explain why some sites contain more such tools than you would seem to need—in some cases, thousands scattered over a very small area. (Or perhaps it is a symptom of the fact that there aren't many feminists in paleoanthropology?) The theory is part of Mithen's larger view that the rise of modern consciousness involved a (relatively recent) onset of communication between different parts of the brain— "multitasking"—from which we get art, language, religion, and the rest of the show.[31]

Based on earlier studies by Eileen O'Brien, the neurobiologist William Calvin has argued that the tools might have been *thrown* at animals gathered around a water hole as an effective hunting strategy (as "killer frisbees").[32] The idea here is that the teardrop shape would force a thrown hand ax into a vertically spinning path, which could be made to terminate on, say, the back or rump of an antelope at a water hole. The sharpened edges of the ax would allow it to stick into the animal, inducing a pain-induced flexion response (magnifying how the animal would normally act in response to a thornbush) and causing it to duck or sit down. As the commotion spread in the herd, the animal might then stumble and be trampled, allowing the hunters to rush in and dispatch the animal. Calvin points out that other shapes would work to a lesser degree, but that hunters would eventually learn that the bifacially sharpened ovate form allows the projectile to transfer more of its momentum into the animal, causing a more pronounced (and deadly) flexion response. Four or five hunters simultaneously throwing hand axes could multiply the efficiency of the technique.

Calvin's theory would help explain many of the enigmatic aspects of the hand-ax shape: the sharpened edge all around (which makes it hard to use as a handheld ax), the persistence of the ovate shape (which he says is difficult to explain in other than aerodynamic terms), and the fact that many hand axes appear "unused," lacking edge wear. It would also explain why some Paleolithic sites have literally thousands of such objects, since it is not hard to imagine hunters losing half a dozen on any given day at an oft-visited water hole, especially when the water was high.[33] The theory also has the advantage of not requiring cultural transmission to explain the constancy and ubiquity of the hand ax's shape: its persistence could simply be a consequence of its effectiveness as a hunting tool. Hominids throughout the world might have experimented with throwing rocks at animals where they gather and have found that rocks shaped in certain ways work better than others. The Acheulean hand ax might have been independently invented thousands or even millions of times in different parts of the world; stones from previous hunters might also have been perennially rediscovered, as water holes dried up or erosion caused their reexposure. Hand axes in this sense may have been a constant part of the geo-ecology of the hunting environment.

A rather different approach has been to claim that Acheulean tools are not in fact so uniform as they might at first appear. There are different shapes and sizes (some as large as thirty centimeters in length).[34] And there are, of course, different kinds of materials, the earliest African assemblages being more often basalt or quartzite, while subsequent European tools are more often flint, chert, or jasper. There are Acheulean sites without hand axes (Clacton-on-Sea in England), and Acheulean-like hand axes that persist into the Late Mousterian that were probably used by Neanderthals (these tend to be classed as "Clactonian" rather than Acheulean, and were made from smaller flakes). The selection of appropriate materials may have involved a great deal of skill and connoisseurship lost to us today; the fact that, to most of us, Acheulean tools "all look alike" may be partly an artifact of distance and lack of familiarity, combined with the archaeologist's (or collector's) selectivity in picking up, preserving, displaying, publishing, or even selling only "good examples" of the tool in question.[35]

Theories of hand-ax use are speculative in many ways; one of the interesting aspects of this for the historian of science is how views of their origin and use have multiplied over time. Experimental archaeologists have given plausibility to some theories, and made certain theories less plausible; but there is still a great deal of uncertainty, and it may well be that these tools have had different uses at different points in the Paleolithic—or among different peoples living at any given time, or among any single individual making or finding such a stone. Calvin's theory, for example, is consistent with the growing recognition that a given tool might have had multiple uses, or might even have once been one kind of tool and later cannibalized for a novel use. A hand ax made (or picked up) for use in an antelope hunt, for instance, might have later been used to disembowel or disarticulate an animal killed in such a hunt, or to dig a hole in which the animal might be stashed. The tool might also have been given some ritual or sacred significance, or used in some sexual or social celebration or rite of passage. Reuse and refashioning have become objects of interest in recent lithic studies, with Paleolithic peoples being credited as more flexible and opportunistic than once thought. Large flakes (axes?) are thought to have become cores, cores refigured as choppers, choppers were used as cores for smaller flakes, and so forth. Ancient hominids in this sense may have been rather more like us—opportunistic and flexible—than is sometimes thought.

This last-mentioned prospect has made it harder to say for sure what is a core (waste or resource) and what is a flake (tool), giving rise also to the suggestion that many so-called hand axes might actually be discarded cores from which flakes were taken. Nicholas Toth has argued that most Oldowan tools are actually remnant cores, the idea here being that suitable pebbles would be carried around and then struck whenever needed to produce a thin, sharp flake. Such flakes are effective cutting tools, and would serve very well for rapid butchery and excision of flesh.[36] The same could well be true for many of the hand axes found in Europe, the Middle East, and Africa: their marvelous symmetry might simply indicate that the core has been exhausted, flakes having been taken from all around the edge. Archaeologists for more than two centuries may have been celebrating the earliest preserved form of human waste: not *tools*, in short, but *trash*.[37]

To return to the question of human recency: one interesting explanation for the consistency of Acheulean tools over such vast stretches of time and distance might be that *humans were not making them*. Richard Klein at Stanford and Alan Walker and Pat Shipman at Penn State have put forward this hypothesis—the idea being that who or whatever made them was culturally and intellectually more like a creative chimp than a modern human, hominids without the use of fully symbolic language, in other words.[38]

Such a theory would be consistent with what we (now think we) know about tool use among chimpanzees and other primates: such creatures are known to have invented new forms of tool use (potato washing or fishing for ants with sticks), and may even have transferred such tools from one group to another, but the capacity for innovation is clearly limited.[39] Humans are unique in our ability to recombine tools for novel uses, a faculty that may well spring from our possession of language— our ability to think and act in terms of abstract symbols.[40] Incessant innovativeness is not an obvious prerequisite for being human; that is a modernist prejudice, if not a capitalist presumption. But the total absence of innovativeness over vast spans of time could well be taken as evidence of a rather feeble recombinant symbolic capacity (language), regardless of whether artifacts of the type here under discussion were spread by cultural diffusion or independent invention.

A diffusionist model, for example, could hold that hand-ax design (or habit, or tradition) was passed around the world by (silent) imitation from one individual (or group) to another, keeping constant only by virtue of the (perceived) optimality (or sufficiency) of that particular design for whatever function it did in fact perform. We might find little variance ("drift") in the particulars of hand-ax size or shape, simply because the design was hard to improve on, and there was not yet the ability to express a sense of creative play—in rocks, at least. The same could be true, even if these so-called tools were repeatedly and independently invented. Hand axes might have been independently invented, and forgotten, thousands or even millions of times in different parts of the world. Here again, tool-type designs could have remained stable, if they served their makers well.[41] In neither case, however, is there necessarily a presumption of linguistic or symbolic capacity. Hand-ax use might have been closer to chimp ant dipping or potato washing than to, say, sonnet writing or H-bomb building.

It is hard to say what to think about this view, that the first hominid creations that are genuinely beautiful, displaying symmetry and undeniable skill (albeit perhaps only trash, or perhaps first trash and then adapted to be some kind of tool), might have been produced by people that were not yet fully people. It could even be that it was in perfecting such things that humans became more fully human, although this latter idea ("more fully human") may make no more sense than the idea of a creature being more "fully cockroach" or "fully chimpanzee." If evolution has taught us anything, it is that there is no essence of humanity, no fixed and final form. Narratives of arrival are pervasive in paleoanthropology, reflecting not just our understandable *sapiens*-centrism but also the (questionable?) sense that we alone have managed to leave some important part of nature's authority behind. The difficulty is compounded, as we shall see, by the fact that more than one species of human may have walked the earth, at several different (and simultaneous) points in hominid history.

Racial Liberalism, the UNESCO Statement, and the Single Species Hypothesis

Understandings of hominid diversity have undergone a profound shift in recent decades, from a conception that there could be only one kind of hominid at any given time, to the view that the past thirty thousand years or so are actually rather unusual in having only one. Many paleoanthropologists now believe that there might have been as many as twenty different species of hominids since our last common ancestor with chimps, the apparent peak being circa two million years ago when as many as half a dozen different hominid species coexisted in Africa, just prior to the *Homo erectus* exodus.[42] That is a dramatic change from a common view of the 1960s, defended by C. Loring Brace and others, that the human cultural/ecological "niche" was so narrow that only one kind of hominid could exist at any given time.[43] This older idea was partly a political outcome of the fear of excluding extinct hominid species from the ancestral so-called family of man.[44] But it was also interestingly consistent with older, gradualist, ladderlike phylogenies deriving from the great chain of being—with qualifications that I shall mention in a moment. The single species hypothesis popular in the 1950s and 1960s championed a linear, nonbranching evolutionary sequence according to which *Australopithecus* begat *erectus*, *erectus* begat Neanderthal, Neanderthal begat *sapiens*, and so forth. The newer family trees, by contrast, are often bushy, with many false starts and dead ends (extinctions), and often more than one species living concurrently.

What accounts for the rise of the single species hypothesis and the reluctance to appreciate fossil hominid diversity? Gould and others have stressed the perennial bias of uniformitarianism, with its *scala natura* progressivism and preference for linear "chains" over diversifying "bushes," but changing local sensitivities also have to be taken into account.[45] I have already mentioned Brace's odd ecological rationalization, but there was also the fact that with the exposé of the Piltdown hoax in the early 1950s, paleoanthropologists were suddenly faced with a much narrower range of hominid skeletal morphology. (Piltdown was a modern human cranium attached to an orangutan jaw.) Yet another impulse was the growing concern over the out-of-control proliferation of hominid taxa. "Lumper" Ernst Mayr, for example, contributed to the hypothesis with his effort to reduce the clutter of hominid generic names. In 1950, Mayr maintained that the proliferation of hominid generic names made little taxonomic sense, and he proposed that the zoo of names circulating at that time—such as *Australopithecus*, *Plesianthropus*, *Paranthropus*, *Pithecanthropus*, *Sinanthropus*, *Paleoanthropus*—be reduced to a single genus, *Homo*, defined by upright posture. Mayr also maintained, though, following Theodosius Dobzhansky, and with race clearly on his mind, that "never more than one species of man existed on the earth at any given time."[46]

Mayr's pronouncement has to be read against the backdrop of changing views on race. Ever since Carolus Linnaeus, and interestingly unperturbed by Darwin, racial theorists had squabbled over how many races humanity should be divided into. Darwin had noted the absurdity of such exercises, with Jean-Joseph Virey distinguishing two races of humans, Immanuel Kant four, Johann Friedrich Blumenbach five, Buffon six, John Hunter seven, Louis Agassiz eight, Charles Pickering eleven, Samuel George Morton twenty-two, Edmund Burke sixty-three, and so forth.[47] Long into the twentieth century, human phyletic trees often showed a

jungly bush of racial diversity, as when Grafton Elliot-Smith distinguished separate branches for Negroes, Mongols, Mediterraneans,
Nordics, Alpines, Australians, and the now-extinct Neanderthals and
Rhodesian Man. German anthropologists did likewise—rather distress-
ingly late into the century.[48]

The history of ideas of diversity cannot, however, be seen as a slow
and steady triumph of "bushiness" over "linearity." Diversity has come
and gone, and come again, keeping different kinds of political company.
Racial diversity had become unfashionable after the revelation of the
crimes of the Nazis (and eventually with the campaign to end racial
segregation), but *fossil hominid* diversity was also interestingly under-
played as attitudes toward the ancestral (or extinct) hominid "other" got
caught up in race relations. The 1950s was not a time to exclude certain
types of fossils from the fold of humanity. So even though "gracile" and
"robust" australopithecines had both been found in South Africa by the
end of the 1930s, it took some time to dispel the notion that these were
simply males and females of one and the same species (the original
version of the single species hypothesis). Interesting also is the fact that
it was not until after the Second World War that these small-brained
creatures were recognized as hominids. Part of the problem was the widespread notion that early humans must have developed in Asia; African
australopithecines were more often seen as apes than as early hominids.
Their elevation to hominid status may have been helped by the inclusive
atmosphere of the postwar era; a cynic could also wonder, though,
whether the global calamities of the 1940s and postwar nuclear foolish-
ness may have helped spawn the view that humans could have very small
brains.

The single species hypothesis was dealt its first solid blow in 1959,
when Mary Leakey discovered the 1.8-million-year-old *Zinjanthropus* at
Olduvai Gorge in Tanzania, a fossil (now known as *Australopithecus
boisei*) with such hyperrobust features (including large, flat, grinding
molars) that it was difficult to imagine these were just the males to the
female gracile australopithecines. *Homo habilis* ("handy man"), found
in the early 1960s at Olduvai, further undercut the assumption of a
single-stalk, non-branching evolutionary tree: *habilis* was clearly more
"human-like" than *Australopithecus*, yet quite a bit older than had previously been imagined for our genus (about 1.75 million years from

radio-dated volcanic ash) and the first real evidence that *Homo* must have lived contemporaneously with the Australopithecines. The reigning assumption had been that early, ape-like hominids were fully replaced by more human-like hominids, but here was a new and disturbing idea— multiple co-existing hominid genera—that took some time to assimilate. The nail in the coffin came in 1975, when Richard Leakey announced the discovery of a *Homo erectus* skull old enough to have coexisted with *Australopithecus boisei.*[49]

Could this be possible? Might two or three different kinds of ape-men have lived at the same time? If so, how did they interact? Could they have conversed with one another? Traded with one another? Fought with one another? The idea of multiple coexisting human lineages seemed to some a rather unsettling prospect—albeit fertile ground for sci-fi, as writers for more than a century had already realized.[50]

The story was made still more complex when it became clear that there were more than two kinds of *Australopithecus*. A key discovery here came in 1974 when Donald Johanson, a graduate student working at a dig near Hadar, in Ethiopia, discovered a 3.2-million-year-old hominid soon regarded as the first-found member of a new species, dubbed *Australopithecus afarensis* (southern ape of Afar), better known as "Lucy" from the fact that the paleoanthropologists were rocking to the Beatles song "Lucy in the Sky with Diamonds" (LSD), as they returned to camp. The skeleton was only 40 percent complete, but clearly showed that "humans" walked upright more than three million years ago.

It eventually became apparent that there were several different species of these apelike humans (or humanlike apes) of Africa, including *Australopithecus anamensis*, a fossil hominid found in 1995 by Meave Leakey of the National Museum of Kenya and Alan Walker of Johns Hopkins, and *Ardipithecus ramidus*, an enigmatic and fragmentary creature (a piece of a jaw and several other bits) found in 1994 by Tim White in Ethiopia. The former is 4.2 million years old and the latter is about 4.4, which is not so long after the point when the ancestors of (what are now) chimps and humans branched off from one another. The new millennium has seen a flood of other early finds, including the 6-million-year-old *Orrorin tugenensis* unearthed by Martin Pickford and Brigitte Senut, and the 3.5-million-year-old *Kenyanthropus platyops* dug up by Meave Leakey, both found in Kenya in 2001.[51] No one knows whether *anamensis*, *ramidus*, *tugenensis*, or *platyops* is our direct ancestor: in a rather trivial sense they almost certainly are not, given the bushiness of the hominid lineage and the fact that almost all lineages eventually perish. You always know that a fossil had parents, but you never know whether it left any offspring.[52] The new finds may eventually do more to clarify the puzzling paucity of chimpanzee fossils, since many may turn out to be closer to the ancestors of chimps than of humans.

How have such finds impacted theories of human recency? In an earlier section, I mentioned the strong professional pressures now favoring "splitters": it is surely better for your career to have found a new hominid species than yet another example of some other scholar's already-discovered sort. Taxonomic modesty favors lumping; hubris sanctions splitting.[53] Similar pressures influence the humanity of one's finds, since it is clearly better to have found an early human than a rather late or precocious ape. The pressure to speak in such terms is enormous: witness Ian Tattersall's most recent book, *Extinct Humans*, whose very title brandishes a concept he himself has admonished against. Perhaps his agent cautioned him that a book titled *Extinct Hominids* would not sell as well.

The trend since the 1970s, however, has been to argue that hominids prior to *Homo sapiens* were not as human as once was thought. I've already noted several causes for this shift, but let me add to this here: (1) a retreat from some of the more optimistic assessments of chimpanzee cognitive capacities of the 1960s and 1970s, and (2) the view that it was not such a bad thing to be "not fully human."

There was also the growing sense, though, that it was not necessarily racist to believe that nonsapient hominids were radically different from "us." Here, it is important to appreciate the ideological obstacles faced by those who wanted to emphasize fossil hominid diversity. The most prominent among these was the liberal antiracialist sentiment of many postwar anthropologists—especially in the Anglo-American world, where shock and horror over the events of Nazi Germany combined with concerns that racial prejudice was still a potent force in other parts of the world as well. Concerns such as these culminated in the first decade after the war, when fears of a resurgence of racial prejudice led liberal activists in the newly founded UNESCO to draft a *Statement on Race* denouncing racial theory and racial prejudice. The resulting document, published in 1950 and in various revised versions ever since, became the canonical liberal resolution of the race issue: race as usually conceived does not exist; people are equal throughout the world in terms of intellectual and cultural worth; the most important differences that you find among peoples are due to nurture rather than nature; and so forth. The Boasian position was vindicated and strengthened. Franz Boas in the nineteenth century had said that race, language, and culture were separate and independent variables.[54] The new view, at least in popular academic translation, was that race does not exist at all.[55]

Historians of science are familiar with the obstructive impact of ill-willed ideologies on science, but less familiar are examples of political goodwill stifling science. On the question of fossil hominid phyletic diversity, however, the impact of the UNESCO statement on race and the larger population-genetics critique of racial typology must be regarded as somewhat stifling. The most common fear seems to have been that by allowing multiple lineages of humans, one would open the door to racism, by excluding one or another lineage from the mainline ancestral sequence leading to modern humans. This was clearly the case in Brace's rejection of multiple lineages, one of his fears being that Neanderthals would be dehumanized (and excluded from the human ancestral line) by what he called "hominid catastrophism."[56] Antilinearity, in his view, was tantamount to antievolution. Tattersall has suggested that the emphasis on population thinking in these peak prestige years of the New Synthesis also helped foster the idea that "no amount of variation" was too great to be contained within a single species.[57] The emphasis on genetic diversity in this sense may have retarded the acceptance of new hominid lineages; it may also have made it difficult to believe that some lineages had perished without issue. The seeds for this myopia were already sown in 1944, when Dobzhansky argued that "no more than a single hominid species existed at any one time level," a view that was taken to an extreme in 1959, when Emil Breitinger argued that hominid evolution was punctuated by "only one single a priori certain case of a complete speciation and splitting"—the divergence of hominids from tertiary primate species.[58] Implicit in such assertions of hominid unity was also the idea that "our" branching point from the other apes was remote— eleven or twelve million years even in the most conservative estimates.[59]

Morphologists also had their blinders, albeit coming from quite different technical and conceptual traditions. Paleoanthropologists in England in the 1960s, for example, could be heard muttering about how "there simply wasn't enough 'morphological space' between *Australopithecus africanus* and *Homo erectus* to shoehorn in a new species."[60] Gould would later argue for a more "bushlike" hominid lineage, in harmony with his punctuated equilibrium model of phyletic morphology and his celebration of evolutionary contingency.[61] In this sense, Gould was an important transitional figure, being one of the first to clearly accept the UNESCO redefinition (or abandonment) of race, while also maintaining that an overly ladderlike phylogeny had straitjacketed human evolution and underestimated the morphological diversity of human (and other) lineages. Multilinearity after Gould became acceptable again, when purged of its earlier racialist overtones.

The liveliness of this issue has to be understood in light of the fact that even as late as the 1960s, human *racial* diversity was still being routinely characterized as taxonomically significant by many physical anthropologists. Carleton Coon at University of Pensylvansia for example, as president of the American Association of Physical Anthropologists, in 1962 claimed that African *Homo erectus* populations ("Congoids") had actually crossed the threshold to fully human *Homo sapiens* two hundred thousand years later than other hominid populations (Europeans, of course, led the way). Africa, as he put it, "was only an indifferent kindergarten" for humanity. Coon also used this prejudice to work secretly, behind the scenes, to undermine the *Brown v. Board of Education* civil rights ruling of the U.S. Supreme Court, which declared that separate was *not* equal and thus mandated desegregation.[62] Franz Weidenreich, a Jewish émigré anthropologist from Germany, had carried over an implicit polygenism into U.S. physical and paleoanthropology, the idea being that humans had diverged into separate racial groups prior to the transition from *erectus* to *sapiens*. De facto polygeny continued also in Germany: a 1965 book edited by the former SS officer Gerhard Heberer, for instance, included a chart showing racial differentiation beginning at the end of the Pleistocene, about one million years ago.[63]

Molecular Anthropology

The idea of modern humans developing slowly and separately in different parts of the world is today known as multiregionalism; this is the infamous alternative to what is often called the replacement or out-of-Africa model, the idea that fully modern humans emerged rather suddenly in Africa about 135,000 years ago and spread from there throughout the world, "replacing" (without interbreeding with) the *Homo erectus* populations they encountered.

The two sides are loosely represented by different instrumental traditions: multiregionalists, led by Milford Wolpoff of the University of Michigan, tend to be physical anthropologists; several of the most prominent out-of-Africanists, by contrast, have been molecular geneticists—notably the diaspora from Allan Wilson's Berkeley lab in the 1980s, including Mark Stoneking, Rebecca Cann, and Svante Pääbo, just to name some of the more distinguished.[64] Multiregionalists tend to stress continuities in physical type as evidence of regional continuity; out-of-Africanists tend to stress rates of nucleotide divergence as evidence of bottlenecks and human biorecency.

Apart from these disciplinary differences, however, there are also intriguing ideological divides, though not always those that make it into the popular press. The tendency has been to gloss the debate as "we're all Africans" versus "racial divisions are really deep," when that is not necessarily the most interesting or accurate fracture plane in the debate (Wolpoff is not Coon). One thing going on is a deep difference over how to grant the Neanderthals dignity. Wolpoff and the multiregionalists basically maintain the UNESCO line that to deny them a biological link to the present is to exclude them from the family of man, a move that smacks of racism.[65] Critics of this view, like Tattersall, say that the Neanderthals are no less respectable for having gone extinct, or for not having been able to breed with *Homo sapiens*; their dignity should not hinge on their biocompatibility with successor populations.

What is also noteworthy, though, are the different rhetorical strategies used by the two groups, multiregionalists and mitochondrialists. These are interesting since each has tried, at various points, to accuse the opposing camp of being more racist. Out-of-Africa theorists have accused multiregionalists of exaggerating racial divisions (conceived of as going back as long as a million years in some of the still-used "candelabra models"). Multiregionalists, in turn, have accused out-of-Africa advocates of implying a total and perhaps violent (genocide-like?) replacement of *Homo erectus* or Neanderthal by *Homo sapiens*.[66] Such a misconception is fueled by silly and sensationalist articles in the popular press.[67] Each side has also managed to brand the opposing camp as old-fashioned. The

Wolpoffians see in the out-of-Africa idea echoes of the rather imperial replacement model going back to W. J. Sollas circa 1911 or even Nicolaas Witsen in the 1600s.[68] The "African Eve" or "Garden of Eden" supporters find in Wolpoff's multiregional model vestiges of the hoary specter of polygenesis—the idea occasionally expressed in the nineteenth century, for example, that white people descended from chimps, Africans from gorillas, and Asians from the orangutans. Multiregionalists see the debate in terms of cooperation versus violence, and the mitochondrialists see a world of recent unity versus deep divisions.

So far, it seems that the geneticists are winning the field. Multiregionalists have no comparable technical wonder, and the original mitochondrial evidence for recency has been joined by nonmitochondrial evidence—for instance, from the Y chromosome. Then, of course, there are the other spectacular successes that the molecularists have enjoyed: Svante Pääbo's extraction and sequencing of DNA from the arm bone of a Neanderthal, suggesting a last common ancestor with humans circa six hundred thousand years ago; the sequencing of the Ice Man of the Alps, the Czar Nicholas II's family remains, the offspring of Thomas Jefferson's liaison with his slave-lover, Sally Hemings, and so forth. You really can no longer do phylogeny and ignore molecular tools.

The politics of human genetic recency, though, have been complex. On the inegalitarian right, Vince Sarich showed in the late 1960s that humans and apes shared a common ancestry with chimps only five to six million years ago. On the egalitarian left, Richard Lewontin showed about this same time that racial differentiation was relatively recent.[69] Sarich's innovation can be seen as part of an effort to reemphasize the animal in our humanity, and Lewontin's the opposite, to de-emphasize whatever biological differences may divide us. Sarich moved up the break with apes; Lewontin moved up the separation of races from one another.

Confusion and Projection

The idea of human recency comes from many different directions, only a few of which have been mentioned here.[70] The ideological aspects are interesting, because people seem to be getting different things out of recency. Some people seem to like the fact that "we are all Africans"; there is a kind of "black Athena" resonance in the molecularist account of the Paleolithic, especially in its popularization by the media. The political resonances of the out-of-Africa idea are not so simple, however.[71] There is also a sometimes rather subtle implication that Africa is a good place *to be from*. I call this "Out-of-Africa: Thank God!" insofar as there is an implication that hominids became *Homo sapiens* in the process of leaving Africa, a slight that seems always to be unintentional, yet is surprisingly common. Just to give one example: In his otherwise-astute paper critiquing (inter alia) "Proto-World" paleo-linguistic theories for the 2001 Summer Academy on Human Origins in Berlin, Jürgen Trabant of Humboldt University wrote that Proto-World "would be the language of that group of humans which made it out of Africa." His intention was simply to characterize (and critique) the assumption by Luigi Luca Cavalli-Sforza and others that all the languages of the world might share some common distant root, but the accidental implication was that in the process of becoming modern, everyone left Africa.[72]

There also appears to be support for recency from those who reject the single species hypothesis. Hominid bushiness seems to reopen one of the questions at the root of the UNESCO statement: How deep can human biodiversity go? Hominid bushiness not only raises the difficult question of what it must have been like to have multiple species of humans living at the same time but also the question, How far back into the hominid past can one reasonably project human qualities?

There are two things that we can be sure of: (1) the history of science is often a history of confusion, and (2) ideologies often come in cumbersome packages. Arguments developed for dealing with racial differences and prejudices have been projected onto dealings with fossil hominid diversity; that was true before the UNESCO statement on race, but it is also true afterward. There are those who feel that it is morally wrong to claim that the Neanderthals, for example, were anything less than fully human.[73] No one can deny that the bestial impregnation of this species in the early part of the twentieth century was wrong in many respects, but their refitting with flowers (say, in 1969 at the Shanidar site in Iraq, where pollen was found in a grave, whence the "flower child of Shanidar") may eventually seem just as quaint, if rather more pleasant. The Neanderthals may or may not have bred with "us" (the molecular evidence suggests they didn't); their replacement by "us" may have been peaceful or bloody (there is no evidence one way or the other). What we can safely assume, though, is that no matter how much evidence we get, the prehistory of tools, bodies, and beliefs will forever remain a fertile field for projection and wishful thinking.

Notes

1. This sentiment can be found in many different sciences of prehistory: witness the recent skepticism with regard to the formerly rock-hard claims for human-generated fire at the 500,000-year-old site of Zhoukoudian, south of Beijing (S. Wiener, Q. Xu, P. Golderg, J. Liu, and O. Ban-Yosee, "Evidence for the Use of Fire at Zhoukoudian," *Science* 281.5374 [1998]: 251–253). Hominid control of fire had been pushed back to 1.5 or even 1.8 million years ago in Britain and Africa, though there is the perennial problem of how to distinguish human-made from accidental fire. Scholars have looked for, but not yet found, the telltale carbon signatures of anthropogenic fire in the seabeds downwind from the hominid sites of East Africa; see M. I. Bird and J. A. Cali, "A Million-Year Record of Fire in Sub-Saharan Africa," *Nature* 394 (1998): 767 ff.

2. See Frans B. M. de Waal, "Cultural Primatology Comes of Age," *Nature* 399 (1999): 635–636; and William C. McGrew, *Chimpanzee Material Culture: Implications for Human Evolution* (New York: Cambridge University Press, 1992).

3. Louis Leakey had suggested *Ramapithecus*'s tool use in a 1968 article in *Nature*. Elwyn L. Simons had earlier granted *Ramapithecus*'s hominid status and bipedalism, based solely on his reconstruction of its jaws and teeth ("The Early Relatives of Man," *Scientific American*, July 1964, 50–62). Richard Leakey signaled the demotion of this fossil in 1982, shortly after his film series *The Making of Mankind*, in a lecture wherein he stated that the "conventional wisdom" tracing humans back through *Ramapithecus* was probably wrong; *Ramapithecus* had been a "red herring" (cited in John Gribbin and Jeremy Cherfas, *The Monkey Puzzle: Reshaping the Evolutionary Tree* [New York: Pantheon Books, 1982], 12). Simons and the elder Leakey were not unusual in upholding this view; Pat Shipman, who did her PhD on the Kenya *Ramapithecus* site, notes that in the mid-1970s, "everybody thought *Ramapithecus* was a hominid" (personal communication).

4. Adrienne Zihlman and Jerold Lowenstein, "False Start for the Human Parade," *Natural History* (August–September 1979): 86–91.

5. Allan C. Wilson and Vincent M. Sarich, "Immunological Time Scale for Hominid Evolution," *Science* 158 (1967): 1200–1203.

6. Frédéric Joulian, "Techniques du corps et traditions chimpanzières," *Terrain*, March 2000, 37–54. Joulian has found sites where nut cracking has gone on for at least two hundred years, estimated from the number of nutshells and wear on the stone anvils at such sites. William H. Calvin speculates that early hominids may have begun deliberately chipping stone after having accidentally caused stones to flake in the course of chimplike hammering (*The Throwing Madonna: Essays on the Brain* [New York: McGraw-Hill, 1983], 27, and "Rediscovery and

the Cognitive Aspects of Toolmaking: Lessons from the Hand Axe,"
http://faculty.washington.edu/wcalvin/2001/handaxe.htm).

7. See M. Kawai, "Newly-Acquired Pre-cultural Behavior of the Natural Troop of Japanese Monkeys on Koshima Islet," *Primates* 6 (1965): 1–30. For a critique, see B. G. Galef, "Tradition in Animals: Field Observations and Laboratory Analyses," in *Interpretation and Explanation in the Study of Animal Behavior*, ed. Marc Bekoff and Dale Jamieson (Boulder, CO: Westview Press, 1990).

8. Calvin, *Throwing Madonna*, 22–23.

9. The argument—spurious in my view—has been made that human linguistic diversity is too shallow to be very old, and that human languages diverged from a common origin only about thirty thousand years ago (Merritt Ruhlen, *The Origin of Language: Tracing the Evolution of the Mother Tongue* [New York: Wiley, 1994]). On the "creative explosion," see John E. Pfeiffer, *The Creative Explosion: An Inquiry into the Origins of Art and Religion* (New York: Harper and Row, 1982). On the "great leap forward," see Jared Diamond, *Guns, Germs, and Steel: The Fates of Human Societies* (New York: W. W. Norton, 1997). Richard G. Klein points out that it is not until about fifty thousand years ago that you find the first evidence of religion, representational art, ornamentation, new and changing tool styles, and perhaps even the first boats (*The Human Career: Human Biological and Cultural Origins*, 2nd ed. [Chicago: University of Chicago Press, 1999], 512–517, 590–591).

10. See, for example, Carleton S. Coon, *The Origin of Races* (New York: Knopf, 1962).

11. I mean "the textual turn in anthropology" more in the sense explored by Brinkley Messick in his *Calligraphic State: Textual Domination and History in a Muslim Society* (Berkeley: University of California Press, 1993), and not so much in the sense intended by Clifford Geertz, Hayden White, and others that "all the world is text."

12. See Robert N. Proctor, *The Nazi War on Cancer* (Princeton, NJ: Princeton University Press, 1999).

13. John Frere, "Account of Flint Weapons Discovered at Hoxne in Suffolk," *Archaeologia* 13 (1800): 204–205.

14. See Donald K. Grayson, *The Establishment of Human Antiquity* (New York: Academic Press, 1983); and Claudine Cohen and Jean-Jacques Hublin, *Boucher de Perthes, 1788–1868: Les origines romantiques de la préhistoire* (Paris: Belin, 1989).

15. See Martin J. S. Rudwick, *Georges Cuvier, Fossil Bones, and Geological Catastrophes: New Translations and Interpretations of the Primary Texts* (Chicago: University of Chicago Press, 1997), 232–234. Cuvier's denial of human antiquity can be found in his 1812 *Discours préliminaire*, translated into English in 1813 as *Theory of the Earth* with an elaborate preface by Robert Jameson, who gave the book a natural theological flavor, equating Cuvier's last revolution with the biblical flood.

16. Grayson, *Establishment of Human Antiquity*, 168–223.

17. A good visual display can be found at http://www.personal.psu.edu/users/w/x/wxk116/axe.

18. See Ann Gibbons, "Chinese Stone Tools Reveal High-Bichard Potts, Yuan Baoyin, Tech *Homo erectus,*" *Science* 287 (2000): 1566; and Hou Yamei, Richard Potts, Yuad Badyin, et al., "Mid-Pleistocene Acheulean-like Stone Technology of the Bose Basin, South China," *Science* 287 (2000): 1622–1626.

19. See Charles W. King, *The Natural History of Gems, or Semi-Precious Stones* (London: Bell and Daldy, 1870), 80, reporting on the views of Anselm Boetius de Boodt in his 1609 *De Gemmis et Lapidibus.*

20. Martin J. S. Rudwick dates the recognition of "prehistory" to the 1830s ("The Antiquity of Man before *The Antiquity of Man*" (unpublished manuscript, 2001)).

21. Cited in Grayson, *Establishment of Human Antiquity*, 65.

22. See Charles Lyell, *The Geological Evidences of the Antiquity of Man* (Philadelphia: George W. Childs, 1863), 112–117. Lyell distinguished two types of stone tools found in the pits at St. Acheul: a "spear-headed form" and an "oval form," the latter being "not unlike some stone implements, used to this day as hatchets and tomahawks by natives of Australia"—the difference being only in the fact that the edge on the Australian "weapons," like European "celts," had been "produced by friction" and was generally "sharpened at one end only." Lyell speculated that such tools were "probably used as weapons, both of the war and of the chase, others to grub up roots, cut down trees, and scoop out canoes." He also mentioned Joseph Prestwich's suggestion that such tools might have been used for "cutting holes in the ice both for fishing and for obtaining water," an idea consistent with the notion that former times might have been much colder (113–116).

23. Louis Figuier, *L'homme primitif* (Paris: Hachette, 1870), Figure 16. See also Stephanie Moser, *Ancestral Images: The Iconography of Human Origins* (Ithaca, NY: Cornell University Press, 1998), 127.

24. See Moser, *Ancestral Images*, 135.

25. Gabriel de Mortillet, *Formation de la nation francaise* (Paris: Alcan, 1897). Mortillet in 1872 coined the term *Acheuléen* to designate the culture using his *coups de poing*; see his *Les premiers francais* (circa 1872). Workers digging up the tools in the 1860s for early archaeologists called them *langues de chat* ("cat tongues"); see Louis Figuier, *L'homme primitif*, 3rd ed. (Paris: Hachette, 1873), 64.

26. The only known exceptions to the absence of combined tool use are a couple of enigmatic grooved wooden objects found in 1997 in four-hundred-thousand-year-old lignite (coal) deposits near Schoningen, Germany. The objects are about forty centimeters long and have a notch for what might have been a blade. See Hartmut Thieme, "Altpaläolithische Holzgeräte aus Schöningen," *Germania* 77 (1999): 451–487. This same site is where Thieme found the world's oldest-known spears, 185 and 225 centimeters long javelin-like objects made from spruce heartwood. These remarkable finds have been used to restore a certain credence to

the "hunting hypothesis," prompting also a reevaluation of two earlier finds that had once been seen as spears, and later discounted. (A spear tip found inside an elephant carcass at Lehringen, for example, and a wood fragment found at Clacton had both been reinterpreted as "digging sticks" or "snow probes" in the 1970s and 1980s). The new finds have also been used to suggest a previously undocumented depth of foresight and planning. See Hartmut Thieme, "Palaeolithic Hunting Spears from Germany," *Nature* 385 (1997): 807.

27. Kathy D. Schick and Nicholas Toth, *Making Silent Stones Speak: Human Evolution and the Dawn of Technology* (New York: Simon and Schuster, 1994), 258–260.

28. See Schick and Toth, *Making Silent Stones Speak*, 258–259. The Kariandusi Museum in Kenya has a nice series of posters attempting to explain the uses of hand axes, said to include "butchering," "digging up roots," "scraping animal hides," and so forth. For a critique, see William H. Calvin, *A Brain for All Seasons* (Chicago: University of Chicago Press, 2002).

29. See Bob Holmes, "The Ascent of Medallion Man," *New Scientist*, May 9, 1998, 16.

30. Most hand axes are so old as to have experienced substantial weathering, including river tumbling, wind faceting, and deposition of desert varnish (if exposed). It is therefore difficult to gauge edge wear. See Lawrence Keeley, *Experimental Determination of Stone Tool Uses: A Microwear Study* (Chicago: University of Chicago Press, 1980).

31. Steven Mithen, *The Prehistory of the Mind* (London: Thames and Hudson, 1996). There are many other proposed uses for hand axes, ranging from ground mounting to hurling at birds, using slings; see the literature cited in John C. Whittaker and Grant McCall, "Handaxe-Hurling Hominids: An Unlikely Story," *Current Anthropology* 42 (2001): 566–572.

32. Eileen M. O'Brien, "The Projectile Capabilities of an Acheulian Hand-Axe from Olorgesailie," *Current Anthropology* 22 (1981): 76–79, and "What Was the Acheulean Hand Ax?" *Natural History* 93 (July 1984): 20–24.

33. Calvin's theory can be found in his "Rediscovery and the Cognitive Aspects of Toolmaking: Lessons from the Hand-Axe," http://faculty.washington.edu/wcalvin/2001/handaxe.htm. Calvin also claims to have confirmed O'Brien's earlier observations that thrown axes shift to vertical spinning, but my tests were not so clear-cut. It is not hard to throw such a tool to ensure a vertical spin, however. A recent critique of Calvin's theory can be found in Whittaker and McCall, "Handaxe-Hurling Hominids."

34. Figuier reports one hand ax from St. Acheul exhibited in the *galerie préhistorique* of the *Exposition universelle* of 1867 that was twenty-nine centimeters long and thirteen centimeters wide (*L'homme primitif*, 3rd ed., 64). The smallest-known Acheulean axes may be those found at Beeches Pit in England, which are four to five hundred thousand years old and only about two inches long (John Gowlett, personal communication).

35. Nineteenth-century scholars and collectors typically chose canonically beautiful, "perfect" examples of teardrop hand axes to reproduce in their texts. This stemmed partly from a concern to convince the reader that these were in fact objects formed by human hands: Charles Lyell in his 1863 *Antiquity of Man*, for example, began his discussion with a refutation of "the doubt [that] has been cast on the question whether the so-called flint hatchets have really been shaped by the hands of man" (112). The book also sports a prominent, gold-embossed relief of a handsome hand ax on its back cover, right above a similarly ornamented image of the surface of a mammoth tooth.

36. Nicholas Toth, "The Oldowan Reassessed: A Close Look at Early Stone Artifacts," *Journal of Archaeological Science* 12 (1985): 101–120.

37. A. J. Jelinek put forward this theory in "The Lower Paleolithic: Current Evidence and Interpretation," *Annual Review of Anthropology* 6 (1977): 11–32. The argument against what has been called the "blade dispenser theory" is that there are also Acheulean forms that resemble picks or cleavers, which one would not expect if the objects in question were simply used-up cores. There is also the difficulty that most hand axes are not in fact exhausted; you can still get blades from them (personal communication, John Gowlett).

38. Richard Klein, *The Dawn of Human Culture* (New York: John Wiley and Sons, 2000); and Alan Walker and Pat Shipman, *The Wisdom of the Bones* (New York: Knopf, 1996). An interesting piece of anatomical evidence here, developed by Walker and Ann MacLarnon, is the narrowness of the vertebral canal of the *erectus* spinal column, which suggests that this creature may not have had the chest-cavity nervous links and musculature required for language. The implication: *Homo erectus* was unable to speak. See Ann MacLarnon, "The Vertebral Canal," in *The Nariokotome Homo Erectus Skeleton*, ed. Alan Walker and Richard Leakey (Cambridge, MA: Harvard University Press, 1993).

39. See Kawai, "Japanese Monkeys"; Galef, "Tradition in Animals"; Andrew Whiten and Christophe Boesch, "The Cultures of Chimpanzees," *Scientific American*, July 2001, 60–67; and Christophe Boesch and Michael Tomasello, "Chimpanzee and Human Cultures," *Current Anthropology* 39 (1998): 591–614.

40. The literature here is vast. Some key texts would include: Derek Bickerton, *Language and Species* (Chicago: University of Chicago Press, 1990), and *Language and Human Behavior* (Seattle: University of Washington Press, 1995); and William Noble and Iain Davidson, *Human Evolution, Language, and Mind* (Cambridge: Cambridge University Press, 1996).

41. The end of the Acheulean is as puzzling as its persistence; it might well be that the evolution of "modern" humans (*Homo sapiens*) circa 150,000 years ago was made possible by the making and use of new tool types (the opposite might just as well be true). It is also possible that the transition from only one type of tool to tool-kit "choice" was connected to the rise of language about this time. This is very much terra incognita.

42. See Ian Tattersall, "Once We Were Not Alone," *Scientific American*, January 2000, 38–44. See also Ian Tattersall and Jeffrey H. Schwartz, *Extinct Humans* (New York: Westview, 2000).

43. C. Loring Brace, "The Fate of the 'Classic' Neanderthals: A Consideration of Hominid Catastrophism," *Current Anthropology* 5 (1964): 3–43. Milford Wolpoff, Brace's student and then colleague at the University of Michigan, was another exponent of the single species hypothesis; see his "Competitive Exclusion among Lower Pleistocene Hominids: The Single Species Hypothesis," *Man* 6 (1971): 601–614. Compare Ernst Mayr's 1950 assertion that humans had stopped speciating because "all the niches that are open for a Homo-like creature" had been filled ("Taxonomic Categories in Fossil Hominids," *Cold Spring Harbor Symposium on Quantitative Biology* 15 [1950]: 112).

44. Elements of this idea are echoed in Jonathan Marks's argument that since we cannot know whether Neanderthals bred with humans, we should assume they did out of a spirit of "inclusiveness" ("Systematics in Anthropology: Where Science Confronts the Humanities [and Consistently Loses]," in *Conceptual Issues in Modern Human Origins Research*, ed. G. A. Clark and C. M. Willermet [New York: Aldine De Gruyter, 1997], 46–59).

45. Stephen Jay Gould, "Unusual Unity," *Natural History*, April 1997, 20–23, 69–71.

46. Mayr, "Taxonomic Categories," 109–118. Dobzhansky had lumped Neanderthals with modern humans in a 1944 paper in the *American Journal of Physical Anthropology*. Jonathan Marks points out that European anthropologists tended to "other" the Neanderthals, excluding them from their own ancestry, while U.S. anthropologists tended to bring them in: "American anthropologists were busy othering the Indians, who were excluded from their ancestry" (personal communication).

47. This is from an even longer list in chapter 7 of Darwin's *Descent of Man*.

48. See, for example, Gerhard Heberer, ed., *Menschliche Abstammungslehre* (Stuttgart: Gustav Fischer Verlag, 1965). See also Robert N. Proctor, "From *Anthropologie* to *Rassenkunde*: Concepts of Race in German Physical Anthropology," in *Bones, Bodies, Behavior: Essays on Biological Anthropology*, ed. George W. Stocking Jr. (Madison: University of Wisconsin Press, 1988), 138–179.

49. See Walker and Shipman, *The Wisdom of the Bones*, 140–147.

50. Three of the best multiple hominid species novels are: J. B. Vercors, *You Shall Know Them* (1953, from the French); William Golding, *The Inheritors* (1955); and Bjorn Kurten, *Dance of the Tiger* (1995), all of which are essentially "encounter" or "first-contact" narratives. Vercors's book imagines the discovery of a band of australopithecines ("Tropis") living in a remote Javanese jungle— a sort of paleoanthropological version of Conan Doyle's *Lost World* with added subplots of hominid enslavement and interspecies breeding. Jean-Jacques Annaud's popular sci-fi fantasy film, *Quest for Fire*, was based on J.-H. Rosny's *La guerre du feu: Un roman des ages farouches* (Paris: E. Fasquelle, 1911), a

World War I–era novel with Neanderthal versus Cro-Magnon love/war themes. Desmond Morris orchestrated the gestures for the 1981 film, which includes a lot of sniffing and head smashing. Clive Gamble suggests that the finding of Neanderthal sites near the Somme in the early part of the twentieth century, around the time of the First World War, may have prompted associations of these creatures with a bestial and violent past that humans had supposedly transcended (personal communication). More general critiques of Paleolithic imagery and narrative cliché can be found in Moser, *Ancestral Images*; and Misia Landau, *Narratives of Human Evolution* (New Haven, CT: Yale University Press, 1991).

51. See John Noble Wilford, "On the Trail of a Few More Ancestors," *New York Times*, Section 1, p. 8, April 8, 2001.

52. Alan Walker attributes this to Vince Sarich (personal communication). The odds that any given organism will contribute genes to subsequent generations become vanishingly small as time marches on; the use of the term ancestor with reference to an individual hominid fossil is therefore misleading, since there is only a remote possibility that it would have contributed anything to the genetics of modern *Homo sapiens*.

53. Cladistics can also be regarded as culpable in this regard: Willi Hennig's 1966 *Phylogenetic Systematics* (translated from the German text of 1950) moved an entire generation of paleontologists in the direction of splitting—as one might expect from a man whose expertise was beetles. The coleoptera order contains an estimated three hundred thousand separate species, whose articulated joints offer an excellent opportunity for quantitative digital distinction, as per the method of cladistics.

54. Franz Boas's 1911 *Mind of Primitive Man* contains a canonical formulation of the U.S. culturalist paradigm.

55. United Nations Educational, Scientific, and Cultural Organization, *The Race Concept: Results of an Inquiry* (Paris: UNESCO, 1952).

56. Brace, "Fate of the 'Classic' Neanderthals." Brace's argument is curious: he maintains that since Neanderthals possessed culture, they could not have been overwhelmed by another species practicing culture. He also argues, again, that there was no ecological space for more than one cultural species.

57. Ian Tattersall, *The Fossil Trail: How We Know What We Think We Know about Human Evolution* (New York: Oxford University Press, 1995), 116.

58. Cited in Richard Delisle, "Human Paleontology and the Evolutionary Synthesis," in *Ape, Man, Apeman: Changing Views since 1600*, ed. Raymond Corbey and Bert Theunissen (Leiden: Department of Prehistory, Leiden University, 1995), 217–228.

59. See, for example, Günther Bergner, "Geschichte der menschlichen Phylogenetik seit dem Jahr 1900," in *Menschliche Abstammungslehre*, ed. Gerhard Heberer (Stuttgart: Gustav Fischer Verlag, 1965), 49.

60. See Tattersall, *Fossil Trail*, 116.

61. Stephen Jay Gould, "Bushes and Ladders in Human Evolution," in *Ever since Darwin* (New York: W. W. Norton, 1977).

62. Coon, *Origin of Races*, 656; See William H. Tucker, *The Science and Politics of Racial Research* (Urbana: University of Illinois Press, 1994), 162–168; and John Jackson, "In Ways Unacademical: The Reception of Carleton S. Coon's *The Origin of Races*," *Journal of the History of Biology* 34 (2001): 247–285.

63. Bergner, "Geschichte," 49. The changing graphic conventions used to portray human phyletic development are interesting in this context, especially when compared to countervailing trends in the portrayal of human racial diversity. Hominid species diversity has increased, at the same time that racial diversity has been progressively downplayed. The concurrence is not a coincidence: the same stress on genetic diversity that helped put an end to the idea that human races constitute separate species was also implicated in the idea that the (singular) human population must have been diverse in the distant past—whence the single species hypothesis. Human racial unity seemed to preclude hominid phyletic diversity.

64. There were also important physical anthropologists championing the out-of-Africa notion prior even to the development of genetic sequencing tools—Christopher Stringer of London's Natural History Museum, for example, who had already made a good case for Neanderthal replacement when the molecular evidence became available. See Erik Trinkaus and Pat Shipman, *The Neanderthals* (New York: Vintage, 1992), 360–419. Other out-of-Africa physicalists include Gunter Brauer and (arguably) Clark Howell. Rebecca Cann's molecular work in the 1980s allowed the two models, described by William Howells in 1976 as "Noah's Ark" and "Candelabra," to be distinguished on the basis of genetic data. See William Howells, "Explaining Modern Man: Evolutionists vs. Migrationists," *Journal of Human Evolution* 5 (1976): 477–496.

65. Kenneth Weiss of Penn State argues that the issue here is not racism but rather differing views on the "specialness" of modern humans—that is, the extent to which modern humans are unique vis-à-vis the rest of the animal kingdom and our own ancestral past (personal communication).

66. See Milford H. Wolpoff and Rachel Caspari, *Race and Human Evolution: A Fatal Attraction* (New York: Westview Press, 1997).

67. See, for example, "Der Krieg der Easten Menschen," the cover story in *Der Spiegel*, February 2000, 240–255.

68. See Wil Roeboeks, "'Policing the Boundary?' Continuity of Discussions in 19th and 20th Century Palaeoanthropology," in *Ape, Man, Apeman: Changing Views since 1600*, ed. Raymond Corbey and Bert Theunissen (Leiden: Leiden, 1995), 173–180.

69. Richard C. Lewontin, *The Genetic Basis of Evolutionary Change* (New York: Columbia University Press, 1974). See also the earlier work of Luigi Luca Cavalli-Sforza.

70. See also Margaret W. Conkey and Sarah H. Williams, "Original Narratives: The Political Economy of Gender in Archaeology," in *Gender at the Crossroads of Knowledge: Feminist Anthropology in the Postmodern Era*, ed. Micaela di Leonardo (Berkeley: University of California Press, 1991), 102–139.

71. The people who migrated out of Africa circa 135,000 years ago cannot be regarded as being closer to modern "Africans" than any other population in the modern world.

72. Jürgen Trabant, "Origins of Language I: Thunder, Girls, and Sheep, and Other Origins of Language" (paper, Summer Academy on Human Origins, Max-Planck-Institute for the History of Science, Berlin, August 13–24, 2001), 15.

73. My personal view as of this writing is that humanness should carry a symbolic/moral (and/or linguistic/cultural) sense separable from its biological (or phyletic-typological) sense—and that if intelligent creatures are discovered in some other part of the universe, they should probably be accorded some kind of human rights. Humanity in this sense (or personhood, if you prefer) is a moral category that transcends biological specifics. It also implies that humans could find closer moral kinships with unrelated creatures (that is, non-DNA based) than with nonhuman species here on earth. There are obvious ethical conundrums in such a view (for example, with regard to the humanity of nonlinguistic *Homo sapiens*). There is also the intriguing question of what kind of answer we should give if and when machines of human construct begin to ask for rights of one sort or another. On machine consciousness, see Igor Alexander, "The Self 'Out There,'" *Nature* 413 (September 6, 2001): 23; Raymond Kurzweil, *The Age of Spiritual Machines: When Computers Exceed Human Intelligence* (Cambridge: MIT Press, 1990); also Rodney A. Brooks, *Flesh and Machines: How Robots Will Change Us* (New York: Pantheon, 2002).

10
Human Nature in a Post–Human Genome Project World

Thomas A. Shannon

If anything would generally characterize our current situation, it is the prefix "post" attached to an ever-growing number of nouns to form an adjective describing our world, our civilization, and our relation to them. Among the first postgeneration in more modern times was the post-Galileo generation that experienced the decentering of the earth in its vision of the solar system. Another postculture was that of the post-Reformation with both the affirmation of religious freedom and the rise of nation-states each with its own religious identity. Then came the post-Darwinian culture with its removal of humanity from the apex of the great Aristotelian chain of being and the striking of a near-lethal blow to hierarchy, both biological and social. Perhaps more significant was the consequent introduction of the concept of change into our notion of reality. For Darwinian thought did provide a devastating, if not fatal, blow to the tree of stability or stasis. Another contribution to the post-civilization was that of Freudianism, which decentered our concept of the self from both its medieval and Enlightenment position of ahistorical privilege and located it in the midst of a struggle for dominance with the forces of the id. Not only is evolution present in the species but also within the bosom of each human. Currently, we have postmodernity with its affirmation of process, dynamism, and the decentering of the text as well as the self, resulting in almost boundless reconstructions of text and self.

Given all these seismic cultural shifts, one would think we might be entitled to a period of integration or at least recuperation from the challenge of making sense of all this. Such is not the case. We are now the postgenomic age that will be the recipient of the fruits of the completion of the Human Genome Project (HGP). While the current focus of the

HGP has been its medical implications, the HGP also has implications for our understanding of ourselves, our very human nature, and our relation to others with whom we share our genome, as well as those whose genome differs from ours by perhaps only three or four percentage points.

The story of the HGP began of course with the discovery in 1953 of the structure of the DNA molecule by James Watson and Francis Crick, and continued through the next decades with one discovery after another almost at the proverbial warp speed introduced by the popular television series *Star Trek*. Such discoveries also gave us the capacity, in the words of the same show, to go where no one had gone before. Now we are on another voyage of self-discovery, a part of which will be difficult for it will involve leaving a comfortable harbor or at least a known harbor. But another part of the voyage may be even more difficult—the reconstruction of a new vision of human nature in light of our new and ever-increasing understanding of the human genome. As the great U.S. philosopher Woody Allen has noted, while the unexamined life may not be worth living, the examined life is no bowl of cherries either.

Before taking some first steps on this journey, I want to make some comments about methodology. With respect to the HGP, much of its success, as well as the success of science in general, is due to the method of reductionism. This method succeeds by breaking components into ever-smaller units and examining them. The whole is explained in terms of the parts and their interaction. This method has been and will continue to be extremely successful, and thus is not to be rejected. A point I would stress is not to confuse the method with a philosophy. That is, to argue that one needs to understand the workings of an organism by understanding its parts—its genetic structure, for example—is not necessarily to argue that an understanding of the genetic structure is a sufficient explanation of the operations of the organism as a whole. One can commit oneself to the use of reductionism as a method without necessarily committing oneself to a philosophy of materialism. This point will recur throughout this chapter, and I wanted to highlight it here.

A second point is what is referred to in the Roman Catholic tradition as *ressourcement,* a method developed by German and French theologians in the 1950s that sought to reappropriate concepts and ideas from the tradition and apply or use them to illuminate contemporary discussions.[1] This is not a matter simply of a language change or a method of "We used to say that, but now we say this, but it really doesn't make any difference because both really mean the same." I want to affirm that while our reality is different, particularly given the substantive cultural shifts we have experienced, insights and ideas from the tradition may provide a different angle of vision or bring a critical question to a contemporary discussion. I am not arguing that we can impose the conceptual framework of the past on the present. Rather, I am seeking to bring the best of the past with me as I seek to understand what we share with so many people, past and present: our human nature. And part of that nature is surely our past, both genetically and culturally.

Finally, the recently completed HGP has given us a map of the human genome. We now know the location of most individual genes, and the next task is to learn the function of these genes and their interaction with each other and the environment. Only when we begin to understand this dimension of our genetic structure will we be in a better position to achieve a more critical understanding of ourselves. But until then, and I want to emphasize this strongly, we are at the level of knowing the location of the genes and the biological or medical function of only a few of these genes. In spite of all the articles and hype that surrounds the routine announcement of a gene for this or a gene for that, very little of the actual effects of a particular gene, gene-gene interaction, or gene-environment interaction is actually known. This is particularly the case when the behavior involved is a complex one such as intelligence, sexual preference, or aggression. Thus at present, we can make only limited comments about human nature based on information from the genetic map we have at our disposal. What we do have, however, are perspectives from current developments in genetics as well as synthetic perspectives such as sociobiology. Even though sociobiology is quite controversial—both with respect to the theories themselves and the perspectives of the critics—information from this field, combined with some information from current genetics, points us in various directions and gives us important information to consider.

To ask the question of the nature of human nature, then, is to enter a whole series of philosophical, scientific, and, for some, theological questions. It is also to enter the complexity of the disciplinary issues within each of these general disciplines and the internal disputes endemic to each. Then there is the problem of any sort of integration of one's knowledge and the validity of the methodological claims on which one rests the validity of such integration.

To choose a context is to choose a viewpoint, and to choose a viewpoint is to choose not to see from other viewpoints. This does not mean that other viewpoints are invalid or wrong, but that a multiplicity of viewpoints cannot be simultaneously maintained. This is why the metaphor of triangulation from biological, philosophical, and cultural perspectives is, I think, critical in this chapter. One needs to think of human beings and human nature from a variety of viewpoints so that one can eventually gain some perspective and some overlap of perspective. By sighting ourselves from different perspectives, we can gradually gain a deeper understanding of our nature. In particular in this chapter, I will be focusing on issues of freedom, altruism, and transcendence because of their centrality in both philosophical and biological discussions.

But to do this is to enter into a variety of controversies: creationism versus evolution, the sociobiology wars, the mechanisms of evolution debate, philosophical debates, and theological controversies. I think this cannot be avoided. Simultaneously, we must also be aware of the provisional nature of our method and argument. Today's commonly accepted facts are tomorrow's erroneous theories.

In what follows, then, I wish to present several perspectives on developments in contemporary genetics to help learn who we are as humans and what implications these perspectives might have for understanding our place in our common cosmos, as well as the implications for religion and ethics.

General Perspectives on Human Nature from Genetics

Evolution

Although perhaps something like 30 to 40 percent of Americans and the school board of the state of Kansas might disagree, the dominant scientifically accepted explanation for the development of life on this planet—from viruses to humans, and everything in between—is some form of Charles Darwin's theory of evolution. This theory has been united with elements of Mendelian genetics to form what is referred to as the Modern

Synthesis. Part of this agenda is to explain the precise mechanisms of evolution—population genetics, kin selection, adaptationism, punctuated equilibriums, sociobiology—but another part of the agenda is to understand the implications of these explanations for understanding ourselves and how we behave, in short, understanding human nature.

A major battle in the 1950s, for example, was the implicit prohibition of hereditarian explanations for human behavior and a focus on cultural or social explanations. The cultural explanation was given official status by the "UNESCO agreement in 1952, which effectively put a ban on biological research in human behavior."[2] Socially, Ullica Segerstråle relates this to the influence of immigrant groups in the United States and the Great Depression that made establishing a relation between economic success and biological fitness harder to maintain. Additionally, the anthropologists Franz Boaz, Ruth Benedict, and Margaret Mead made a successful argument for the prominence of culture over biology. Finally, biological or hereditarian explanations of differences were seen as racist, a view made easier by the excesses of the uses of genetics in Nazi Germany as well as at least the rhetoric of the eugenics movement.

In the 1980s, however, genetic or behavioral explanations gained ascendancy, a position for which Segerstråle gives several reasons. A major share of the credit for this goes to the HGP, which focused attention again on the role of genetics. The field of anthropology also focused on the commonalities of human behavior rather than the diversity, and this gave more credence to some biological explanations. Language was understood as an adaptive response rather than a purely cultural artifact. And we humans were more frequently described as being in continuity with animals than before, with the emphasis on nonverbal communication and emotions, particularly the emotion of morality.[3]

A second shift is in the perspective on genetics: from nature-nurture to gene and environment to gene-environment (including culture) interaction. The critical issue here is a shift from the role of single genes and their frequency in a population or their random recombination (in which evolution is mainly an additive phenomenon) to a perspective that sees multifaceted feedback loops between and among genes and their environment—a perspective that highlights the complexity of the interaction as well as decreases the role of single genes (except for some diseases).[4]

The shift over the last decades focused on the complexity of the makeup of organisms. Even synthetic approaches such as sociobiology appreciate the complexity of the organism, and the critical interaction between its genome and the environment in which it exists. Ironically, as a result of the mapping of the human genome, some have used the results to emphasize the role of the single gene for determining particular diseases, traits, or behaviors, regardless of their complexity. Thus, in addition to constant announcements of discoveries of genes for any number of diseases, we also have the concomitant announcement of a single or a small number of genes for complex behaviors such as homosexuality, alcoholism, intelligence, shyness, aggression, and all manner of other behaviors. We seem to be returning to an earlier genetic essentialism, a genetic explanation of behavior that focuses exclusively on the role of the single gene rather than gene-gene interaction and/or the interaction of the genome as a whole with the larger environment. This often-unacknowledged shift will have profound implications for how we understand ourselves, and we need to keep this perspective in mind as we think about human nature.

Biological Solidarity

One of the most critical discoveries of modern genetics is the communality of the DNA of all organisms. This biological solidarity is extremely interesting as well as quite threatening. Studies of mammals, primates, lesser vertebrates, and other organisms reveal a striking complementarity of genetic structure. It is clear that humans differ genetically from orangutans and other chimps by perhaps only 1 or 2 percent. The mouse is becoming a major model for the study of human diseases because its genetic profile overlaps considerably that of humans.

The question is whether to focus on differences or solidarity. Obviously the differences are critical, and 1 or 2 percent of DNA in the right place and in relation to specific environments does make a critical difference, as the history of human culture reveals. As Jonathan Marks notes, "The fact that our DNA is 98 percent identical to that of a chimp is not a transcendent statement about our natures, but merely a decontextualized and culturally interpreted datum." Thus, by looking at both chimps and humans, we can differentiate them quite easily as well as spot several common characteristics. Marks observes that "the apparent paradox is simply a result of how mundane the apes have become, and how exotic DNA still is."[5] A critical question emerging from both solidarity and diversity is, Do shared genes act differently in humans than in other mammals? This, of course, is one of the key questions in the sociobiology wars, for E. O. Wilson defined sociobiology as the "systematic study of the biological basis of social behavior," and he suggests a high degree of continuity between mammalian and human behavior.[6] But on the other hand, Wilson exhibits a degree of ambiguity in his argument. For example, he states that genes hold culture on a leash. Yet Segerstråle notes that Wilson suggests the possibility of aggression being a recently acquired trait in which a "learned behavior may be 'tracked' genetically. Here, then, we may have the protostatement of his famous pronunciation that 'the genes hold culture on a leash'—this time run in the *opposite* direction, however, that is: culture holding the *genes* on a leash, or the genes tracking culture."[7] And then there is the famous sentence in Richard Dawkins's *The Selfish Gene*: "We alone on earth can rebel against the tyranny of the selfish replicators."[8]

Is animal behavior a model or a predictor of human behavior? How do we understand the term altruism as applied to animals and humans? Finally, we have the question implicitly raised by Dawkins: If we can rebel against our genes, what is the basis for this?

Race and Human Origins

One of the causes of contention among humans has been the phenomenon of racism. The perception of the superiority of a set of physical characteristics, a specific trait, or even the assumption of the possession of a superior genotype has been the source or cause of racism, war, public policy, and much individual and social pain and sorrow. The perception of advantage has been the cause of enormous grief. Contemporary biology and genetics, however, have taught us something important: "The careful study of hidden variations, unrelated to climate, has confirmed that homogeneous races do not exist. It is not only true that racial purity does not exist in nature; it is entirely unachievable, and would not be desirable."[9]

On the other hand, it is clear that groups differ from each other, for example, with respect to skin color, eye shape, hair texture, height, and so on. Luigi Luca Cavalli-Sforza argues that the primary explanation for such characteristics is environmental. He offers four arguments. First, he maintains that "exposure to a new environment inevitably causes an adaptation to it." Variations in skin color as well as body shape and size are adaptations to temperature and humidity. Second, explains Cavalli-Sforza, "There is little climatic variation in the area where a particular population lives, but there are significant variations between the climates of the Earth. Therefore, adaptive reactions to climate must generate groups that are genetically homogeneous in an area that is climatically homogeneous, and groups that are very different in areas with different climates." His third point is that "adaptations to climate primarily affect surface characteristics." Fourth, "We can see only the body's surface, as affected by climate, which distinguishes one relatively homogeneous population from another."[10] Others note that perhaps .01 percent of our genes are responsible for our external appearance and that we differ "from one another only once in a thousand subunits of the genome."[11]

It is clear that there are many differences between humans and human groups. But these differences do not constitute a race: "a group of individuals that we can recognize as biologically different from others," in Cavalli-Sforza's words. Such differences would have to be statistically significant and biological. He continues "Because genetic divergence increases in a continuous manner, it is obvious that any definition or threshold would be completely arbitrary."[12] And while such information might logically demonstrate the uselessness of classification—for example, efforts to establish some sort of superiority—Cavalli-Sforza does indicate one justification for genetic classification: to identify groups with a genetic similarity that, because of common ancestry, increases their probability of having similar diseases and, therefore, the possibility of developing drugs responsive to these diseases. Here the motive for classification is therapeutic and justified by the humanitarian need to cure disease.

Another argument against the concept of race and racism is the common origin of all modern humans from a population in Africa. The separation of chimps and humans occurred about five million years ago, and modern humans arose in Africa about one hundred thousand years ago. The age of this so-called African Eve or, more precisely, mitochondrial Eve was calculated by counting "the number of mutations that differentiate two living individuals, and identify when their last common ancestor lived." Such calculations gave rise to the notion of an African Eve: "the woman whose mitochondria were the last common ancestors of all surviving mitochondria today" and who lived around 190,000 years ago.[13] A similar African Adam was found by developing techniques to trace nucleotide mutations of the Y chromosome, and this African Adam's age was dated at around 144,000 years ago. Thus modern genetics, in addition to modern anthropology, demonstrates what seems to be a significant human reality: "The continents were settled by Africans in the expected order. Modern humans appear first in Africa, then in Asia, and from this big continent they settled its three appendices: Oceania, Europe, and America."[14] Such migrations began eighty thousand to one hundred thousand years ago. And as the populations grew and migration occurred, so began the process of adaptation to new environments and climates that in turn led to the differences we currently observe between and among modern humans. Such differences are environmental adaptations by groups, but they are not genetic, and can neither override the reality of our common origin nor provide any justification for any claims to superiority, genetic or otherwise.

Individuality

Populations are essentially homogeneous with some variations—a function of the distance from the original ancestor. But even these differences slow down as geographic distance increases. Scientifically, then, it is irresponsible to use the term race to denote some sort of biological superiority or the primacy of some genotype or some group. Such homogeneity, however, is not the case in looking at individuals. The argument for this comes from the various technologies involved in DNA fingerprinting that identifies the probability of a DNA specimen coming from a particular individual. "The chance of two [unrelated] individuals on average having the same DNA profile is about one in a million billion," according to one researcher in the forensic application of this technology.[15] And as Cavalli-Sforza observes, "Regardless of the type of genetic markers used (selected from a very wide range), the variation between two random individuals within any one population is 85 percent as large as that between two individuals randomly selected from the world's population."[16] Additionally, through migration and increasing intermarriage, we have a greater mixing of genes that will have two effects: first, decreasing any genetic differences between groups and, second, increasing the differences between individuals of the same population.

The medieval champion of individuality John Duns Scotus anticipated something of Cavalli-Sforza's insight into the significance of individuality:

In the universe as a whole, order is mainly considered according to types or species where their inequalities or differences pertain to order. According to Augustine, however, in the *City of God* [bk. 19, chapter 13] "order is an arrangement of like and unlike things whereby each of them is disposed in its proper place." That is why this Agent who primarily intended the order of the universe (as the principle good, intrinsic to Himself) not only intended this inequality that is one requirement for order (among species) but also desired a parity of individuals (within the same species), which is another accompaniment of order. And individuals are intended in an unqualified sense by this First One insofar as he intended something other than himself not as an end, but as something oriented to that end. Hence to communicate his goodness, as something befitting his beauty, he produces several in each species. And in those beings which are the highest and most important, it is the individual that is primarily intended by God.[17]

Summation

This general orientation lays out some critical insights into our considerations of human nature from the perspective of modern genetics. We are a dynamic, evolving species with a common genetic as well as geographic origin. We have a genome that is adaptive and responsive to a variety of environments. Cavalli-Sforza neatly summarizes this: "Anthropometric characteristics, including skin color, demonstrate the selective effects of the different climates to which modern humans have been exposed in the course of their migrations over the Earth's surface. They vary especially with latitude. By contrast, genes are considerably more useful as markers of human evolutionary history, especially migrations. They vary more with longitude."[18]

The differences between populations are skin deep and essentially irrelevant socially or politically. Nevertheless, within the population of humans as a whole, each individual presents with a unique genotype. Even so-called identical twins have some genetic differences. Thus, within an essentially genetically homologous group, the individual stands out. As humans we therefore exist as individuals within a dynamic environment, our physical evolution speeded up dramatically by culture. What is a clear and significant factor in understanding human nature is that it is impossible to present a fixed model of it as has traditionally been done in many religious and philosophical theories. But we are not left hanging, so to speak, for we can reflect on our selves, our situation, and our experiences. We know that we are a species that engages in symbolic discourse and communicates efficiently and profoundly through language as no other organisms can. Most important, we seek to find systems of meaning for our lives that help us to make sense of our experiences as well as to transform them.

The shift to genetics and genetic understandings of both evolution and human origins, as well as the HGP itself, has given rise to a variety of explanations of human nature and behavior loosely grouped under the heading of sociobiology. In the next section of this chapter, I will examine both general sociobiological claims as well as various philosophical perspectives that ground these claims, focusing thematically on freedom, altruism, and transcendence, for the sake of offering insight into our elusive, dynamic, and changing human nature.

Human Nature in the Context of Modern Biology

Here, moving from the general considerations about humans in relation to modern biology discussed earlier, I wish to consider three specific questions that have historically been associated with human nature, but that have been challenged or seen as irrelevant in light of modern biology. As mentioned above, these are the questions of freedom, altruism, and a capacity for transcendence or religion.

These three characteristics of humans have typically been understood as qualities that separate us from other animals, that give us a particular relation to our own actions and other beings, as well as provide a sense of meaning that transcends our biological fate. Contemporary commentators have also singled out these characteristics for analysis. I wish to join this debate by incorporating aspects of other philosophical traditions as well as aspects of contemporary thought to help develop some insights into our human nature.

Sociobiological Perspectives

In what follows, I will present a sampling of sociobiological perspectives on two core problems historically associated with an understanding of human nature. I do this, first, to set a general context for our discussion, and second, to identify particular problems that can then be addressed in light of other philosophical perspectives.

Freedom   The question of freedom and determinism is an ancient philosophical concern, but it is also proving to be a critical scientific one. Knowledge of the action of specific genes as well as the action and interaction of hundreds of genes has focused on the question of freedom in an especially sharp way. The discipline of sociobiology in particular has helped to refocus our attention on this issue. A general problem in sociobiology is the tendency to assume that what is true of animal behavior is also true of human behavior. Hence, one could assume that since a large part of the human genome is shared with other animals, we are simply following our genetic programs as they do. Some respond to this by noting the presence of culture, understood broadly in a social and biological sense, as a mediating force on our genome. So we need to attend carefully to the question of whether or not there is direct evidence of a genetic or cultural foundation for a particular trait or behavior, and to what degree that foundation determines that behavior.

Another part of the problem is definitional. For example, Wilson (and coauthor C. L. Lumsden) responded in the following way to the question of whether the fact that the brain is programmed by the genes destroys free will: "The biases in mental development are only biases; the influence of the genes, even when very strong does not destroy free will. In fact, the opposite is the case: by acting on culture through the epigenetic rules, the genes create and sustain the capacity for conscious choice and decision."[19] This is a clear rejection of determinism and a good example of gene-environment interaction. But it also identifies freedom as choice. While that is a common understanding of freedom, we need to reflect on whether it is a fully adequate one. Lumsden and Wilson qualify freedom by stating that "while [humans] exercise free will in moment-by-moment choices, this faculty remains superficial and its value to the individual is largely illusory," and "real freedom consists of choosing our masters by a procedure that allows us to master them."[20] This statement presents freedom as illusory, and in fact, we have this illusion of freedom only because we choose what will determine our actions. But the resolution is unsatisfactory. While we seem to make ourselves genetically, which results in our genes controlling our actions, we also seem to be choosing the particular genes that do the controlling. This correlates with Wilson's position, noted above, that while sometimes genes hold culture on a leash, interestingly enough, culture also holds the genes on a leash. How human freedom would fit here is quite unclear, for a leash, is still a leash, and in this perspective it sets clear limits.

Wilson goes on to specify the nature of freedom: "To the extent that the future of objects can be foretold by an intelligence which itself has a material basis, they are determined—but only within the conceptual world of the observing intelligence. And insofar as they can make decisions of their own accord—whether or not they are determined—they possess free will."[21] He uses the example of a bee. If we were to know all the properties of small animals—for instance, the bee's nervous system, its behavioral characteristics, and its personal history—and if this information could be put into a computer program, we could predict the bee's flight. To the circle of human observers watching the computer readout, the future of the bee is determined to some extent. But in the bee's own "mind," the bee, who is isolated permanently from such human knowledge, will always have free will.[22] The same is true for humans, insofar as their behavior can be specified. Yet because of the complexity of human behavior, technical limitations, and perhaps, the capacity of intelligence in general, such specification and prediction of human behavior is practically impossible. Wilson concludes: "Thus because of mathematical indeterminacy and the uncertainty principle, it may be a law of nature that no nervous system is capable of acquiring enough knowledge to significantly predict the future of any other intelligent system in detail. Nor can intelligent minds gain enough self-knowledge to know their own future, capture fate, and in this sense eliminate free will."[23]

For Wilson, free will is either indeterminacy or unpredictability, and it is a function of a technical inability either to know all the variables or—should they be known—to program them in a meaningful way.

Dawkins also contends that there is no clear relation between a particular trait's being under genetic control and the possibility of its modification. While this argues against a particular kind of genetic determinism and lack of freedom, the question of how such modification occurs still remains. Dawkins states as well, especially in *The Selfish*

Gene, that he is describing how things evolved, not how humans ought to act. He is interested not in humans and human behavior but rather animal behavior. So again, one must be careful how one reads and parses his observations. But, having been tarred with the brush of genetic determinism in critiques of the first edition of his book, Dawkins is quite blunt in his rejection of it: "It is perfectly possible to hold that genes exert a statistical influence on human behaviour while at the same time believing that this influence can be modified, overridden, or reversed by other influences. . . . We, that is our brains, are separate and independent enough from our genes to rebel against them."[24]

The interesting part of this sentence is the identification of the self with the brain. How one understands that will also suggest something about freedom and how it functions. And we must remember that Dawkins, like Wilson, maintains that we have the capacity to rebel against our replicators, as he notes in *The Selfish Gene*. But again, one must seek for the foundation or basis of such a capacity. Is this a capacity found generally in all animals, the focus of his study, or is it unique to humans?

One important part of the argument of both these authors is that any discussion of freedom must occur within a context, one that is both genetic and cultural. No one stands apart from such an environment, and this environment must at least condition or qualify both our understanding of freedom as well as its exercise. But since both argue for some capacity to transcend one's genetic program, we need to look carefully for the basis of that capacity.

Altruism   Altruism is a word describing a noble tendency in humans: actions on behalf of another with little or no regard for oneself or one's interests. In the literature of sociobiology, however, it is the near equivalent to a fighting word. Generally, altruism refers to some form of behavior that promotes the fitness of another organism at the expense of its own fitness. On the one hand, this is a *behavioral* term that portrays how natural selection occurs, not a depiction of *motives*. On the other hand, Wilson, for example, argued that altruism is the central problem of sociobiology. With this, he also brought a "particular philosophical style: the coupling of scientific and moral notions;" he thus looked for holistic explanations of behavior, leading him occasionally to commit the naturalistic fallacy of describing moral norms from biological descriptions.[25] For Dawkins, discussing this from the gene's perspective, the point is not the survival of the individual but the survival of copies of the genes. Since relatives are the ones who share these genes, altruistic behavior toward relatives is to be expected.

As if this were not problematic enough, the term also is involved in a dispute over the workings of natural selection, with the debate falling roughly between group selection and kinship selection, and with the phrase "inclusive fitness" being introduced for good measure as well. Historically, most claimed that natural selection proceeded through group selection—that is, through behavior that was to the advantage of the group. In this model, altruistic behavior was self-sacrificial behavior for the good of the group. The late William Hamilton developed a complex mathematical argument for kin selection. This was altruistic behavior on the part of the individual "towards relatives with whom they have genes in common." Inclusive fitness, again a concept developed by Hamilton, "explains how natural selection can favor altruism. This can happen if the benefits of altruism can be made to fall on individuals who are likely to be altruist rather than random members of the population."[26] Thus from Hamilton's perspective, inclusive fitness is a broader notion that can include both kin and group selection as mechanisms for the evolution of altruism.

Now the problem: Is this explanation relevant to human behavior? Is this mechanism of natural selection operative in our nature as well? Are we genetically predisposed to favor our relatives over others? In a controversial paper, Hamilton argued the following:

It can even be suggested that certain genes or traditions of the pastoralists revitalize the conquered people with an ingredient of progress which tends to die out in a large panmietic population for reasons already discussed. I have in mind altruism itself or the part of altruism which is perhaps better described as self-sacrificial daring. By the time of the Renaissance, it may be that the mixing of genes and cultures (or cultures alone, if these are the only vehicles, which I doubt) has continued long enough to bring the old mercantile thoughtfulness and infused daring into conjunction in a few individuals who then find courage for all kinds of inventive innovation against the resistance of established thought and practice. Often, however, the cost in fitness of such altruism and sublimated pugnacity to the individuals concerned is by no means metaphorical, and the benefits to fitness, such as they are, go to a mass of individuals whose genetic correlation with the innovator must be slight indeed. Thus civilization probably slowly reduces its altruism of all kinds, including the kinds needed for cultural creativity.[27]

The line of argumentation certainly suggests that when the benefits of an altruistic act do not go to relatives, the benefits tend to disappear over time. Additionally, it seems to indicate that acting against natural selection or one's genes decreases the number of such genes in the population as well as the overall fitness of society.

Wilson phrases the issue this way:

Can the cultural evolution of higher ethical values gain a direction and momentum of its own and completely replace genetic revolution? I think not. The genes hold culture on a leash. The leash is very long, but inevitably values will be constrained in accordance with their effects on the human gene pool. The brain is a product of evolution. Human behavior—like the deepest capacities for emotional response which drive and guide it—is the circuitous technique by which human genetic material has been and will be kept intact.[28]

For Wilson, the genetic program is key to understanding human development on all levels. Thus, while a culture may move in a particular direction, eventually and ultimately, it will be conformed to the genetic program, and group and kin selection will win out.

Wilson makes altruism the central theoretical problem of sociobiology. This is so because in a "Darwinist sense the organism does not live for itself. Its primary function is not even to reproduce other organisms; it reproduces genes, and it serves as their temporary carrier." This occurs through natural selection, "a process whereby certain genes gain representation in the following generations superior to that of other genes located at the same chromosome positions."[29] Thus the organism is but DNA's way of making more DNA, and the individual but the vehicle for the genes.

In this context, the question is how can altruism—"self-destructive behavior performed for the benefit of others"—possibly evolve through natural selection.[30] This behavior obviously reduces personal fitness and would seem to lead to the loss of the gene or genes responsible for that behavior. Wilson finds the answer to this question in kinship: "If the genes causing the altruism are shared by two organisms because of common descent, and if the altruistic act by one organism increases the joint contribution of these genes to the next generation, the propensity to altruism will spread through the gene pool. This occurs even though the altruist makes less of a solitary contribution to the gene pool as the price of its altruistic act."[31]

Wilson argues that "the impulse need not be ruled divine or otherwise transcendental, and we are justified in seeking a more convenient biological explanation."[32] Though Wilson notes that specific forms of altruism are culturally determined, he argues that the sociobiological hypothesis "can explain why human beings differ from other mammals and why, in one narrow aspect, they more closely resemble social insects."[33]

Wilson further distinguishes two forms of cooperative behavior. First is what he terms hard-core altruism: "the altruistic impulse can be irrational and unilaterally directed at others; the bestower expresses no desire for equal return and performs no unconscious actions leading to the same end." Here, the responses are unaffected by social reward and punishment, and tend to serve the "altruist's closest relatives and to decline steeply in frequency and intensity as relations become more distant."[34]

Second is soft-core altruism: the altruist, in Wilson's words, "expects reciprocation from society for himself or his closest relatives. His good behavior is calculating." Thus, soft-core altruism is essentially selfish in a traditionally moral sense as well as being influenced by cultural evolution. For Wilson, the psychological vehicles for this behavior are "lying, pretense, and deceit, including self-deceit, because the actor is most convincing who believes that his performance is real."[35]

In Wilson's perspective, soft-core altruism is crucial for human society because it broke the constraints on the social contract imposed by kin selection. Reciprocity is crucial for the formation of society. Hard-core altruism, on the other hand, is the "enemy of civilization." This favors kin selection, the favoring of one's own relatives, and permits only limited global cooperation. Hence Wilson says, "Our societies are based on the mammalian plan: the individual strives for personal reproductive success foremost and that of his immediate kin secondarily; further grudging cooperation represents a compromise struck in order to enjoy the benefits of group membership."[36]

This gives Wilson a basis for optimism, for he thinks humans are "sufficiently selfish and calculating to be capable of indefinitely greater harmony and social homeostasis. This statement is not self-contradictory. True selfishness, if obedient to the other constraints of mammalian biology, is the key to a more nearly perfect social contract." Moreover, these other constraints are learning rules and emotional safeguards. Thus, honor and loyalty are reinforced while cheating, betrayal, and denial are universally rejected. Thus it seems that learning rules, based on innate, primary reinforcement, led human beings to acquire these values and not others with reference to members of their own group. . . . I will go further to speculate that the deep structure of altruistic behavior, based on learning rules and emotional safeguards, is rigid and universal. It generates a set of predictable group responses.[37]

Soft-core altruism therefore provides the basis for various social allegiances, shifting though they may be. The critical distinction is the ingroup and the out-group, the line between which fluctuates continually. But this is our social salvation for if hard-core altruism were the basis for social relations, our fate would be a continuous "intrigue of nepotism and racism, and the future bleak beyond endurance." Soft-core altruism provides an optimistic cynicism that can give us the basis for a social contract. Such behavior has been "genetically assimilated and is now part of the automatically guided process of mental development." Thus, genes hold culture on a leash, and though the leash is long, "inevitably values will be constrained in accordance with their effects on the human gene pool."[38]

Dawkins, who is most popularly associated with a narrow reading of altruism through the publicity and controversy surrounding *The Selfish Gene*, explicitly rejects any direct application of his explanation of evolution to human behavior. Two things work against him, however. First, he describes the evolutionary mechanism from the perspective of the gene and highlights the interest of the gene in producing replicas of itself rather than the individual as such. The choice of the metaphor of selfishness, as opposed to cooperation perhaps, suggested a motive rather than a behavior—a motive that could easily be applied to human behavior. Second, as the preface to the first edition written by Richard Trivers stated, "In short, Darwinian social theory gives us a glimpse of an underlying symmetry and logic in social relationships which, when more fully comprehended by ourselves, should revitalize our political understanding and provide the intellectual support for a science and medicine of psychology. In the process it should also give us a deeper understanding of the many roots of our suffering."[39]

For those who wanted to read a theory of human behavior into *The Selfish Gene*, such an opportunity was handed to them on a silver platter. Yet the question remains: Are we on a genetic leash? Do we act to benefit primarily our relatives? Is action beyond the group possible or, as Hamilton suggested, will civilization gradually erode self-sacrificial behavior? This point is complicated by the absence of Trivers's preface in the 1989 edition of *The Selfish Gene*, together with these sentences by Dawkins in the first chapter: "My purpose is to examine the biology of selfishness and altruism.... Apart from its academic interest, the human importance of this subject is obvious. It touches every aspect of our social lives, our loving and hating, fighting and cooperating, giving and stealing, our greed and our generosity."[40]

Even though Dawkins affirms that his focus is behavior, not motive— the effects of one's act, not one's subjective dispositions—the language here certainly is open to a discussion of motives, even though there is a strong attempt to redefine such terms. Thus, in the definition of altruism as behavior "to increase another such entity's welfare at the expense of its own,"[41] welfare is understood as one's chance of survival. One looks at outcome, not motives. A selfish gene therefore tries "to get more numerous in the gene pool. Basically the gene does this by helping to program the bodies in which it finds itself to survive and to reproduce." Nevertheless—and this is a critical issue for my argument here—"a gene might be able to assist *replicas* of itself that are sitting in other bodies. If so, this would appear as an act of individual altruism but it would be brought about by gene selfishness."[42]

The key way in which such genetically altruistic acts occur is through kin selection or within-family altruism, one that increases the greatest net benefit to one's genes—that is, ensures the highest success rate for a particular gene. As Dawkins phrases it:

A gene for suicidally saving five cousins would not become more numerous in the population, but a gene for saving five brothers or ten first cousins would. The minimum requirement for a suicidal altruistic gene to be successful is that it should save more than two siblings (or children or parents), or more than four half-siblings (or uncles, aunts, nephews, nieces, grandparents, grandchildren), or more than eight first cousins, etc. Such a gene, on average, tends to live on in the bodies of enough individuals saved by the altruist to compensate for the death of the altruist itself.[43]

And so Dawkins concludes, "I have made the simplifying assumption that the individual animal works out what is best for his genes."[44]

This is essentially what Wilson calls hard-core altruism, and he describes such behavior as "the enemy of civilization." Soft-core altruism, recall, is what makes society possible, though to a limited degree only. Hence for Wilson, the

> most elaborate forms of social organization, despite their outward appearance, serve ultimately as the vehicles of individual welfare. Human altruism appears to be substantially hard-core when directed at closest relatives, although still to a much lesser degree than in the case of the social insects and the colonial invertebrates. The remainder of our altruism is essentially soft. The predicted result is a mélange of ambivalence, deceit, and guilt that continuously troubles the individual mind.[45]

This perspective seems to leave us in a rather melancholy state at best and total despair at worst. From a biological perspective, both Wilson and Dawkins seem to have placed us squarely in the middle of a Hobbesian world. This view was promulgated most clearly in Dawkins's *The Selfish Gene,* the main argument of which was that "a predominant quality to be expected in a successful gene is ruthless selfishness. . . . Much as we might wish to believe otherwise, universal love and the welfare of the species as a whole are concepts which simply do not make for evolutionary success." Indeed as Dawkins says, "I think 'nature red in tooth and claw' sums up our modern understanding of natural selection admirably."[46]

Summation   So where do these considerations leave us in exploring human nature? First, I think in a very confusing place. In part, this is because terms and their meanings vary from author to author. But it is also because authors are attempting to develop integrating theories of human behavior without appealing to motives. Nonetheless, there is an appeal to some kind of an ethical theory on which people can be held accountable. Second, the authors operate out of an evolutionary framework that shapes their perspectives. They correctly note that we simply cannot speak of human behavior without simultaneously speaking of genes and their effect on the total organism. But third, the primacy seems to be on the role of the genes. Though the authors explicitly affirm the role and significance of culture, they return to the role of the gene. Wilson is most explicit when he says that culture is held on a genetic leash. Dawkins is more ambiguous when he says we can rebel against our culture, but the basis for that is not clear. Additionally, one would wonder if there was a genetic consequence for straying from our genetic program. Connections between these perspectives and the HGP's tilt toward genetic essentialism are also easy to make. The HGP will reinforce the search for the role and the consequences of single genes. In turn, this will heighten the search for genetic programs that control our behavior.

The questions for examination are complex. Are we simply matter? Are we at the disposal of our genes? Is there a basis for a kind of rebellion against our genes? Is there a human nature? Is freedom an illusion, or do we have the capacity to transcend our nature? These questions press us from the perspective of the HGP as well as contemporary studies in genetics.

Perspectives from the Philosophy of John Duns Scotus

In keeping with my methodological interest in *ressourcement*, I would like to turn to John Duns Scotus to examine a surprisingly fruitful perspective from which to consider these issues. The move from contemporary genetics to a medieval philosopher may seem strange or bizarre to some (or many). Yet I have become convinced that some of the ideas that Duns Scotus developed in his writings can shed light on some aspects of our contemporary problem. Given that Duns Scotus died in 1302, it is obvious that he had neither knowledge of the theory of evolution nor any concept of what sociobiologists refer to as a reproductive strategy. Thus, I am not attempting to bootleg any such theories into his thought. Nor will I use his ideas as a procrustean bed with which to shape contemporary ideas. Rather, my sense is that Duns Scotus has some insights that can help clarify the conundrum into which the sociobiologists seem to have gotten themselves. I wish to focus in particular on his concepts of nature, freedom, and transcendence as a way to help think through some of the problems posed in the sociobiology debate.

Duns Scotus's Concept of Nature   Sociobiologists, I would argue, have made a major mistake in their use of the term altruism. My issue is the term, not the behavior—although my concern is not exclusively semantic. That is, while the behaviors described are biologically accurate— insofar as they stick to biology—the significance of these behaviors also has been misinterpreted primarily because of the sociobiologists' almost idiosyncratic use of the term altruism. And it is because of this that they have gotten themselves into what many consider to be a Hobbesian world.

Duns Scotus begins with two distinctions. First is the concept of a nature: a principle of activity by which an entity acts out or actualizes its reality. A being's nature is the reason why an entity acts as it does. Or as he says, "The potency of itself is determined to act, so that so far as itself is concerned, it cannot fail to act when not impeded from without."[47] A nature essentially explains why an entity acts as it does.

A will, on the other hand, "is not of itself so determined, but can perform either this act or its opposite, or can either act or not act at all."[48] Hence, the reason why this act was done as opposed to another is that the will is the will and can elicit an act in opposite ways. Following Saint Anselm, Duns Scotus distinguishes two movements in the will as the *affectio commodi*—the inclination to seek what is advantageous or good for one self—and the *affectio justitiae*—the inclination to seek the good in itself.

Here, I focus on the affectio commodi, the will to do what is to our advantage, perfection, or welfare. This affection or inclination is a nature seeking its own fulfillment. For Duns Scotus, this affectio commodi is not an elicited act. Rather, it is a natural appetite necessarily seeking its own perfection. As Duns Scotus explains:

That it does so *necessarily* is obvious, because a nature could not remain a nature without being inclined to its own perfection. Take away this inclination and you destroy the nature. But this natural appetite is nothing other than an inclination of this sort to its proper perfection; therefore the will as nature necessarily wills its perfection, which consists above all in happiness, and it desires such by its natural appetite.[49]

Allan B. Wolter provides an interesting commentary on this concept:

All striving, all activity stems from an imperfection in the agent. As the etymological derivation of the word itself suggests, nature [from *nasci*, to be born] is literally what a thing was born to be, or more precisely, born to become, for nature as an active agent is essentially dynamic in a Faustian sense. It is restless until it achieves self-perfection. Since what perfects a thing is its good and since this striving for what is good is a form of love, we could say with Socrates that all activity is sparked by love.[50]

This love, however, is neither objective nor directed to the good of another, regardless of whether or not this other being might be a kin. It is self-centered and directed to seeking its own welfare. As Wolter further remarks, "If at times we encounter what seems to be altruistic behavior in the animal world, for instance, it is always a case where the 'nature' or 'species' is favored at the expense of the individual. But nature, either in its individual concretization or as a self-perpetuating species, must of necessity seek its own perfection. Such is its supreme value and the ultimate goal of all its loves."[51]

As Wolter interprets Duns Scotus here, when an individual entity or a nature acts, it seeks its own good or what is to its advantage. This is not cause for surprise for this is what a nature does, whether looked at as an individual representative of the species or the species as a whole. The affectio commodi drives the being "to seek his perfection and happiness in all he does."[52]

What is significant about this perspective—particularly in the context of the sociobiologists—is that for Duns Scotus, and indeed for the entire classical philosophical tradition from Plato forward, seeking one's own perfection is a *good*. It is "not some evil to be eradicated. For it too represents a God-given drive implanted in man's rational nature which leads him to seek his true happiness."[53] In fact, to ignore our perfection or give it no standing in our actions is an act of injustice to oneself.

I maintain that what Wilson and Dawkins refer to as genetic selfishness is what Duns Scotus labels the affectio commodi. The importance of the Scotistic position is, on the one hand, that he too sees the same kind of tendency present in human nature as do the sociobiologists, but on the other hand, he, together with the entire philosophical tradition up to that time, sees that behavior as a good because it achieves the perfection of the individual and the species. That is, the affectio commodi is that dimension of human nature that leads us to seek our fulfillment or perfection as a human. This affection is a good precisely because it leads to our perfection.

There is, however, a critical difference between Duns Scotus and the sociobiologists. For the sociobiologists, the behavior comes from evolutionary success, whereas for Duns Scotus, the cause is the creative will of God expressed in creation. Nonetheless, though the origin is quite different, the behavior is the same. Part of the difference surely lies in both philosophical and theological frameworks. Yet another part of the difference is that Duns Scotus sees self-perfecting behavior as a good, while the sociobiologists describe this as selfish—which even in their framework has a negative connotation.

But there remains this issue raised by the sociobiologists: Is such genetically selfish activity the only possible mode of human activity? Or as Duns Scotus would phrase it, can we see and actualize a good beyond ourselves and our perfection, beyond the affectio commodi? Scotistic thought would agree with the sociobiologists that as natures, we, like any other nature, seek our good and our individual perfection, and that we do so necessarily. But it would disagree that this is selfish in the pejorative sense of sociobiology. In fact, I think from a Scotistic perspective, the sociobiologists' discussion of genetic selfishness makes no sense at all and is a significant distortion of human existence, as I will argue below.

Duns Scotus on Freedom and Altruism   Duns Scotus calls the affectio justitiae or the affection for justice the source of true freedom or liberty of the will, and this is the basis for his claim that true freedom goes beyond freedom understood as choice. Additionally, the affectio justitiae is the means by which we can transcend nature and go beyond our individually defined good and ourselves to see the value of another being. As Duns Scotus observes, "To want an act to be perfect so that by means of it one may better love some object for its own sake, is something that stems from the affection for justice, for whence I love something good in itself, thence I will love something in *itself*."[54]

Wolter notes four characteristics of the affectio justitiae. First, it gives us the capacity to love a being for itself rather than for what it can do for us. Second, it enables us to love God for who God is rather than for the consequence of God's love on us. Third, the affectio justitiae allows us to love our neighbor as ourselves, thereby making each individual of equal value. Finally, such a seeking for the good in itself leads to a desire to have this good beloved by all rather than being held to oneself.[55] This leads Wolter to the conclusion that the affectio justitiae amounts to a "freedom *from* nature and a freedom for values."[56] Or as Duns Scotus puts it, "From the fact that it is able to temper or control the inclination for what is advantageous, it follows that it is obligated to do so in accordance with the rule of justice that it has received from a higher will."[57]

Such an understanding of will as affectio justitiae frees the will from the constraints of the necessity of human nature's act of self-realization or the seeking of its own good *only*. For Duns Scotus, then, when a free agent acts according to nature to realize itself or seek its own good, it paradoxically acts *unnaturally* since to seek what is *"bonum in se* is not to seek something that 'realizes the potential of a rational nature.' It is somehow to transcend 'the natural' and thus to have a mode of operation that sets the rational agent apart from all other agencies."[58]

This understanding of will grounds, for Duns Scotus, the possibility of our being able to transcend our own self-interest or self-benefit (what sociobiologists call genetic selfishness)—a topic to be addressed later.

Duns Scotus also proposes a view of freedom that is not limited to the choice of alternatives or freely elicited acts. Rather, in keeping with his mentors Saints Augustine and Anselm, Duns Scotus views freedom as "a positive bias or inclination to love things objectively or as right reason dictates."[59] The proper focus of freedom, and by implication moral analysis, is not the individual act of choosing but the inclination as a whole. And such an inclination focuses on fidelity to the good in itself, not the specific act of choosing that good or the necessary appreciation of what is good for the fulfillment of the nature of the agent. Here, Duns Scotus follows the older Catholic tradition of Anselm when he says, "Whoever has what is appropriate and advantageous in such a way that it cannot be lost is freer than he who has this in such a way that it can be lost."[60] From a psychological point of view, Duns Scotus argues that our awareness of the limitation of any particular act of will means that we experience freedom as choice. That is, we are aware that we could have chosen otherwise and that such a choice would have given a different degree of perfection. Thus, "choice is simply basic freedom in inferior conditions"—that is, human finitude.[61] When we will or make a choice, our will is never fully actual or fully expressed, for it is contingent—we can in fact choose this or that option. Yet for all that, we can approach our perfection through our steadfastness or constancy in cleaving to the object of our love. "The perfection of freedom connotes a perseverance and stability in the will's adherence to the good," comments William Frank.[62]

Duns Scotus presents both a critical and a positive perspective on freedom that is of particular importance. He discounts the significance of choice, understood as any particular choice or any choice considered as an isolated event. To say this, of course, flies totally in the face of certainly the normative U.S. experience of freedom and perhaps the Enlightenment tradition as well. For we revel in individual choice and assume that this is the essence of freedom. Such freedom is the core of autonomy, our expression of self-determination. From early in our lives, we are taught that ahead of us lies a series of decisions that will shape our lives and for which we alone will be responsible. For those of us in the United States, we have taken to heart existentialism's perspective that our existence precedes our essence and that one becomes oneself only through particular, individual choices. And if such choices are absent, one remains inauthentic.

Yet Duns Scotus fashions his development of freedom "from above," from a theological perspective that grapples with the question of how God can be free if love for the divine essence—for only an infinite being can fulfill an infinite being—is necessary. Duns Scotus develops two formulations of freedom to respond to this. The first looks to love for finite objects and, in Frank's words, is the ability *"not to limit* oneself to limitedly perfecting objects." The second envisions love for God and freedom as, to cite Frank again, the "ability to *continually adhere* to the unlimitedly perfecting object." The point common to both formulations is the will's ability to achieve perfection "through active union with its beloved."[63] This holds true regardless of whether the will is infinite and de facto there is no other intentional object or whether the will is finite and there are multiple intentional objects. Thus, for Duns Scotus, the essence of freedom is not choice but what he calls *firmitas*, or what we could call fidelity or constancy.

What follows from this is that the finite will can never fully express its basic freedom, because for humans there will always be another intentional object, another "what if I would have done this?" that would lead to another version of myself. For us to choose one goal, then, is to abandon others together with the perfection they could have given us. And given that we are finite, we are not able—as is God—to choose that which would ultimately perfect us. Freedom therefore manifests itself in choice: "basic freedom in inferior conditions"—that is, in the context of finitude.[64]

For Duns Scotus, however, free will is not limited only to the fact of choice or even appropriately characterized by it. Rather, as Frank notes, choice is "reflective of a deeper structure at work in a specific situation."[65] And this deeper structure is steadfastness, which constitutes the perfection of the will: "a perseverance and stability in the will's adherence to the good."[66] It is in this steadfastness of commitment that we attain our perfection, not in particular choices, regardless of their relation to the good.

The affection for justice is the capacity to love something or someone for their own selves, regardless of whether this happens to be a good for me or not. As Wolter phrases it, this is a "freedom from nature and a freedom for values." The conclusion is the paradox that "what differentiates the will's perfection as nature from the perfection of all other natural agents is that it can never be attained if it be sought primarily or exclusively: only by using its freedom to transcend the demands of its nature, as it were, can the will satisfy completely its natural inclination."[67]

Duns Scotus's affirmation here is that we have the capacity to value an entity for its own sake, independent of its personal or social utility. As Duns Scotus would put it, we have the ability to transcend the capacity to do justice to ourselves by doing justice to the good itself. The strong claim is that we are capable of recognizing goods distinct from our self-perfection and independent of our interests, and capable of choosing them even though such a choice may run counter to our personal self-interest or what does justice to my own nature. Or as Valerius Messerich remarks,

The will by freely moderating these natural and necessary tendencies to happiness and self-perfection is able to transcend its nature and choose Being and Goodness for their own sake. . . . Thus the free will is not confined to objects or goods that perfect self, but is capable of an act of love. . . . [L]ove is the most free of all acts and the one that most perfectly expresses the will's freedom to determine itself as it pleases.[68]

The conclusion is that one can distinguish at least a good and a better in human life. What is good in human life is a life that perfects us, that brings our being to a greater actualization. This is the realization of the affectio commodi. But what is better is the transcendence of self either to appreciate goods independent of us or even curb our legitimate interest in self-perfection to seek the good of others for their own sakes. This is the realization of the affectio justitiae. In Messerich's existentialist terminology, "A free choice, then, is the meaning of existence and the total initiative is left to man to rightly moderate his natural tendencies in the pursuit of being for its own sake. And in this sense one's existence is one's own responsibility and depends on one's causal initiative as an ultimate response to Being or Nothingness."[69] Put ethically, Wolter, says, "Right reason also recognizes that our self-perfection, even through union with God in love, is not of supreme value. It enables man, in short, to recognize that the drive for self-perfection paradoxically must not go unbridled if it is to achieve its goal, but must be channeled lest it destroy the harmony of the universe intended by God."[70]

What is most helpful about this perspective is that while it affirms self-perfection, ultimately such perfection is not an end in itself. To be all that we can be, we must step beyond the confines of self and actualize that most free of all acts, an act of love. For only then do we find ourselves open to the depths of reality. And in the steadfast adherence to that beloved, we realize the fullness of freedom.

Religion

I now turn to the general topic of religion, particularly with respect to the idea of its very possibility. In exploring the foundations that could make such a reality possible, I will also examine the adequacy of the philosophy of scientific materialism in capturing the sufficiency of matter as well as attitudes about religion expressed by various authors.

Scientific Materialism   Although the phrase "scientific materialism" appears late in Wilson's *On Human Nature*, it is a key principle that provides the overarching framework for many of the ideas in sociobiology. Scientific materialism, according to Wilson, is "the view that all phenomena in the universe, including the human mind, have a material basis, are subject to the same physical laws, and can be most deeply understood by scientific analysis." The core of scientific materialism is the evolutionary epic whose minimum claims are "that the laws of the physical sciences are consistent with those of the biological and social sciences and can be linked in chains of causal explanation; that life and mind have a physical basis; that the world as we know it has evolved from earlier worlds obedient to the same laws; and that the visible universe today is everywhere subject to these materialist explanations."[71]

Scientific materialism is a mythology, and Wilson asserts that "the evolutionary epic is probably the best myth we will ever have." It can be "adjusted until it comes as close to truth as the human mind is constructed to judge the truth." notes Wilson.[72]

Of critical importance is a discussion of matter, the ultimate grounding—so to speak—of evolution. In Wilson's theory, matter is all that is, it is also all that is needed to account for all activity—insect or animal, private or social. For Wilson, matter is most creatively expressed in the gene, the basic unit of heredity and "a portion of the giant DNA molecule that affects the development of any trait at the most elementary biochemical level." Thus, we need to examine human nature through biology and the social sciences. This will lead us to an understanding of the mind "as an epiphenomenon of the neuronal machinery of the brain. That machinery is in turn the product of genetic evolution by natural selection acting on human populations for hundreds of thousands of years in their ancient environments."[73]

The Transcendent Potential of Matter   But is matter only matter, inert particles interacting according to the laws of physics and/or chemistry, or is there another level?

One traditional theory explaining the interaction of particles of matter such as electrons and positrons is hylo-systemism, which as Wolter explains, holds that "all bodies, or at least nonliving bodies, are composed of elementary particles or hylons which are united to form a dynamic system or functional unit." In this context, system refers to "a functional nature, possessing new powers."[74] When put into various combinations or actualized under various conditions, these elementary particles form new systems educed from the matter and the properties of this new system. Wolter notes that they "are not simply the arithmetical sum of the actual properties manifested by these hylons in isolation for the property of any given system such as the nucleus or the hydrogen atom . . . is rooted proximately in the new powers of the respective system, powers which, though ultimately reducible to the two or more hylons that function as essentially ordered causes, exist only virtually in the individual hylons."[75]

Consequently, the properties of individual particles seen in isolation can never tell us the full range of these particles when combined into a system. Therefore, within matter lies a range of possibilities that emerge or are actualized only when these particles are put into a system or a previous system is restructured.

What are the implications of such a theory? Karl Rahner argues that we are the beings "in whom the basic tendency of matter to find itself in the spirit by self-transcendence arrives at the point where it definitely breaks through." For Rahner, "Matter develops out of its inner being in the direction of spirit."[76] This becoming—a becoming more, rather than a becoming other—must be "effected by what was there before and, on the other hand, must be the inner increase of being proper to the previously existing reality." This notion of becoming more is a genuine self-transcendence, a "transcendence into what is substantially new, i.e., the leap to a higher *nature*."[77]

While Rahner does not argue that life, consciousness, matter, and spirit are identical, he does maintain that such differences do not exclude development:

Insofar as the self-transcendence always remains present in the particular goal of its self-transcendence, and insofar as the higher order always embraces the lower as contained in it, it is clear that the lower always precedes the actual event of self-transcendence and prepares the way for it by the development of its own reality and order; it is clear that the lower always moves slowly toward the boundary line in its history, which it then crosses in actual self-transcendence.[78]

For Rahner, then, the human is the "self-transcendence of living matter." On the one hand, Rahner describes this as the cosmos becoming conscious of itself in the human. On the other hand, this self-transcendence of the cosmos reaches

its final consummation only when the cosmos in the spiritual creature, its goal and its height, is not merely something set apart from its foundation—something created—by something which receives the ultimate self-communication of its ultimate ground itself, in that moment when this direct self-communication of God is given to the spiritual creature in what we—looking at the historical pattern of this self-communication—call grace and glory.[79]

Lindon Eaves and Lora Gross offer another presentation of matter as the ground for new potentialities. They argue for a dynamic, holistic conception of matter that emphasizes the "unity of matter, life, and energy and understands nature as a profoundly complex, evolving system of intricately interdependent elements."[80] They suggest a vitality in matter that gives it depth and intensity, value, and the inclination toward organization.

Eaves and Gross operate from a biological and specifically genetic perspective that "seeks a new framework for its comprehension that does justice to all the so-called higher aspects of human consciousness in a phylogenetic and ontogenetic framework." This perspective focuses on the mechanisms of inheritance, which "have within themselves the probability of presenting new transcendent possibilities for action within history."[81] Thus, they argue that surprise is inherent in nature and then develop a view of nature itself as gracious. And like Rahner, Eaves and Gross contend that "genetics provides *a basis for grace within the structure of life itself.*"[82]

This position serves as the basis for a rejection of crude determinism for "the material processes of life have produced a person who transcends all conventional definitions of personhood to the point where the term *freedom* is the best we have available."[83]

This gives rise to two consequences: first, that "culture creates conditions for completion in community that would otherwise be impossible in a mere aggregation of individuals," and second, the "recognition that the conditions of life are such that the process that produces pain, in the sense of genetic disease, is also the process that maintains life in the cosmos."[84]

This second point is critical in that it highlights the value of genetic diversity and provides the ground for criticizing simplistic models of genetic waste, unfitness, and disease. Additionally, this point recognizes a fundamental ambiguity in the nature of reality. Cancer is a result of the extremely rapid division and growth of cells, the very same process that allows life to continue. In the process of genetic recombination in sexual reproduction, copying errors sometimes occur that result in disease. Yet it is this very same process that allows reproduction to occur at all. These biological processes are the means through which life is transmitted from one generation to another, yet it is through these very same processes that life can be transformed in ways that are sometimes new and helpful and sometimes new and harmful.

A similar point emerges from a consideration of the multiplicity of forms and species. As Eaves and Gross contend, "There are many forms which do not constitute a value or an advantage in the struggle of life;

they are useless in this sense, and for that reason they are beautiful. Beauty is a factor that is not necessitated by lower needs, but is something that supposes the liberty of artistic creation."[85] Considerations such as these regarding the chemical composition of life expressed in the wonderously complex DNA molecule cannot help but also push us in the direction of a radical reconsideration of the nature of matter from both a religious and a scientific perspective. For example, the theologian Zachary Hayes expresses it this way: "The biblical tradition is a religious tradition that is convinced of the deep religious significance of the material world and of its profound potential for radical transformation into a form so different from its present form in space and time (that is, the idea of the incarnation and the metaphor of resurrection as the final condition of 'becoming flesh')."[86]

This is an echo of the medieval Franciscan theologian Saint Bonaventure who said: "Again, the tendency that exists in matter is ordained toward rational principles, and there would be no perfect generation without the union of the rational soul with the material body."[87] Although expressed in what we would consider dualistic language, Bonaventure suggests that matter has within it the potential to transcend itself. John Paul II also articulates this in an address on evolution when he speaks of an ontological leap in which something profoundly different appears within the material reality out of which humans evolve.[88] Such discussions of necessity force us into a more critical dialogue with contemporary physics, particularly quantum mechanics, with its take on the nature of matter. While such a discussion is beyond the scope of this chapter, I recognize the necessity for such dialogue as captured in this question by Hayes: "Do we have a spiritual substance such as a 'soul,' or are soul functions such as consciousness, etc., really symptoms of chemical complexification of matter that is still in the process of moving to its final, fulfilling form?"[89]

Whatever the outcome of such a debate, the view of matter and evolution suggested here is in the tradition of Augustine and his follower Bonaventure, who saw history as a most beautiful song, or as Philotheus Boehner put it, a *"pulcherrimum carmen* which has been played by the divine Wisdom since the first organisms were called into existence, and of which our present forms are but one scene."[90] Or as the *Book of Proverbs* (8.30) says of wisdom: "I was by his side, a master craftsman, delighting him day after day, ever at play in his presence, at play every-where in his world."

Specific Religious Issues   Religion is an interesting test case in an examination of human nature, for what one says about religion also reveals a commitment to a particular ideology and perhaps a methodology. Especially problematic is the frequent assumption that a commitment to methodological reductionism also implies a commitment to metaphysical reductionism, which does not necessarily follow. Here, above all, one's prior commitments to specific positions need to be attended to and examined carefully.

For example, Dawkins adopts an explicitly antireligion position. He sees religion as superstition and/or myth (understood as a false statement) whose purpose is to hide scientific truths from the unsuspecting or the naive. Faith, Dawkins declares, "is such a successful brainwasher in its own favour, especially a brainwasher of children, that it is hard to break its hold." And in addition to faith's being an arbitrary belief—otherwise, one could give reasons for one's position—faith for Dawkins leads to fanaticism: "It is capable of driving people to such dangerous folly that faith seems to me to qualify as a kind of mental illness. It leads people to believe in whatever it is so strongly that in extreme cases they are prepared to kill and die for it without the need for further justification."[91]

Dawkins defines the idea of God as a meme (Dawkins's term for a cultural unit of replication) and part of the meme pool. Thus, the meme "God" gains its survival in this pool through its appeal to our psychology: "It provides a superficially plausible answer to deep and troubling questions about existence."[92] For Dawkins, God exists, but only as a meme within the culture.

Dawkins's *The Blind Watchmaker*, in addition to being a sustained argument for the randomness of evolution, is also an explicit attack on the proof of God based on design in nature. Here, he is "advocating Darwinism not only as a candle in the dark against pseudo scientific beliefs, but also as a direct substitute for personal religion."[93] As Dawkins sees it, evolution has no purpose other than the survival of particular genes, and which ones survive cannot be predicted in advance. As such, there is no design in the process of evolution.

Dawkins also says the following: "You scientists are very good at answering 'How' questions. But you must admit you are powerless when it comes to 'Why' questions. . . . [B]ehind the question there is always an unspoken but never justified implication that since science is unable to answer 'Why' questions there must be some other discipline that *is* qualified to answer them. This implication is, of course, quite illogical."[94] The question is on what basis does Dawkins make such a claim. Is this on the basis of scientific methodology? If so, what is it? On what basis does one determine that the differentiation of "why" and "how" questions is illogical? Is this a prejudice resulting from a precommitment to a metaphysical reductionism? It is one thing to reject religion—for whatever reason; it is quite another to argue that the rejection of religion follows directly from the acceptance of a scientific or Darwinian perspective.

Recall also that Dawkins argues that humans alone among all other species have the capacity to rebel against our genes. The basis on which one might do this is not clearly spelled out. Dawkins recognizes that we do this—the practice of artificial contraception is one of the stock examples of such behavior—but the justification for it is not completely or satisfactorily explained. It seems that there is some ambiguity in the nature of reality that escapes a totally scientifically materialist explanation.

Wilson comes at the religion question from quite another perspective. First, he was raised as a Southern Baptist and underwent a conversion experience as a youth. But Wilson later underwent another conversion experience, one to evolution and against his own religious upbringing. This led him, according to Segerstråle, to want to "prove the (Christian) theologians wrong. He wanted to make sure that there could not exist a separate realm of meaning and ethics which would allow the theologians to impose arbitrary moral codes that would lead to unnecessary human suffering."[95] Important here is the strong identification of religion and ethics, which is not necessarily the case, as well as the desire to show that religion is not a privileged locus of knowledge for right and wrong. Wilson seems quite close to Dawkins in adopting a position of metaphysical reductionism.

On the other hand, Wilson, unlike Dawkins, is sympathetic to the "Why" questions that humans ask, for he recognizes that humans have deep emotional needs that must be satisfied. Wilson argues that "our metaphysical quest is an evolutionary one: religious belief can be seen as adaptive. The submission of humans to a perceived higher power, in the case of religion, derives from a more general tendency for submission behavior which has shown itself to be adaptive. By submitting to a stronger force, animals attain a stable situation."[96] In other words, Wilson here used ethological insight to argue that we cannot eliminate our metaphysical quest—it is part of our nature. For Wilson, the choice is between empiricism and transcendentalism, whether philosophical or religious. His own preference is the empiricist view because it is objective—that is, scientific. It proceeds by "exploring the biological roots of moral behavior, and explaining their material origins and biases."[97] And ultimately, the evolutionary myth of origins will replace the religious one.

Yet Wilson leans toward deism, since he states that there could exist a cosmological God whose existence could be proved by astrophysics. On the other hand, "a biological God, one who directs organic evolution and intervenes in human affairs . . . is increasingly contravened by biology and the brain sciences." For all this, though, Wilson says we need our transcendental beliefs: "*We cannot live without them*. People need a sacred narrative. They must have a sense of larger purpose in one form or another, however intellectualized."[98] A transcendental form of this narrative neither will nor can endure, however, for it eventually will not withstand scientific scrutiny. Our guiding narrative will therefore need to be taken from "the material history of the universe and the human species." But that is not to our or religion's disadvantage, since as Wilson adds

the true evolutionary epic, retold as poetry, is as intrinsically ennobling as any religious epic. Material reality discovered by science already possesses more content and grandeur than all religious cosmologies combined. The continuity of the human line has been traced through a period of deep history a thousand times older than that conceived by the Western religions. Its study has brought new revelations of great moral importance. It has made us realize that *Homo sapiens* are far more than a congeries of tribes and races. We are a single gene pool from which individuals are drawn in each generation and into which they are dissolved the next generation, forever united as a species by heritage and a common future. Such are the conceptions, based on fact, from which new intimations of immortality can be drawn and a new mythos evolved.[99]

So although disagreeing with Dawkins about the need for raising "why" questions, Wilson essentially lands in the same place: metaphysical reductionism and materialism, for science ultimately will answer all questions. And the answer to the question "Why religion?" is that it is adaptive and leads to social stability.

In a concluding perspective on this, Wilson said in an interview,

I just believe, to put it as simply as possible, that science should be able to go in a relatively few decades to the point of producing a humanoid robot which would walk through that door. The first robot would think and talk like a Southern Baptist minister, and the second robot would talk like John Rawls. In other words, *somehow I believe that we can reconstitute, re-create, the most mysterious features of* human *mental activity*. That's an article of faith but it has to do with expansionism. That's expansionism!"[100]

Hence, every element of mental and physical behavior will have a physical basis, and ultimately there will be a materialist explanation for everything. For science will continue to test every religious assumption and claim about God and humans, and will in the end come to the foundation of all human moral and religious sentiments. Wilson Asserts, "The eventual result of the competition between the two worldviews, I believe, will be the secularization of the human epic and of religion itself."[101] According to Segerstråle, "One would then test, in the sociobiological mode, whether the peculiarities of the human brain are inferred to have taken place. If such matching does exist, then the mind harbors a species god, which can be parsimoniously explained as a biological adaptation instead of an independent, transbiological force."[102] Thus, God and religion are products of the brain, itself a product of evolution, which leads us to various adaptive behaviors, of which religion is one. And we are back again to biology as the full explanation of all behavior—Wilson's original point in developing his theory of sociobiology. But is this the whole story?

A problem here might be the lack of distinction between three types of "why" questions. A scientific why question seeks to answer how one could account for a particular outcome: why do bodies fall, for example. A philosophical question tries to seek out inner relations and ultimate principles—Aristotle's seeking out of final causes, for instance. Religion pursues its why question in terms of ultimate meaning—say, for what may we hope. Each of these disciplines has a particular set of rules and a framework in which its particular why question can be answered along with a set of criteria for evaluating the adequacy of the answer. A problem arises when one asks the why question of one discipline from within the perspective of another. Or when one insists on the criteria from one discipline as being the only criteria acceptable for verification. While it is the case that the boundaries of these disciplines more frequently resemble semipermeable membranes rather than fixed borders, one continually needs to be sensitive to what kind of question one is asking and what are acceptable criteria for evaluating an answer. Border crossings are to be expected in our interdisciplinary world, but one must also remember to respect the customs and culture of the territory we visit.[103]

Conclusions

Dawkins is totally transparent in his disdain for religion. At best, religion is a holdover from a past filled with ignorance. At worst, it is false security for the desperate and immature. Wilson recognizes the need for mythology and grandeur in human life. And he says this need will be fulfilled admirably by our evolutionary myth, the grandest myth we have. Yet he too, like Dawkins, winds up with a form of philosophical materialism that admits no transcendence, no reality other than matter.

Dawkins argues against a form of genetic predestination or determinism. He states that we are the only creatures who can rebel against our genes. Wilson also argues for a type of distance from the genes in that we can build various cultures, though he adds that the genes will always keep the culture on a leash of varying length.

We have here two central philosophical claims that have specific applicability to human nature: materialism and freedom. The claims serve as working hypotheses of the analytic framework for both of these men, but they are not given any full examination or defense. For both Dawkins and Wilson, the claims of philosophical materialism are strongly made, yet both seem to want some slack cut in their conclusions. We continue to live in our world of "as if": as if we were free, as if belief made a difference, as if meaning mattered. In cold, hard reality, however, none of this may be true. For evolution is without direction, matter began and it will end, species evolve and go extinct, the world eventually ends. If anything, the human species is cursed because through consciousness, it sees this and knows reality's inherent meaninglessness. Humans create myths, but they are groundless, adult "just so" stories to hide the impersonal march of natural selection, which is ultimately indifferent to anything.

"Science tells us that we are creatures of accident clinging to a ball of mud hurling aimlessly through space. This is not a notion to warm hearts or rouse multitudes."[104] This quote from Paul Ehrlich is an interesting rephrasing of Wilson's noble myth of evolution that helps put one's finger on the nub of the problem: if rational explanations such as quantum physics and evolution are fully adequate explanations of our origins and our reality, why do we continue to read, create, and reformulate myths? Why have not *The Epic of Gilgamesh, Beowulf,* Exodus, Bhagavad Gita, *The Pilgrim's Progress,* and the American Dream all vanished? Why has religion shown such a dramatic rebound following the breakup of the Soviet Union? Why is there such resistance to any form of transcendence in China?

It is facile simply to allege that this is clear and indisputable evidence for the reality and truth of religion. Yet the counterclaim that scientific explanations for the realities of birth, death, and tragedy suffice is equally facile. In contrast, Ehrlich points to an interesting opening or way to think about transcendence and freedom.

In his recent book *Human Natures,* Ehrlich refers to a theory developed by Jared Diamond called the "great leap forward," referring specifically to the shift in toolmaking that occurred at the end of the age of the Neanderthals. "The change to that Upper Paleolithic technology which appeared first in the Middle East about 40,000–50,000 years ago, was the start of the most rapid and radical cultural change ever recorded in the hominid line. . . . It is a leap into new technologies, art, and population growth—perhaps even into a new mode of speaking." What is interesting, according to Ehrlich, is that at a certain point while brain size remained fairly constant, "cultural changes took place at astonishing speeds with no significant change in the physical appearance of people or in the characteristics of their brains that can be divined from fossil skulls." The question, then, is, "Did the physical evolution of our ancestors' brains cause the Great Leap Forward—or did only the 'software' of culture change, not the 'wetware' of brain structure?"[105]

Here, I want to reengage several of the ideas introduced earlier as a way of thinking about a basis for this great leap forward to suggest an alternative reading of the interpretations of Dawkins and Wilson.

In their discussion of evolution, Eaves and Gross focus on a view of matter, evolution, and genetics that seeks to do justice to the reality of human consciousness. Their focus looks to suggestions within the mechanisms of inheritance that indicate a capacity within historical nature for self-transcendence. They then argue that such mechanisms are the basis for surprise and graciousness within nature, suggesting that grace is found within life itself.[106]

This type of position is also articulated by Rahner, who echoes a much earlier tradition expressed in the writings of Bonaventure. In his second book of the *Sentences*, Bonaventure phrases the insight this way: "Thus nature, according to the Philosopher, always desires what is better; matter, which is composed of elementary forms, desires to be under mixed forms and that which is under mixed forms desires to be under complex forms."[107] While this language is clearly dualistic, it also takes seriously the reality of matter and expresses, in the language of medieval philosophy, a dynamic that is present within matter, a dynamic that carries matter beyond itself to a point of transcendence. Matter is not content to be itself but strives for ever-greater complexity.

Further, Eaves and Gross note, as mentioned earlier, that culture produces conditions for community that are not possible in aggregates, and that the very same conditions of life that produce tragedy also maintain life itself. One example of such conditions could be the previously discussed great leap forward in culture. But importantly, this was followed by the great axial age that lasted from about 800 to 400 B.C.E. This was the age that saw the rise of the great religions of the East, particularly Hinduism, Buddhism, and Confucianism. The West saw the rise of Zoroastrianism and Judaism. In Latin America, we had the religions of the Aztec and Mayan civilizations. Additionally, in Greece, the first philosophical speculations were being advanced. Although the axial age lasted but a few centuries, much was compressed into it—the foundations of classical religions and philosophy. And as in the great leap forward of culture that preceded it, the question is why. Homo sapiens had been present for several centuries, and civilizations had begun to flourish. But here was a new development—a focus on the transcendent, the other, the metaphysical, a world other than this one, but for many a world no less real than the one available to our senses.

One suggestion, of course, is that such efforts were but the first, feeble steps of what would become scientific explanations of the mysteries of the world. Another was that such speculations helped to shelter people from the terrors of nature or the fickleness of chance. And indeed in many cases this is probably a reasonable explanation. But the problem still remains—the same kinds of concerns, speculations, and searchings arose relatively simultaneously in separate geographic areas.

In these perspectives, we have another development of the evolutionary process that both gives a foundation for these culture-altering events and a response to the materialism of Dawkins and Wilson. The key point is that both our experience and our very culture suggest another dimension of life, another quality that helps explain our drive for mythmaking, our drive to transcendence. Neither the great leap forward nor the great axial age can be dismissed. The point of contention is their basis. Complexity brought to a higher level is certainly one valid interpretation. But another dimension that has to be incorporated is the reality of genuine difference. Ehrlich notes this by observing that we share genes, but not cultures, with chimpanzees.[108] We create a culture that grounds the further creations of art, music, philosophy, and religion. Our larger brain and its enormous complexity provide the biological substrate necessary for such a leap. Yet the continuing question of the brain is, Is it necessary, or is it necessary but not sufficient? The alternative reading that I suggest argues that such capacities are not added from without; in fact, they are the supreme fulfillment of matter manifested not only in a great leap forward but also in moments of self-transcendence such as those expressed in the great axial age as well as in moments of individual transcendence.

One element in this is Ehrlich's rather straightforward admission that even though he is not a mind-matter dualist, his version of human nature "finds a strictly materialistic interpretation of the world unsatisfying." While neither denying a form of materialism influenced by quantum physics nor the value of methodological reductionism, Ehrlich concludes that "we seem to be always forced back to the larger view to find a degree of satisfaction not provided by dissection of a problem into its smallest parts."[109] While this leads Ehrlich to a kind of practical dualism, the problem is still there: the parts do not adequately explain the whole.

The examination of freedom from Duns Scotus's perspective also forces to us look beyond materialism, but without denying our own biological nature. Here, we can reexamine Duns Scotus's distinction between the affectio commodi and the affectio justitiae with complementary insights from Ehrlich. The affectio commodi states that a given nature will seek its own good. What this good is will be understood through an examination of this nature. The concept is open, in my judgment, to being understood in light of our knowledge of the nature of a particular organism in view of the best of our interdisciplinary or multidisciplinary knowledge. This would include, for example with human nature, how both biological and cultural evolution shape who we are—that is, how we define our nature. To say that we act according to our nature is to say that we act as we do because we have evolved into beings of a particular kind. Ehrlich refers to the experience of values that are connected to such direct feelings as "perceived values." These are the immediate motivations or goods that guide our daily lives and actions, and are tied closely to our evolutionary past. Ehrlich remarks,

Whereas the motivation to get our genes into the next generation may be the distant cause of much of our behavior the immediate motivations are more familiar. We rarely mate to reproduce ourselves; we ordinarily mate because it feels good. We don't dodge an approaching car to preserve our ability to raise our children; we do it to avoid anticipated pain or death. We don't eat to gain energy; we eat to assuage hunger or for pleasure.[110]

This is about as clear a restatement of Duns Scotus's affectio commodi as one would want. It affirms both the biological and cultural dimensions of the formation of our nature, but it also avoids a genetic reductionism by not suggesting a gene for each action. We act as we do because of who we have become.

But for Duns Scotus this is not the end of the story, for we also experience another dimension to ourselves. In addition to the experience of pursuing our good to fulfill or complete ourselves, we also experience the desire to seek the good of another. This is Duns Scotus's affectio justitiae—a check on our nature, if you will. This desire moves us in a different direction, not contrary to our nature, but transcending it. This affection leads to a pursuit of the good, in Duns Scotus's perspective, for its own sake or for the sake of one's neighbor. The affectio justitiae initiates a basic move beyond the parameters of our own nature to the situation of another.

Ehrlich calls such an experience empathy and relates this to the development of what he labels "conceived values"—values evolved to help deal with the social environment.[111] This is also the arena of ethics, an evolved system of culturally shared understandings of right and wrong. Critical here is altruism, which sociobiology explains on the basis of inclusive fitness (for one's relatives) or reciprocity (for strangers). Ehrlich makes two interesting observations in relation to this. First, the origin of ethics cannot be traced to chimpanzees: "Chimps have no way to share values; ethics had to await at least the evolution of language, of an efficient method of sharing the ideas that were presumably generated by notions of empathy. There appears to be an unbridgeable gap between the ethical capabilities of human beings and those of chimpanzees." Second, explains Ehrlich, "empathy and altruism often exist where the chances for any return to the altruist are nil. Indeed, careful psychological experiments suggest that much of human helping behavior is divorced from any real prospect of reproductive or other reward."[112]

The basis of such behavior, Ehrlich argues, is empathy, and it "would seem a necessary prerequisite for such altruism, and many of our empathetic feelings are unrelated to personal advantage."[113] Empathy is an evolved capacity to feel for others, and while it will have a high degree of variability in its expression and may indeed have some limits to its expression, its presence is another fact of our experience not satisfactorily explained by appeal to our genome. What Ehrlich calls empathy is at least analogous to Duns Scotus's concept of affectio justitiae.

The point of differentiation, of course, is the source of such an affection. For Ehrlich, empathy comes from the process of gene-culture coevolution. For Duns Scotus, the affectio justitiae is ultimately a result of our being created in a certain way by God, though Duns Scotus is not a literalist in his understanding of how that creation occurred. But the more critical point, in my judgment, is that both have identified an extremely similar behavior in humans based on experience. Humans in fact can transcend their nature by stepping beyond themselves and acting for the benefit of another. Both affirm that humans have the capacity to see a good outside of themselves and to pursue it or use it as the basis for constructing an ethic. And here is the foundation that Dawkins needs to ground his claim that humans alone can rebel against their genes.

The presence of the affectio commodi and the affectio justitiae in the same person gives rise to a paradox—one noted earlier, but that now will be developed a bit more. The presence of both affections makes morality possible, but as John Boler observes, Duns Scotus "cannot accept a theory such as Aristotle's where the moral is analyzed in terms of self-perfection or self-realization, i.e., in terms of the rational agent's inclination to realize the perfection of its nature."[114] That is, a morality based exclusively on the good of the individual agent cannot be the whole story for it is a morality limited to my own human nature. To pursue the affectio justitiae or to experience empathy is to transcend one's human nature and, in a paradoxical way, act against one's nature. Thus, in a free act—though not free in any unbounded or totally arbitrary sense— the agent can seek the good of another—as opposed to seeking one's genetic advantage only. I raise this issue not only to engage in a discussion of a critical experience on which we can begin to construct an ethic but also to question whether such an experience of the affectio justitiae might be a grounding of another transcendent experience—a religious one. Can the experience of a good beyond oneself lead to an experience of some yet-higher or perhaps ultimate good? Can such an experience be a transcendent point of opening for an encounter with the presence of another, or another dimension of, reality? Reality seems to be open enough for such a reading, particularly when we recall Ehrlich's own dissatisfaction with a strictly materialist reading of human experience. An expression of such a reflection on this possibility is the poem "God's Grandeur" by the Jesuit poet Gerard Manley Hopkins:

The world is charged with the grandeur of God.
It will flame out, like shining from shook foil;
It gathers to a greatness, like the ooze of oil
Crushed. Why do men then now not reck his rod?
Generations have trod, have trod, have trod;
And all is seared with trade; bleared, smeared with toil;
And wears man's smudge and shares man's smell: the soil
Is bare now, nor can foot feel, being shod.
And for all this, nature is never spent;
There lives the dearest freshness deep down things;
And though the last lights off the black West went
Oh, morning, at the brown brink eastward, springs
Because the Holy Ghost over the bent
World broods with warm breast and with ah! bright wings.[115]

Notes

1. See Etienne Fouilloux, "The Antepreparatory Phase: The Slow Emergence from Inertia (January 1959–October 1962," in *History of Vatican II*, ed. Giuseppe Alberigo, trans. Joseph A. Komonchak (Maryknoll, NY: Orbis Books, 1995), 1:85–87.

2. Ullica Segerstråle, *Defenders of the Truth: The Battle for Science in the Sociology Debate and Beyond* (New York: Oxford University Press, 2000), 30.

3. Ibid., 307–308.

4. E. O. Wilson, *Consilience: The Unity of Knowledge* (New York: Alfred Knopf, 1998), 125.

5. Jonathan Marks, "98% Alike? What Our Similarity to Apes Tells Us about Our Understanding of Genetics," *Chronicle of Higher Education*, May 12, 2000, B7.

6. Wilson, *Consilience*, 163.

7. Segerstråle, *Defenders of the Truth*, 94.

8. Richard Dawkins, *The Selfish Gene* (New York: Oxford University Press, 1989), 201.

9. Luigi Luca Cavalli-Sforza, *Genes, Peoples, and Languages*, trans. Mark Seielstad (New York: North Point Press, 2000), 13.

10. Ibid., 11–12.

11. Natalie Angier, "Do Races Really Differ? Not Really, Genes Show," *New York Times*, 22 August 2000, F6.

12. Cavalli-Sforza, *Genes*, 23, 27.

13. Ibid., 78, 79.

14. Ibid., 81.

15. Andrew Watson, "A New Breed of High-Tech Detectives," *Science* 289 (August 11, 2000): 851.

16. Cavalli-Sforza, *Genes*, 29.

17. Ordinatio II.3.251 (Vat. 7:513–514), cited in Allan B. Wolter, "Scotus' Eschatology: Some Reflections," in *That Others May Know and Love: Essays in Honor of Zachary Hayes, OFM*, eds. Michael Custado and F. Edward Coughlin (St. Bonaventure, NY: The Franciscan Institute, 1997) 336.

18. Cavalli-Sforza, *Genes*, 65.

19. E. O. Wilson, cited in Segerstråle, *Defenders of the Truth*, 395.

20. Cited in ibid., 398.

21. E. O. Wilson, *On Human Nature* (Cambridge, MA: Harvard University Press, 1978), 71.

22. Ibid., 73.

23. Ibid., 73–74.

24. Richard Dawkins, cited in Segerstråle, *Defenders of the Truth*, 395.

25. Segerstråle, *Defenders of the Truth*, 37.

26. William Hamilton, cited in Segerstråle, *Defenders of the Truth*, 472.

27. Ibid., 147.

28. E. O. Wilson, cited in Segerstråle, *Defenders of the Truth*, 39.

29. E. O. Wilson, *Sociobiology: The New Synthesis* (Cambridge, MA: Belknap Press, 1975), 3.

30. Wilson, *On Human Nature*, 213.

31. Wilson, *Sociobiology*, 3–4.

32. Wilson, *On Human Nature*, 152.

33. Ibid., 153–154.

34. Ibid., 155, 155–156.

35. Ibid., 156, 157.

36. Ibid., 157, 199.

37. Ibid., 157, 162–163.

38. Ibid., 164, 167.

39. Richard Trivers, preface to Dawkins, *The Selfish Gene*, cited in Segerstråle, *Defenders of the Truth*, 78.

40. Dawkins, *The Selfish Gene*, 1–2.

41. Ibid., 61.

42. Ibid., 95.

43. Ibid., 100.

44. Ibid., 105.

45. Wilson, *On Human Nature*, 157, 159.

46. Dawkins, *The Selfish Gene*, 2–3, 2.

47. John Duns Scotus, *Quaestiones in Metaphysicam* 1.15.2, in *Duns Scotus on the Will and Morality*, ed. Allan B. Wolter (Washington, DC: Catholic University of American Press, 1986), 151.

48. Ibid.

49. Duns Scotus, *Ordinatio* 4.49.9–10, in *Duns Scotus*, 185.

50. Allan B. Wolter, "Native Freedom of the Will as a Key to the Ethics of Scotus," in *The Philosophical Theology of John Duns Scotus*, ed. Marilyn McCord Adams (Ithaca, NY: Cornell University Press, 1990), 150.

51. Ibid.

52. Ibid., 151.

53. Ibid.

54. Duns Scotus, *Ordinatio* 2.6.2.12, cited in Wolter, "Native Freedom of the Will," 155.

55. Wolter, "Native Freedom of the Will," 151.

56. Ibid., 152.

57. John Duns Scotus, *Reportatio Parisiensis* 11.6.2.9, in Wolter, "Native Freedom of the Will," 152.

58. John Boler, "The Moral Psychology of Duns Scotus: Some Preliminary Questions," *Franciscan Studies* 28 (1990): 4.

59. Wolter, "Native Freedom of the Will," 152.

60. John Duns Scotus, cited in Felix Aluntis and Allan B. Wolter, trans., *John Duns Scotus: God and Creatures* (Princeton, NJ: Princeton University Press, 1975), 378.

61. William Frank, "Duns Scotus' Concept of Willing Freely: What Divine Freedom beyond Choice Teaches Us," *Franciscan Studies* 42 (1982): 87.

62. Ibid., 98.

63. Ibid., 83.

64. Ibid., 87.

65. Ibid., 85.

66. William Frank, "Duns Scotus' Quodlibetal Teaching on the Will" (PhD diss., Catholic University of America, 1982), 77.

67. Wolter, "Native Freedom of the Will," 152, 154.

68. Valerius Messerich, "The Awareness of Causal Initiative and Existential Responsibility in the Thought of Duns Scotus," in *De Doctrina Ionnis Scoti* (Rome: Acta Congressus Scotistici Internationalis, 1968), 2:630–631.

69. Ibid., 631.

70. Wolter, "Native Freedom of the Will," 153.

71. Wilson, *On Human Nature*, 221, 201.

72. Ibid., 201.

73. Ibid., 216, 195.

74. Wolter, "Native Freedom of the Will," 98, 105.

75. Ibid., 105.

76. Karl Rahner, "Christology within an Evolutionary View," in *Theological Investigations*, trans. Karl-H. Kruger (New York: Crossroad, 1983), 160, 164.

77. Ibid., 164, 165.

78. Ibid., 167.

79. Ibid., 168, 171.

80. Lindon Eaves and Lora Gross, "Exploring the Concept of Spirit as a Model for the God-World Relation in the Age of Genetics," *Zygon* 27 (1992): 226.

81. Ibid., 274, 278.

82. Ibid., 274.

83. Ibid., 275.

84. Ibid., 277, 278.

85. Ibid., 157.

86. Zachary Hayes, "letter to author, January 15, 2001.

87. Saint Bonaventure, *On the Retracing of the Arts to Theology*, in *The Works of St. Bonaventure*, ed. Jose De Vinck (Paterson, NJ: St. Anthony Guild, 1966), 3:28–29.

88. John Paul II, "Message to Pontifical Academy of Sciences" on Evolution," *Origins* 26.22 (November 14, 1996) 350, 351–352.

89. Hayes, letter to author.

90. Philotheus Boehner, "The Teaching of the Sciences in Catholic Colleges," *Franciscan* Educational Conference, (1955): 157.

91. Dawkins, *The Selfish Gene*, 330.

92. Ibid., 193.

93. Richard Dawkins, cited in Segerstråle, *Defenders of the Truth*, 400; See also *The Blind Watchmaker: Why the Evidence of Evolution Reveals a Universe Without Design* (New York: W. W. Norton and Company, 1996).

94. Ibid., 401.

95. Segerstråle, *Defenders of the Truth*, 38.

96. E. O. Wilson, cited in Segerstråle, *Defenders of the Truth*, 402.

97. Wilson, *Consilience*, 240.

98. Ibid., 241, 264.

99. Ibid., 265.

100. E. O. Wilson, cited in Segerstråle, *Defenders of the Truth*, 160.

101. Wilson, *Consilience*, 265.

102. Segerstråle, *Defenders of the Truth*, 160.

103. Zachary Hayes, *A Window to the Divine* (Quincy, IL: Franciscan Press, 1999), 11–13.

104. Paul R. Ehrlich, *Human Natures: Genes, Cultures, and the Human Prospect* (Washington, DC: Island Press, 2000), 214.

105. Ibid., 104, 106, 107.

106. Eaves and Gross, "Exploring the Concept of Spirit," 278, 274.

107. Bonaventure, cited in Alexander Schaeffer, "The Position and Function of Man in the Created World according to St. Bonaventure," *Franciscan Studies* 20 (1960): 318 (my translation).

108. Ehrlich, *Human Natures*, 204.

109. Ibid., 317, 318.

110. Ibid., 310.

111. Ibid., 311.

112. Ibid., 311, 312.

113. Ibid., 313.

114. Boler, "Moral Psychology," 4.

115. Gerard Manley Hopkins, "God's Grandeur," in *The Poems of Gerard Manley Hopkins*, W. H. Gardner, ed., 2nd ed. (New York: Oxford University Press, 1953), 27.

11

Telos, Value, and Genetic Engineering

Bernard E. Rollin

Legend has it that when Alexander the Great conquered North Africa, he remembered his old teacher, Aristotle, fondly and sent him a gift, an elephant, escorted by a legion of troops. The legend unfortunately stops there and fails to record what Aristotle did with the elephant. Of two things, however, we can be morally certain: first, as a practicing biologist, and as a philosopher infused with biology as his root metaphor, Aristotle was doubtless delighted. Second, we can affirm that he did not favor his own former teacher, Plato, by passing the gift on.

Aristotle had little tolerance for Plato's contempt for the world we live in and correlative penchant for seeking truth beyond the world. For Aristotle, truth was, for the most part, in the world of ordinary experience, and humans were built to find it.

"All men by nature desire to know," is the first line of Aristotle's *Metaphysics* (1.1.980a22). Our biology makes us capable of knowing, and the proper object of this desire is the dynamic world we find through sense experience, not an extraworldly, frozen realm of Platonic objects. Contrary to Plato, the real world is a world of change, flux, coming to be, passing away, although such change is not chaotic; there are consistent patterns in change, that which happens for "the most part." Change is lawlike; patterns repeat.

Telos and Biology

It is wrong, for Aristotle, to look at the world the way the atomists did then or the mechanists have done since the Newtonian revolution—as a *machine*. The world is more like a living thing than it is like a clock. Plants, animals, birds, fish, tools, and even rocks have *natures*, regular functions that they perform, and correlatively, virtues (*aretai*) that enable them to perform these functions. "Fish gotta swim, birds gotta fly; rocks gotta go to the center of the earth, the natural place for rocks." The science of biology is the study of how different kinds of organisms respond to the tasks constitutive of life itself; nutrition, growth, sensation, reproduction, locomotion, and, in the case of humans alone, complex thought. The way each sort of living thing answers each of these challenges determines its *telos*, its nature, its final cause, what it does.

In Aristotle's commonsense worldview, then, living things are the paradigm for all things. There is no one set of rules or laws that governs the behavior of all things, as the mechanists suggest, so even if everything is in fact made of atoms, atomic explanations do not explain function; to think otherwise is to commit a category mistake. At best, mechanistic explanations are only one "cause" or principle of explanation—the efficient—and certainly not the most important for understanding nature. Biology, in its recognition of a vast array of natural kind functions, is the master science; physics is a subspecies of biology. Aristotle would totally reject René Descartes'—and modern molecular biology's—acceptance of the other paradigm, where biology is a subspecies of physics—he correctly realized that such a way of thinking ultimately ends up trivializing the world we know directly through experience.

Telos is thus a fundamental metaphysical category for seeing the world, based in biology and an attempt to understand living things, and growing out of a commonsense worldview. It encapsulates a worldview we should realize has been largely rejected by modern science, ever since Benedict de Spinoza's blistering—and unfair—attack on teleology. But it has been rejected, not disproved. For what could disprove the claim that it is better or more reasonable in an explanatory sense to look at the world, particularly the world of living things, in terms of functions, purposes (conscious and nonconscious), and telos than to look at it as a mechanical assemblage of dead particles? Similarly, of course, one cannot disprove the opposite claim—namely, that talk of functions and organismic sorts are better abandoned in favor of physicochemical explanations operative at the molecular level. In the end, metaphysical worldviews are not empirically disproven, for they in fact partly determine what counts as an empirical disproof. Molecular biology does not *disprove* talking of "why" questions (Why does the adrenal gland secrete adrenalin? Why do the swallows return to Capistrano?), it *disapproves* of them. We shouldn't say that mechanistic worldviews, however powerful, falsify teleological ones; rather they reject them. Commitment to either of these metaphysical worldviews is going to be a valuational commitment based on one's preference of "how" to "why," or in one's predilection for control of nature, rather than awe for it.

Thus, for Aristotle, telos is a foundational concept for looking at the world. It is the cornerstone of biology, which in turn is the paradigm for all fully legitimate explanation. In dealing with the nonhuman world, it seems to have no ethical import for Aristotle; it is rather a template for scientific investigation. But that does not mean it cannot have ethical significance, and I will shortly demonstrate that it does, or rather has come to enjoy such significance.

There is, in Aristotle, no overt ethic for treating nonhuman beings, despite his recognition that many animals feel pleasure and pain and have desires.[1] This is not surprising for a variety of reasons. In the first place, given Aristotle's belief in a natural hierarchy, certain things are inferior, and the inferior exists to be used by the superior.[2] Hence his notion of "natural slaves." Indeed, he affirms that "the use made of slaves and of tame animals is not very different." On the other hand, as he says in *De Anima*, "All tame animals are better off when they are ruled by man; for then they are preserved" (1.5).

From this passage, it would appear that Aristotle believed that proper (ethical) care for domestic animals naturally follows from domestication, and for this reason, we may infer, it is not an issue. What can he mean by this? I believe he anticipates the fact that, from antiquity until the mid–twentieth century, *husbandry* was key to the successful keeping of animals—be it for food, fiber, locomotion, or power—in all agrarian societies. Husbandry, a word derived from the old Norse word *hus/bond*, "bonded to the household," meant that domestic animals existed in a state of symbiotic unity with their human owners. In husbandry, a human put an animal into the optimal conditions possible for which that animal had biologically evolved, and then augmented the animal's natural ability to survive and thrive with additional care—provision of food during famine, water during drought, medical attention, help in birthing, protection from predators, and so on. Both the human and the animal were better off by virtue of the "contract": animals benefited from our ministrations; we benefited from their products, toil, and sometimes their lives. But animals lived better with us than without us.

Consider a lamb in ancient Judea, where the Bible tells us predatory animals such as lions, jackals, and velociraptors abounded. Without a shepherd, the animal would live a Hobbesian life—nasty, miserable, brutish, and short. In fact, so powerful is the husbandry image, that when the psalmist wishes to create an ideal metaphor for God's ideal relationship to humans, the shepherd metaphor in Psalm 23 is employed:

The Lord is my shepherd, I shall not want; He leadeth me to green pastures; He maketh me to lie down beside still water; he restoreth my soul.

We want no more from God than the shepherd provides to his sheep!

Harming an animal was sanctioned by the greatest and most powerful sanction—self-interest, which assured proper care. We know, for example, that rough treatment of animals reduces milk production and reproductive success. Thus, no explicit ethic for animal treatment was needed in husbandry societies, save perhaps for injunctions against those unconcerned with self-interest, the ethical edicts against deliberate, purposeless, willful, intentional cruelty, aimed at deviant sadists: "The wise man cares for his animals."

The very logic of animal use created its own self-evident ethic, not requiring much philosophical analysis. The telos of an animal in a husbandry context was an implicitly normative concept. If you wished an animal to be happy and healthy so it is productive, respect its telos. And it is probably for this reason that we find virtually no moral discussion of animal treatment until the mid–twentieth century. For it was at this historical juncture that husbandry was abandoned in favor of *industry*, with the rise of intensive confinement agriculture, symbolically betokened by the change of name in university departments from animal husbandry to animal science. Whereas husbandry was about putting square pegs into square holes, round pegs into round holes, and creating as little friction as possible while you did so, in industrial agriculture, thanks to "technological sanders" such as antibiotics, vaccines, bacterins, air-handling systems, and hormones, one could force square pegs into round holes and keep animals productive, albeit not happy. Whereas before such high-tech fixes anyone who attempted to raise one hundred thousand chickens in one building would have dead chickens in a month due to uncheckable disease spread, today's drugs prevent this, while not preventing the animals' misery in having their *teloi* violated. Animal productivity was severed from well-being; and what Aristotle took for granted was shown to be violable.

Those of us alarmed by the violation of the ancient symbiotic contract with animals obviously needed a new ethical vocabulary to ground our concerns. Peter Singer's work in *Animal Liberation* (1975) employed pleasure- and pain-based utilitarian notions, but these seemed inadequate. While it is true that keeping a sow in a $2\frac{1}{2} \times 7 \times 3$ foot enclosure for her entire life surely occasions misery, it seems odd to use the same term—pain—as we do to talk about the misery created by branding, or castration without anesthesia, which is also different from the social isolation experienced by, say, veal calves. So the British Brambell Commission, created in 1964 as a response to public concern about "factory farming," spoke about the basic "freedoms" farm animals ought to enjoy. Later, the Swedish Law of 1988 abolishing confinement agriculture referred to needs following from the animals' biological natures. And in my own philosophical articulation of a moral theory for animals in the late 1970s, I appropriated Aristotle's notion of telos—the "pigness of the pig," the "cowness of the cow," and generally much the same across a species—as a basis for legally codified rights for animals. If respect for animal nature no longer naturally followed sound agricultural practice, it needed legal articulation, even as legal protection for fundamental aspects of *human nature* from the general welfare was encoded in the U.S. Bill of Rights. Thus, emerging social concern for animal treatment is being plausibly couched in the language of rights, which are themselves based on the idea of protecting the animals' telos, the satisfaction of which constitutes happiness. So, in the face of modern animal use, telos emerges as a basic normative notion guiding our obligations to and protections of animals. Animals' rights should flow from animal telos as human rights flow from what we perceive as human telos.

In some cases, we are guided more accurately in our ethical behavior toward animals we live with by looking at the more specific telos of subspecies or breeds of animals. Hence, in addition to a greyhound or an Australian shepherd having the general telos of a dog, a greyhound has a greater need to run than an ordinary dog, a shepherd has an urge to work herding, and so forth.

With the advent of genetic engineering, the concept of animal telos was again cast into prominence, for we can certainly in principle change telos by genetic engineering. One argument against doing this proceeds as follows: given that emerging social ethics affirms that human use of animals should respect and not violate animal telos, we therefore should not *alter* animal telos. Since genetic engineering is precisely the deliberate changing of animal telos, it is ipso facto morally wrong. I suspect that something like this, at least in part, underlies the knee-jerk antipathy that many people have to genetic engineering.

Seductive though this move may be, I do not believe it will stand up to rational scrutiny, for I contend that it rests on a logical error. What the moral imperative about telos says is this: Maxim to Respect Telos: *If an animal has a set of needs and interests that are constitutive of its nature, then, in our dealings with that animal, we are obliged to not violate and to attempt to accommodate those interests, for violation of and failure to accommodate those interests matters to the animal.* It does not follow from that statement, however, that we cannot change the telos. The reason we respect telos is that the interests comprising the telos are plausibly what matters most to the animal. If we alter the telos in such a way that different things matter to the animal, or in a way that is irrelevant to the animal, we have not violated the above maxim. In essence, the maxim says that, given a telos, we should respect the interests that flow from it. This principle does not logically entail that we cannot modify the telos and thereby generate different or alternative interests.

The only way one could deduce an injunction that it is wrong to change telos from the Maxim to Respect Telos is to make the ancillary Panglossian assumption that an animal's telos is the best it can possibly be vis-à-vis the animal's well-being, and that any modification of telos will inevitably result in an even greater violation of the animal's nature and consequently lead to greater suffering. This ancillary assumption is neither a priori nor empirically true, and can indeed readily be seen to be false.

Consider domestic animals. One can argue that humans have, through artificial selection, changed (or genetically engineered) the telos of at least some such animals from their parent stock so that they are more congenial to our husbandry. I doubt anyone would argue that, given our decision to have domestic animals, it is better to have left the telos alone and to have created animals for whom domestication involves a state of constant violation of their telos.[3]

Or to take a simpler example, suppose we genetically engineer animals to be resistant to certain diseases, as has in fact been done with chickens and Marek's disease; we certainly curtail a source of suffering that matters to the animal, and we have changed its telos, yet we have done it no harm and indeed have improved its well-being. By the same token, consider the current situation of the farm animals mentioned earlier, wherein we keep animals under conditions that patently violate their telos so that they suffer in a variety of modalities, yet are kept alive and productive by technological fixes. As a specific example, consider the chickens kept in battery cages for efficient, high-yield, egg production. It is now recognized that such a production system frustrates numerous significant aspects of chicken behavior under natural conditions (that is, violates the telos), including nesting behavior, and that frustration of this basic need or drive results in a mode of suffering for the animals. Let us suppose that we have identified the gene or genes that code for the drive to nest. In addition, suppose we can ablate that gene or substitute a gene (probably per impossibile) that creates a new kind of chicken, one that achieves satisfaction by laying an egg in a cage. Would that be wrong in terms of the ethic I have described?

If we identify an animal's telos as being genetically based and environmentally expressed, we have now changed the chicken's telos so that the animal that is forced by us to live in a battery cage is satisfying more of its nature than is the animal that still has the gene coding for nesting. Have we done something morally wrong?

I would argue that we have not. Recall that a key feature, perhaps *the* key feature, of the new ethic for animals I have described is concern for preventing animal suffering and augmenting animal happiness, which I have maintained involves the satisfaction of telos. I have also implicitly argued that the primary, pressing concern is the former, the mitigation of suffering at human hands, given the proliferation of suffering that has occurred in the twentieth century and continues in the twenty-first. I have also contended that suffering can be occasioned in many ways, from the infliction of physical pain to the prevention of satisfying basic drives. So, when we engineer the new kind of chicken that prefers laying in a cage and we eliminate the nesting urge, we have removed a source of suffering. Given the animal's changed telos, the new chicken is now suffering less than its predecessor and is thus closer to being happy—that is, satisfying the dictates of its nature.

Why, then, does it appear to some people to be prima facie somewhat morally problematic to suggest tampering with the animal's telos to remove suffering? In large part, I believe, it is because people are not convinced that we cannot change the conditions rather than the animal. (Most people are not even aware of how far confinement agriculture has moved from traditional agriculture. A large East Coast chicken producer for many years ran television ads showing chickens in a barnyard and alleging that he raised "happy chickens".) If people in general do become aware of how animals are raised, as occurred in Sweden and as animal activists are working to accomplish elsewhere, they will doubtless demand, just as the Swedes did, first of all a change in the raising conditions, not a change in the animals. It is far more sensible to raise the bridge than to lower the river; it is more reasonable to alter clothes than to surgically remodel a body. And it is quite plausible to do so, since we raised chickens for millennia outside of confinement deprivational conditions.

I have thus argued that it does not follow from the Maxim to Respect Telos that we cannot change telos (at least in domestic animals) to make for happier animals, though such a prospect is undoubtedly jarring. A similar point can be made in principle about nondomestic animals as well. Insofar as we encroach upon and transgress against the environments of all animals by depositing toxins, limiting forage, and so on, and do so too quickly for them to adjust by natural selection, it would surely be better to modify the animals to cope with this new situation so that they can be happy and thrive rather than allow them to sicken, suffer, starve, and die, though surely, for reasons of uncertainty on how effective we can be alone as well as for aesthetic reasons, it is far better to preserve and purify their environment.

In sum, the Maxim to Respect Telos does not entail that we cannot change telos. What it does entail is that if we do change telos by genetic engineering, we must be clear that the animals will be no worse off than they would have been without the change, and ideally will be better off. Such an unequivocally positive telos change from the perspective of the animal can occur when, for example, we eliminate genetic disease or susceptibility to other diseases by genetic engineering, since disease entails suffering. The foregoing maxim that does follow from the Maxim to Respect Telos is what I call the Principle of Conservation of Well-Being. This principle does, of course, exclude much of the genetic engineering currently in progress, where the telos is changed to benefit humans (for instance, by creating larger meat animals) without regard to its effect on the animal. A major concern in this area, which I have discussed elsewhere, is the creation of genetically engineered animals to "model" human genetic disease.[4]

There is one final caveat about the genetic engineering of animals that is indirectly related to the Maxim to Respect Telos and that has been discussed, albeit in a different context, by biologists. Let us recall that a telos is not only genetically based but environmentally expressed. Thus, we can modify an animal's telos in such a way as to improve the animal's telos and quality of life, but at the expense of other animals enmeshed in the ecological/environmental web with the animal in question. For example, suppose we could genetically engineer the members of a prey species to be impervious to predators. While their telos would certainly be improved, other animals would very likely be harmed. While these animals would thrive, those who predate them could starve, and other animals who compete with the modified species could be choked out. We would, in essence, be robbing Peter to pay Paul. Furthermore, while the animals in question would surely be better off in the short run, their descendants may well not be—they might, for example, exceed the available food supply and also starve, something that would not have occurred but for the putatively beneficial change in the telos we undertook. The price, therefore, of improving one telos of animals in nature may well be to degrade the efficacy of others. In this consequential and environmental sense, we would be wise to be extremely circumspect and conservative in our genetic engineering of nondomestic animals, as the environmental consequences of such modifications are too complex to be even roughly predictable.

It is important, then, to clean up some possible questions and misunderstandings regarding my account of telos and the morality of changing telos. In the first place, the question arises as to whether the account of telos and its modification I have given is true to the view of telos promulgated and defended by Aristotle. The answer is clearly that my view is ultimately neither true to nor compatible with a strict and classical Aristotelian account. For Aristotle, of course, telos was fixed and immutable, with the evolution of species or natural kinds ruled out a priori, in part on the grounds that such evolution would make the world unknowable. Aristotle was familiar with the version of evolution by natural selection advanced by Empedocles. When confronted by fossils, Aristotle would simply have dismissed them as another natural kind— stone fish, for example—rather than acquiesce to the possibility of a nature eternally in flux.

Hence, I have not advanced an orthodox Aristotelian view of telos. I have rather adapted the concept to a worldview where it is plain that natural kinds do undergo transformation over time, with biological species being, as it were, stop-time snapshots of what is inherently, in the long run, in flux. And I believe that this is a perfectly plausible move. Whether species change by traditional breeding and artificial selection (as in plants), natural selection done historically over aeons, or rapidly by genetic engineering does not obviate the need I have outlined for the notion of telos to serve as an ethical goal or target for the treatment of individual sentient creatures at human hands. As I have said, the telos of an animal represents the set of needs and wants, genetically encoded and environmentally expressed, that characterize a certain sort of animal at a given period of time. From an animal's nature, we get a sense of what matters to animals of that sort during a certain stage of evolution.

For that reason, the ethical value of the concept of telos in my scheme is to tell us how to best treat individual animals of a certain characterizable kind. Unlike certain environmental ethicists, I believe one's ultimate moral responsibility is to individuals, not to species. One could certainly view species as morally more important than individuals—say, in certain theologically based metaphysical schemes. But in my view, the focus of moral concern is always individuals. The only sense, according to the account I have developed, in talking about moral obligations to species is in terms of the moral effect of what we do to species on the individuals making up that species. For instance, if we insert the gene for some defect into dogs, as we have indeed done in virtue of breeding for show standards, that is wrong because it harms individual animals, not because it does harm to the abstract notion of "dogness." When we speak in ordinary language of harming a subspecies such as bulldogs by breeding animals that cannot breathe or of harming the telos of dogs in general by creating defective breeds such as bulldogs, we mean that we harm the individuals falling under those categories. One cannot harm a species (or telos) except by harming the individuals falling under the concept.

Thus, the problem with creating chickens for current agricultural systems is not a problem of harming "chickenness" in the abstract; it is rather a matter of not meeting the inborn needs and wants of the actual chickens we create. It is for this reason that we can morally condemn confinement agriculture; the animals kept in its systems are *miserable*. Could we genetically change the chickens to be happy under these conditions (probably per impossibile physically, but logically possible), we would not be causing harm because, in my view, abstract entities cannot be harmed.

Telos and Engineering Human Nature

When applying the original Aristotelian concept of telos to human beings, the issue becomes far more complex than those that arise about animals. Obviously, if we look at humans in strictly biological terms, the concept of telos can serve as a basis for the study of human biology as it does for animal biology. There are, after all, certain ways in which humans sense, reproduce, move, grow, metabolize, and so forth—the sorts of things one would learn about in a course on human biology or find in a textbook for such a course. Such a sense of telos, however, would be extremely impoverished because it would not do justice to the high degree of plasticity that can be found in the most significant aspects of human nature, rationality, and sociality, as Aristotle recognized. (In what follows, by the way, I would not claim to be doing Aristotelian scholarship, a task one of my colleagues claims is impossible, since Aristotle moves so quickly he stimulates one to *do* philosophy, not figure out what he meant.)

In any case, it is clear that Aristotle recognizes that there is an enormous range of answers to the human teleological characteristic of sociality. Humans are indeed social, yet the social nature of Spartans is very different from the social nature of democratic Athenians, which again differs from the social satrapy of Persia, which differs from feudal

Europe, tribal Africa (among which there are again huge differences), and so on, indefinitely.

The sociality of wolves, geese, elephants, and other social animals is quite different in that there does not exist anything like such a degree of variation in how they exist socially. Wolves are pretty much wolves; culture plainly plays a far more insignificant role in animal societies, which seem to follow more of an inborn biological imperative.

Similarly with rationality. Even if animals can be said to possess some degree of reasoning (as I believe they do), there is no reason to believe that they possess the huge variation that humans have in rational approaches to issues. We can develop elaborate rational, teleological approaches to biology, and we can develop elaborate rational, mechanistic approaches to biology, both of which claim exclusivity. We can adopt rationally defended naturalistic worldviews, reductionistic worldviews, or theological worldviews.

Thus, rationality and sociality are highly variegated in their instantiation, and to attempt to create a descriptive account that does justice to all of their differing manifestations would seem to be impossible. For this reason, the notions of "is" and "ought" seem to be much more closely connected in a teleological worldview than in a mechanistic one. If humans are by nature rational and social beings, and yet rationality and sociality differ widely in how they manifest themselves, it is natural, as Aristotle might say, to seek to determine "the best," "the highest," the normative notion of rationality and sociality to which all humans ought naturally aspire and work toward. And this seems precisely to be what Aristotle undertakes in his various writings on these issues such as the *Ethics* and the *Politics*. Even if most people, statistically, do not seek happiness as the "rational activity of the soul in accordance with perfect virtue," still Aristotle believes that they ought to—counting heads does not falsify that statement as the telos toward which humans aspire, no more than most of a math class failing to prove a theorem shows that the theorem is unprovable.[5]

In short, on this interpretation (or misinterpretation) of Aristotle, what most people do has no bearing on the interesting sense of human teleology—namely, what they ought to be striving to do.

This same linking of human telos with what people ought to be trying to actualize has persisted even in our modern political theory. For example, the rights enumerated in the Bill of Rights of the U.S. Constitution presuppose a fairly definitive view of human nature—humans are beings who wish to hold on to religious beliefs (or, as has been subsequently interpreted, beliefs that play a similar role to religion in one's life), who wish to express themselves freely, who wish not to be tortured, who wish to hold on to their property, who seek justice, who wish a democratic form of government, and so on.

It is important to note that even if the majority of people at a given time were not rational, did not care about religious freedom or free speech, preferred a corrupt system of justice, or alleged that they were content to live in a tyrannical society, this would not be taken by Aristotle or the framers and interpreters of the Bill of Rights to mean that the human telos had changed. All of these aspects would still remain as ideals, as humanity at its best. For Aristotle, they would still be unrealized potentials that ought to be realized; they would still be human nature despite people's failure to realize it. There are, of course, major differences between our view of human nature and Aristotle's, most notably his belief in natural slaves, the inferiority of women, the superiority of certain peoples over others, and so on (ironically, probably mirrored in the views of the framers of the Constitution, but have been rejected in our ideal for human nature today). The key point is that the idea of human nature or telos, for us or Aristotle, remains as much prescriptive as descriptive, being in the prescriptive sense a goal to aim at that humans potentially can and ought to achieve.

To summarize the discussion thus far, telos is both a metaphysical notion grounding a certain view of biology in particular and reality in general, best expressed in Aristotle. In many ways, this view accords with common sense, though it conflicts with the dominant modern mechanistic approach to science.

With regard to animals, the concept of telos helps to orient us ethically toward our obligations to animals—obligations that followed naturally when animal use was based on husbandry. Now that we need no longer respect telos to use animals successfully, the concept helps articulate our moral obligations to them. Since animal nature is fairly fixed and invariant, understanding animal nature factually is a simple way to orient us ethically in how we ought to treat them.

Human telos, on the other hand, is far more plastic and malleable. Certainly there is a human biological nature, which is fairly straightforward. But the social nature of humans, unlike that of horses, is infinitely variable, and our ratiocinative abilities lead us to highly diverse conclusions and worldviews; as such, the use of the concept of telos in ethical thinking orients us toward what we consider the best and highest in the way humans define themselves. We now believe, contrary to both Aristotle and the framers, that it is more rational and noble to treat everyone equally, not according to an alleged natural hierarchy where there are natural superiors and inferiors. Telos thus articulates an ideal view of humans to aim at.

This, then, provides us with a way to judge the morality of genetically modifying humans by the use of genetic engineering. We must first make a distinction between genetic modifications that are at the "is" level of telos and those at the "ought" level. By the "is" level, I mean those modifications that directly affect mainly the biology of the human telos. Here I have in mind things like genetically engineering increased resistance to cancer or infectious diseases. In my view, such modifications would have little effect on our "ought" sense of telos since being more resistant to certain diseases isn't likely to affect our rationality, sociality, moral concern, and so forth.

On the other hand, consider genetically engineering people in a *Brave New World* sort of scenario, where people are engineered to be acquiescent slaves of the state so that they don't resent enslavement or miss freedom, say, because they have been engineered to produce massive amounts of endogenous opiates. That clearly would affect our "ought" sense of telos since it results in a radical change in what we believe we ought to strive to be—namely, free agents fighting against a repressive regime, not narcotized robots or John Stuart Mill's "satisfied pigs."

As in the case of genetically engineering chickens to be happy in confinement, we first of all have a raise the bridge, don't lower the river perspective, namely, that the repressive society should be changed to fit humans, and not vice versa. But there is a dis-analogy between chickens and people that points us toward a major difference between changing animal and human telos. We do not accept *any* claim that asserts that human society must be structured so that people are totally miserable unless they are radically altered or their consciousness distorted. That is in fact the point of *Brave New World*. Given our historical moral emphasis on reason and autonomy as nonnegotiable ultimate goods for humans, we believe in holding on to them, come what may. Efficiency, productivity, wealth—none of these trump reason and autonomy, and thus the *Brave New World* scenario is deemed unacceptable. On the other hand, were Mill not a product of the same historical values but rather truly consistent in his concern only for pleasure and pain, the *Brave New World* approach or otherwise changing people to make them feel good would be a perfectly reasonable solution.

In the case of animals, however, there are no ur-values like freedom and reason lurking in the background. We furthermore have a historical tradition as old as domestication for changing (primarily agricultural) animal telos (through artificial selection) to fit animals into human society to serve human needs. We selected for nonaggressive animals; animals that depend on us, not only on themselves; animals disinclined or unable to leave our protection; and so on. Our operative concern has always been to fit animals to us with as little friction as possible—as discussed, this assured both success for farmers and good lives for the animals.

If we now consider it essential to raise animals under conditions like battery cages, it is not morally jarring to consider changing their telos to fit those conditions in the same way that it jars us to consider changing humans.

In other words, we would not accept as moral any genetic engineering of humans that conflicts directly with our long-standing and currently strongly held moral traditions regarding what a human ought to be. Though Aristotle might accept genetically engineering more and better natural slaves, we certainly would not.

So I would argue first of all that genetically engineering changes in humans at the "is" level of telos (always assuming no untoward consequences) is morally acceptable if it preserves and increases the well-being of humans. Changing elements of human nature at the "ought" level should be constrained by our strongly held ethical traditions. I also acknowledge that sometimes the distinction is blurred; is increasing human intellectual power an "is" or an "ought" change? It is probably an "ought," but one that may not create any moral concerns.

(Anything proposed at the "ought" level should occasion major *moral* discussion, but genuine moral discussion, not fear or theology posing as morality.)

Are there any other sorts of traits that we can a priori argue would be wrong to genetically engineer? Certainly, I would think, anything that would create a danger to others in society. This might include that favored example from Jean Claude Van Damme or Dolph Lundgren B movies, genetically engineering for a warlike, merciless temperament and enhanced physical ability. It is the former, not the latter, that merits concern.

Or suppose, probably per impossibile, that we could render someone immortal or create a life span of one thousand years in select individuals. There are a variety of reasons this would be prima facie wrong. In the first place, such a person would be effectively alienated from the love and friendship of others. If their secret were known, they would be never-ending targets of resentment. In addition, they would be subject to constant heartbreak, outliving lovers, friends, spouses, and, most cruelly if the trait(s) were not passed down, their own children.

In a deeper, philosophical sense, the absence of death as a constant possibility might well, in a Heideggerian sense, negate the very basis of human existence, that is, the realization of "the possibility of the impossibility of one's being," from whence issues the call for authenticity of one's "project." Given unlimited time, there is no imperative for separating authentic concerns from inauthentic ones.

Moreover, I would argue that it is wrong to genetically engineer traits in people that would radically separate them from the companionship of other humans—for example, if we could engineer people to live only underwater, their forms of life would differ enough from that of other humans that they would be permanently alienated, physically, culturally, and psychologically. Even if they had a peer group of similarly engineered people, they would inevitably suffer fear, loathing, and ostracism from "normal people," and surely one would need to *choose* such a way of life, as opposed to having it thrust upon them. (Vide the monster's arguments in Mary Shelley's *Frankenstein* novel.)

What of correcting genetic diseases at the genomic rather than somatic level? I consider such an action obligatory given the technical ability to accomplish this at an acceptably minimal level of risk. Religious traditions strongly resist such intervention, yet I consider the alternative—supplying the missing enzyme somatically—far more dangerous. If our technology ever breaks down—for instance, due to nuclear winter—people dependent on somatic fixes will perish, and such people will be numerous, as we have fixed the disease manifestations without fixing the underlying heritable defect. I am undisturbed by the claim that this smacks of eugenics, which is an ad hominem, guilt-by-association argument.

At this point, we must engage a vexatious issue that emerges from some of my own earlier work. The discussion thus far presupposes that what counts as genetic diseases is self-evident; such diseases are in the world. Yet in my own work, I have criticized the medical community for treating diseases as if they were simply facts to be read off from the world, self-evident defects in the body machine or mind machine. I have argued (from a base established by Thomas Szasz) that the concepts of disease, sickness, and illness all contain sociovaluational judgments as well as empirical ones. For example, during the 1970s, textbooks of internal medicine and pronouncements of the human medical community began to trumpet obesity as the leading disease problem in the United States. Conceptually, this raised two questions. First of all, while obesity certainly leads to disease—from flatfeet to back problems to heart disease—it is hard to see why it is itself a disease anymore than boxing or football are, since they too lead to disease. Second, what counts as obesity? One can say objectively and empirically of a person that he weighs 250 pounds by putting him on a scale, but what is the objective measure of obesity? Clearly, "too heavy," "fat," or "overweight" are in part at least value judgments. It turns out, of course, that what is called obesity is based on actuarial tables, coupled with the debatable valuational assumption that longevity is the only value reasonably employed to judge lifestyle. (A reasonable person could after all choose to be obese, consume more and tastier food, and enjoy a shorter life.) Similarly, the past few decades have seen child abuse, violence, and alcoholism all confidently labeled diseases, as if that were a factual discovery and not a partly valuational judgment.

I further argued that citizens should not allow the medical community the authority to unilaterally decide what are diseases, but rather that the acceptance of disease appellations should be openly discussed.

All of this is highly relevant to the issue at hand. For what counts as *genetic* disease is also subject to sociovaluational designation. Just as obesity became a disease rather than a cause thereof, so too could shortness of stature or slightness of build in men, or stubbiness in women, or an IQ below 140 in children. People could then demand that such potential "diseases" be treated at the genomic level by genetic engineering.

This is indeed a real possibility, which could in turn lead both to a major expenditure of resources to develop ways of "fixing" things, like body type, that we are not inclined to now think of as diseases and to uniformity in the population. To the first concern, it suffices to say we are already diverting medical money and effort into modalities like breast augmentation and gluteus reduction that are largely based on (historically and culturally) mercurial aesthetic values. We cannot stop wealthy people from underwriting such work. The uniformity argument is of less concern, as different people will, I suspect, always value different things, and even if most want tall progeny, some will inevitably want short ones.

I think we can reach social agreement that the situations currently classified as genetic diseases—Down's syndrome, Huntington's Chorea, and Lesch-Nyhans disease, which all grossly create pain, suffering, and major biological dysfunction—should have research and insurance preference over height, and that this will remain the case whenever medical resources are limited. Furthermore, even if everyone wants tall progeny, and shortness is seen as a disease or deficit, so what? People have grown progressively taller during human history; the extant suits of armor we have inherited from the Middle Ages seem tailored for Yosemite Sam, not Arnold Schwarzenegger. Surely height augmentation will not change the human telos. Augmentation is an "is" change not an "ought" one. And even if, as mentioned earlier, intelligence augmentation is viewed as an "ought" change, it is difficult to see why higher intelligence raises a moral problem. (This assumes, by the way, that intelligence could be augmented by genetics alone, a highly debated notion since we don't even know clearly what intelligence is.)

In sum, then, human genetic engineering at the "is" level to correct obvious defects seems morally acceptable—perhaps obligatory—if it is likely to improve biological function with little or no risk to the person so engineered, or to others. The criteria for adjudicating the morality of effecting genetic alteration at the "ought" level are far more difficult to develop. Aside from the same concerns about potential harm to the person or others, we must also consult our long-standing and nonnegotiable ethical ideals for humans—such as autonomy, freedom, and responsibility—and see if the proposed manipulation does violence to them. (The augmentation of intelligence, or certainly of rationality, if doable, would seem prima facie to be a salubrious change in the human telos.) With a few glaringly obvious exceptions, such as engineering subservience, what we choose to engineer at the "ought" level should be accomplished by a well-crafted ethical dialectic on a case-by-case basis.

This in turn means that we must have a far greater public understanding of what genetic engineering can in fact do. It is one thing to cure a patent genetic defect like cystic fibrosis when we are confident that such a modification will unequivocally effect a cure for pain, suffering, and dysfunction without also creating untoward consequences. It is quite another thing to attempt the modification of some highly complex phenotype trait like "violence" or "intelligence," where we are not even sure what these concepts mean, and are reasonably certain that they are the products of both many genes and environmental factors.

Since genetic engineering is unquestionably the most powerful tool ever discovered by humans, with the greatest potential for effecting enormous and possibly irrevocable change in both our environment and ourselves, we simply cannot be cavalier about its deployment. If we are to make informed, democratic decisions about such technology, we must understand it, or else we will end up making decisions nonrationally, by appeal to half-truths (or less), fear, or hope. This in turn means that scientists (or someone) must educate the public on emerging biotechnological options.

All new technology creates a lacuna in social thought. If the void is not filled by proper information and well-structured discussion of the eventualities, it will instead be filled by the lurid and sensationalistic, essentially aborting what little rational control we might have over our destinies.

Notes

I am grateful to Dick Kitchener, Jane Kneller, Peter Markie, Mike McCulloch, Linda Rollin, Mike Rollin, and Ron Williams for dialogues that helped this chapter.

1. Aristotle, *De Anima* 2.3. 414a29–415a14.

2. Aristotle, *Politics* 1.5. 1254a17–1255a1.

3. Note that a changed telos would be inconceivable to Aristotle, given his cosmology, so we cannot deduce his responses thereto. My guess is that he would be horrified by an "anything goes" universe.

4. See Bernard E. Rollin, *The Frankenstein Syndrome: Ethical and Social Issues in the Genetic Engineering of Animals* (New York: Cambridge University Press, 1995).

5. Aristotle, *Nicomacheas Ethics* 1.7. 1098a16–18.

IV

Social and Political Critiques

12

Nature, Sin, and Society

Lisa Sowle Cahill

The chapters in this volume are attempting to address three questions: Does genetic engineering require a new understanding of human nature? Should there be—and can there be—effective limits to genetic manipulation? Here, I would like to consider these concerns from the standpoint of justice. I shall do this on the foundation of my own discipline of theological ethics, proposing, however, that the Christian ethical commitments and insights I endorse can make an important contribution to public discourse about the ethics of genetics research and the development of genetics-based biotechnology. The basic framework of my analysis will be social ethics, drawing on the Catholic social tradition and the "Christian realism" of the U.S. Protestant ethicist Reinhold Niebuhr. By emphasizing our social nature and the social reasons for controlling genetics, I will argue, first, that the most pressing issues of genetic ethics can be handled on the basis of traditional understandings of human nature, and second, that the moral requirements of human nature urge the limitation of genetic manipulation.

The fundamental ethical premise of inherent and natural human sociality in Western philosophy goes back at least to Aristotle: human beings are social animals, and political existence is constitutive of human nature. As the point is put in the *Nicomachean Ethics*, "No one would choose to have all [other] goods and yet to be alone, since a human being is political, tending by nature to live together with others."[1] Both our happiness and our good depend on the fulfillment of our social nature, and virtue requires society both for its formation and its expression. Human nature is not considered by Aristotle as a set of properties belonging to individuals but as the capacity to live and act politically, to engage in the practices of "living well and doing well" that bring happiness and justice.[2] Social ethics, governed by the norm of justice, is about defining and realizing the practices and institutions necessary to human flourishing.

Now, in the classical conception, justice defined as giving "to each his due" was specified according to a system of hierarchically ordered statuses and roles, in which individual human beings were considered innately to deserve lower or higher places—for example, woman or man, slave or master. The obvious consequences for distributive justice were that not all were entitled to an equal share in the basic necessities of life, much less privileges and luxuries; nor were all entitled to a participatory role in defining the common good of the polis.

Contemporary Christian and Western political theories of justice are influenced by modern, post-Enlightenment ideals of liberty and equality. Christian theories are also shaped by New Testament symbols presenting ideals of inclusive community, such as the "Kingdom of God" and "body of Christ." The Christian social ethics I will propose affirms the intrinsic sociality of the person as a keynote in analyzing the ethics of genetic control, but it will expand the modern affirmation of the equal worth of persons by adopting the biblically informed "preferential option for the poor" found in more recent papal statements as well as in liberation theology. (A secular form of the preferential option might be affirmative action for previously excluded groups.)

Catholic social teaching affirms the goodness and moral demands of human interdependence in a century-long series of papal encyclicals that envisions humans as participants in the common good of society, and enjoins all persons and societies to cooperate in society for the well-being of all. From Niebuhr, we can profitably take the point that however much human fulfillment and happiness may depend on cultivating, in his phrase, "the harmony of life with life," there is a propensity to self-interested behavior in nature *as we find it* that constitutes a strong disincentive to the formation of just social relationships and institutions. The destructive actual propensities of human behavior may be named theologically as "sin." This categorization furthers a more general point, affirmed even more strongly by Catholic social teaching than by Niebuhr, that such tendencies are neither natural, justified, nor ultimately necessary.

Hence, we gain some purchase on the second question: whether limits on genetic manipulation are both advisable and possible. The Christian social position I hope to advance responds to the first option with a resounding confirmation, and to the second with a somewhat less assured but nonetheless hopeful consent. That limits are possible as well as morally desirable is a point I will take some time to develop toward the end of my chapter, offering some historical and political evidence to back up my theological and ethical exhortations.

A Caveat and Two Examples

My approach to human nature will, then, be more focused on human relations and society than on any paradigm case of *the* individual human. One ought not try to discover and enumerate the "natural" and morally compelling characteristics of a human being as such, but rather, look at the ethics of genetic control from the standpoint of the implications of some uses, especially market uses, of genetic knowledge for society. I do not deny in principle the validity of trying to discern what intrinsic characteristics of human beings could be irreparably harmed or violated through genetic alteration. Human physical characteristics or aspects of consciousness, such as intelligence, freedom, and emotion, could be adduced to assess the anticipated effects of genetic interference on what humans have known to date, and to judge whether they constitute a threat to the human as we know it.

The problem is that such approaches meet with difficulty or even founder in trying to define clearly and persuasively exactly what characteristics are essential to human nature, to predict both the immediate and the long-term effects of genetic interventions, and to stipulate the degree of risk required to constitute an actionable threat. Perhaps most especially, the "normative human characteristics" approach finds it hard to get past the fact that, while there are at least some recognizable parameters to "human nature," especially the human body, one of human nature's more salient elements is certainly creative freedom. The humanly defining character of human freedom suggests to many that other human characteristics might be controlled or "engineered," at least in some cases, to serve freedom's aims, and that the most compelling argument against genetic engineering is the diminishment of human freedom itself, either for an individual, a class of individuals, or future generations. But this minimal limit on genetic engineering, while no doubt necessary, seems insufficient.

Finally, the human characteristics approach seems to aim at a definition of "inviolable" human nature that can clearly, decisively, and persuasively rule out certain kinds of genetic intervention as off-limits in virtually all conceivable cases. Again, many of us feel almost instinctively—or on the basis of cumulative moral experience that we find hard to put into the form of a logical argument—that some genetic engineering should be off-limits. Yet the route to that conclusion that goes by way of a definition of the inherent and required characteristics of human nature never seems quite adequate to its objective. Thus, not only do we have a problem in understanding human nature and the respect we owe it, we also have a problem in understanding moral reasoning—in knowing what counts as evidence, what must go to make up a persuasive argument, and how any given evidence and arguments can be introduced into philosophical or public debate in a way that goes beyond mere assertion.

I do not have answers to these problems and questions. But I want to propose another, somewhat different way of going about the task of ethically analyzing genetic engineering, especially in light of justice concerns. I hope this approach will not only reinforce our understanding of human nature as social but also help to locate our ethical analysis of genetic engineering within a more social and historical model of moral reasoning.

In the words of the philosopher and legal scholar Margaret Jane Radin, "There aren't any lock-down logical arguments that compel people to recognize," for instance, that there are some values whose worth cannot be reduced to a monetary equivalent, or that some practices tend to commodify human persons and undermine human society. Sometimes a more pragmatic, inductive approach to ethics and persuasion is required; just like human persons, practical reason is for Radin "irreducibly social" by nature. It does not belong to individuals but to social groups, and is carried out only within the relations of "connectedness" that make the social and the political "possible for us."[3]

Now for my two examples or cases to illustrate some of the main ethical dangers of the new research on genetics and its clinical applications. Both are intended to highlight the importance of a social ethics approach to genetic engineering. The first, a current venture in human reproductive cloning, shows the inconclusiveness of a human characteristics approach, as well as the accessibility and urgency of a social justice one. The second, the use of international patent law by drug companies to control profits by restricting access to lifesaving therapies, is offered as a paradigm for understanding where genetic research and genetic engineering are likely to lead in the near future. As research enters the stage of clinical application, criteria of social justice will have to be applied in a global context.

Cloning

In January 2001, an international consortium of fertility specialists announced its intention to accomplish what most scientists and national governments have forsworn, if not forbidden, up until this time: the creation, gestation, and birth of a human individual grown from the nucleus of a single parental cell. The group, headed by the controversial Italian Severino Antinori, who in 1994 induced pregnancy in a sixty-two-year-old woman with the use of a donated ovum, includes an American, Panos Zavos, cofounder of a fertility clinic in Lexington, Kentucky. While the U.S. government has barred the use of public funds for so-called reproductive cloning (intending to bring a cloned individual to birth), no such ban exists if federal grant money is not used, and only a few states (including California, Michigan, Louisiana, and Rhode Island) have adopted laws barring the creation of cloned human beings.

Reproductive cloning would have appeal to couples who cannot bear children together, but are reluctant to use sperm or eggs from a donor. If cloning were their fertility therapy of choice, they could take the nucleus of a cell from one partner, insert it in the enucleated egg of the woman (or a donor), and implant it in the uterus of the woman (or a surrogate) for gestation. In the closest parallel to sexual reproduction, the resulting child would have only one genetic parent (the father), but would be carried to term by the other parent (the mother). Such cloning could be of interest not only to infertile heterosexual couples but to gay and lesbian couples, single parents, couples seeking to replace a deceased child or other relative, couples seeking to avoid the manifestation of genetic disease in their child, and parents seeking a tissue match for an existing child. Reproductive technologies constitute a largely unregulated industry both in the United States and internationally. Human reproductive cloning is banned in most of Europe, but in many other countries, including China, India, Pakistan, and South Korea, it is not prohibited.

A recent cover story in the *New York Times Magazine* described the "delirious scientism" of an eccentric Canadian sect called the Raelians, whose founder claims to have visited with aliens in a flying saucer in 1973, and who are also deep into the cloning quest. Their company, Clonaid, hopes to normalize reproductive cloning to the extent that procreating through sex will be regarded as just too risky for the prospective child.[4] While cloning entrepreneurs may offer alleviation of the woes of barren or bereaved couples as their motivation, there is also big money to be made in cloning. This is not a technique that researchers are proposing to offer free of cost to all, but one that could draw on a wealthy market and investors, not only on this continent, but especially in cultures where the scions of a fabulously wealthy upper class are expected to produce heirs, and where neither adoption nor pollution of the family bloodlines by donor gametes are regarded receptively. Even now, a cloning research project at Texas A&M is going forward under a multimillion dollar grant bestowed by a pet owner who hopes to eventually acquire an extra copy of his beloved dog. Each step in mammalian cloning research brings closer the day when human cloning will be feasible.[5]

What exactly is it that is objectionable about human cloning? This may be harder to pin down than it would at first seem. Few people still believe that cloning could actually produce exact replicas of parent human beings, much less whole classes or armies of identical persons. The interaction of genetics and environment is too strong for that. Many react to what seems the coldly technocratic approach to bearing children by terming cloning a sort of "manufacture" or "production" of a child. For instance, a statement released by the U.S. National Conference of Catholic Bishops' Secretariat for Pro-Life Activities calls for a stronger, comprehensive ban on reproductive cloning, and asserts that cloning dehumanizes and objectifies a child: "In human cloning, a new human being does not arise from the loving union of a man and woman but is manufactured to specifications."[6] It is hard, though, to show that this is necessarily true in every case. Indeed, cloners may be all too focused on the aim of having their union produce a biological child; they may, if anything, be overinvested in the child's personality and personhood. Their efforts to produce or control a birth are not necessarily any greater than those of couples using other types of therapy, or of couples reproducing "naturally" in traditional societies, where a marriage itself may be arranged in order to produce the right kind of heir. And nothing guarantees absolutely that a cloned child would be loved and nurtured any differently from a sibling produced in the old-fashioned way.

There are a couple of ways in which reproductive cloning would indeed be different from other kinds of procreation. First, the offspring would have only one genetic parent. Second, the child would be the later-born genetic twin of that parent. The novel effects of cloning on the intergenerational, biologically anchored patterns of family and kinship present the most obvious challenge to our understanding of human "nature." If new notions of nature are required to understand this phenomenon, they probably derive from the effects of cloning on the family. For example, parents who clone children from themselves would be raising sons or daughters who are also their twins; their spouses would become the parents of younger versions of their husbands or wives. I believe great caution is to be advised, and a strong "hermeneutic of suspicion" should be aimed at those who downplay the significance of human asexual and replicative reproduction in order to pursue financial gain or as an answer to their personal problems and desires. The fact that at least some would-be cloners and customers are willing to proceed with an untested technology despite the risks to embryos, fetuses, children, and families is another strong moral contraindication.

Nonetheless, the precise immorality of cloning is difficult to specify in "intrinsicist" terms. The novelty of cloning in departing from all known types of parenthood and kinship does not clearly make it immoral. Change does not necessarily equate to harm or violation, and a judgment of the latter is necessary before we can designate any activity as immoral. Philosophically, there is an important distinction between using the term nature in the descriptive or factual sense and using it to indicate the normatively human: those aspects of humanity that should be protected, preserved, valued, or enhanced.[7] For the philosopher Aristotle and the theologian Saint Thomas Aquinas, for instance, human nature denotes not just what in fact humans are or do but an ideal or normative conception of what constitutes human flourishing. Just as the fact that something occurs "in nature" or in practice does not make it morally commendable, so changing human capacities or behavior is not in and of itself either right or wrong. While concerns can be expressed over the bad consequences that might follow from the disruption of known patterns of family relationships that cloning would cause, it is another and more difficult task to argue that such disruptions should necessarily forbid the practice, much less that they make each and every instance of cloning immoral.

I believe that cloning is more amenable to moral analysis when placed in its social context. First, cloning furthers a cultural tendency to view biomedical technology in a simplistic, triumphalist, and uncritical way, placing in it hope for the alleviation of too many human ills—both social and spiritual—that require instead ethical and religious resources. Second, it represents the use of biomedical knowledge in combination with technological expertise, to make profits with too little consideration of the common good and the restraint it requires. Third, it overlooks or represses the gap between rich and poor that throughout the world allows the lucky few access to exotic techniques while depriving many more of basic health care and other necessities. Characterizations like "manufacture" and "produce" have a good deal more force when applied to cloning as a part of a highly remunerative, widely advertised, and increasingly mass-market infertility industry. Individual parents or couples would be appalled to think that they are obtaining manufactured children from a production line, but this does not keep them from being the desperate, naive, or just opportunistic consumers who will ensure that expanding infertility and cloning programs turn a profit by satisfying customers. On such grounds alone, regardless of whether or not cloning is intrinsically evil in itself, cloning should be regulated or even banned. Commercialized, technology-driven reproduction affects the social institutions of family and parenthood in deleterious ways because it makes basic, intimate human relations and communities increasingly subject to individualism, commodification, and exploitation.

Patenting

Cloning babies is not likely to be the most immediate or widespread use of genetic engineering in the biotech industry. Already, genetic information is being put to use to carry out genetic tests on humans, to improve drugs' performance by tailoring them to a variety of diseases, and to splice genes across species of plants and bacteria. All of these techniques are ostensibly aimed at great benefit for humans and the relief of suffering, and all are or have the potential to be highly profitable.

The gateway to profit is the patent. A patent gives its holder the right to exclusive use of an invention for twenty years, during which time royalties are charged for licenses to use the patented information, either for a marketable application or further research. Although patent laws vary nationally and regionally, an international regime of patent law has been established by means of the World Trade Organization's (WTO) requirement that member nations respect intellectual property rights as defined according to North American and European standards. Adherence to the 1995 Trade Related Aspects of Intellectual Property Rights (TRIPS) agreement is part of the price of entry into the global economic market, and noncompliant members will be placed on trade "watch lists" that threaten eventual trade sanctions and discourage investment even in the short term. At least in theory, patents can only be obtained for inventions, not discoveries in nature; and patentable inventions must have clear and specific utility. Enforcement of these criteria has been questionable in practice. Patent applications have been filed for genes and segments of genes, even though these are not inventions, and no useful process or product based on them has yet been proposed in any detail. As of 2000, according to a U.S. Department of Energy report, over three million gene-related patent applications had been filed, mostly in the United States, Europe, and Japan.[8]

In the emergent global market, patented drugs are big international business. It is now clear that the number of functional human genes is much smaller than once anticipated, which may mean that pharmaceutical companies will be able to produce genetically engineered drugs more quickly, even though there may turn out to be fewer of them to produce, and production may depend on further study of the proteins genes code for, not just a knowledge of genes themselves. Human Genome Sciences, based in Rockville, Maryland, already has drugs in clinical trials.[9]

Pharmaceutical development is expected to customize drugs to address both the genetic causes of particular diseases and the genetic profiles of individuals. Among the early targets for new gene-based drug products are asthma and Alzheimer's.

But what kind of social implications will the manufacture of genetically engineered drugs have? International control of currently available drugs through patent laws gives us a preview of a likely scenario. Let us focus on an ongoing controversy over AIDS drugs, involving developing countries, transnational pharmaceutical companies, and the World Trade Organization.[10] According to international trade agreements, companies can "segment" the market for their products, meaning that they can charge different prices for the same product in different countries. National governments, companies, or health care providers, however, are not free to import drugs or their components from foreign countries where prices may be lower. Although TRIPS provides that countries can set intellectual property rights aside in the case of a "national emergency," efforts of the South African government to pass and act on a 1997 law permitting parallel importing to help address its AIDS crisis were fought tooth and nail by a coalition of big pharmaceutical companies. They were led by the world's largest, Glaxo Smith Kline, based in Britain with extensive U.S. holdings. In 1998, the Pharmaceutical Manufacturers Association of South Africa brought a suit against the South African government to the Pretoria High Court, claiming that the new law violated their patent rights.

South Africa has over four million people affected with AIDS. The normal cost of the triple-drug "AIDS cocktail" in the West is $10,000 to $15,000 per patient a year. The companies that hold the patents have agreed to charge about $1,000 a year per patient in Africa, still far beyond what countries on that continent could afford. As the Pretoria trial was about to open, in March 2001, a local generic drugs manufacturer in India, Cipla Ltd., declared that it would provide AIDS drugs for $350 a year to Doctors Without Borders, which runs forty AIDS clinics in Africa, and that it would provide the drugs to government programs for $600.[11] A few days later, the British charity Oxfam began a campaign to force multinational drug companies to cut prices in poor nations, accusing transnationals of waging an "undeclared war" for profits by keeping prices high and using trade sanctions to protect patent treaties that give them a monopoly on life-saving drugs.[12] By mid-April, support for the South African revolution had become widespread, including the European Union, the World Health Organization, and the National AIDS Council of France. On April 19, the thirty-nine drug companies behind the case dropped their suit. In June, the United Nations's "Declaration of Commitment on HIV-AIDS" endorsed the proposal of UN Secretary General Kofi Annan to establish a worldwide $7–10 billion fund to prevent and treat AIDS and other diseases, through a variety of social measures.[13] At its November 2001 summit in Doha, Qatar, the WTO reacted to international pressure by adapting its trade policies to allow members more latitude in determining when to permit the manufacture of generics. Meanwhile, countries such as Thailand and Brazil have demonstrated that local efforts to promote effective use of AIDS drugs can succeed even in very poor populations with little health care access. Brazil's very successful national program of clinics and drug distribution has managed to attain—even among very sick, uneducated, and impoverished patients—a level of compliance with the demanding AIDS treatment regime that approaches that of the United States.[14]

What this case suggests for moral analysis is that genetic engineering is highly likely in the immediate future to lead to egregious injustices that can be identified quite well without any new conceptions of human nature, and that representatives of vastly different cultures can agree to address. If there are relevant challenges here to our present notions of human existence, they derive not from genetics as such but the vastly heightened communication and transportation technologies that magnify and intensify human relationships at the global level, creating the opportunities for global investment, production, and marketing of which the transnational biotech firms are so quick to take advantage. Social, ethical, and policy analysts will be remiss if we do not target the national, international, and global institutions through which genetic engineering in all its forms is being developed and deployed. Possible challenges to our philosophical categories aside, we are confronted here with a human crisis of significant proportions—one that may or may not be novel on the world historical scene, but that is self-evidently grave all the same.

The Catholic Perspective on the Common Good

A first framework of analysis may be provided by Catholic social teaching. Although Catholic social ethics refers at its foundation to a belief in a creating and redeeming God who sustains and judges human societies, it also advances a normative view of social relations that may be shared with other communities of religious and moral belief. The distinctive contributions of this view are that it upholds relatively objective and universal standards of behavior, it emphasizes human solidarity above individualism, it trusts in and relies on a human propensity for cooperative social living, and it evokes imaginative empathy with our fellow human beings by drawing on biblical symbols and commands. In the last half century, this normative view of society has become increasingly global in scope.

This social vision goes back in its essentials to Aquinas and even Saint Augustine; but it makes its signature modern appearance in 1891 in the encyclical letter of Pope Leo XIII, *Rerum Novarum* (*On the Condition of Labor*). An admittedly somewhat conservative response to the abuses of industrialization, this encyclical sought to maintain order and deter Marxist revolution by urging the property-owning classes to use their wealth in responsible ways, and to recognize the basic material and social rights of workers. Some of Leo's main concerns are captured in the following statement of his program for just social reform:

To the State the interests of all are equal whether high or low. The poor are members of the national community equally with the rich; they are real component parts, living parts, which make up, through the family, the living body; and it need hardly be said that they are by far the majority. It would be irrational to neglect one portion of the citizens and to favor another; and therefore the public administration must duly and solicitously provide for the welfare and the comfort of the working people, or else that law of justice will be violated which ordains that each shall have his due.[15]

Later eras modified, if not abandoned, Leo's organic view of society and his assumption that the state and the higher classes shall take the lead in making provision for the lower classes. Yet the lasting contributions of this encyclical include the ideas that the state and all social relations are subject to higher laws of justice and reason; that the state's function is to order and serve society according to the moral law; that members of society enjoy a basic equality; that human persons by nature exist in social relationships; that cooperative social relations work to the benefit of all; and that societies and governments have the duty to ensure for all the basic social and material necessities of life.

The fundamental premises and standards that *Rerum Novarum* lays down have been reappropriated and restated in response to different social situations and with different nuances, agendas, and tones at intervals of about four decades for over one hundred years.[16] After the Second Vatican Council, in the 1960s, two important qualifications introduced were a vision of all nations cooperating in a global society or a "universal common good," and a growing realization that the common good requires full social participation by all members, not just the leadership of the upper classes, government officials, or property owners. The pope of the Council, John XXIII, opened his 1963 encyclical *Pacem in Terris* (*Peace on Earth*) with a hopeful appeal to "all men of good will." He reads in "the signs of the times" that "there is reason to hope . . . [that] men may come to discover better the bonds that unite them together, deriving from the human nature they have in common," and that they may give up the arms race and all threat of war, in order to collaborate in an atmosphere of love.[17]

Beginning in the 1960s, with the encyclicals of Paul VI, and increasing in the 1980s and 1990s, with the pontificate of John Paul II, more and more attention has been devoted to the impact on the universal common good of inadequately regulated capitalism, often couched in or advanced by the cultural values of individualism, materialism, consumerism, and imperialism. Papal social teaching has striven to maintain a balance between the independence and free initiative of social groups and organizations and the government regulation that is sometimes needed to ensure the fair participation of all in the common good. The axis of balance is the "principle of subsidiarity," originally used to protect subordinate bodies from state interference.[18] Later, it was wielded to call on governments (including international organizations) to correct imbalances in the social order.[19] John Paul has certainly never condemned capitalist economic behavior outright or in toto.[20] Yet he has often expressed acute awareness of some of the excesses to which it is liable. In *Sollicitudo Rei Socialis*, John Paul warns that world development is not merely a matter of economics, notwithstanding "the many real benefits provided in recent times by science and technology." Unless economic expansion is "guided by a moral understanding and by an orientation toward the true good of the human race, it easily turns against man to oppress him." Although many possess too much, "there are others—the many who have little or nothing—who do not succeed in realizing their basic human vocation because they are deprived of essential goods." A couple of years later, he links the plight of "the great majority of people in the Third World" with the "human inadequacies of capitalism," noting that they are deprived not only of material goods but the education and skills necessary to gain "fair access to the international market."[21]

In *Evangelium Vitae*, the pope reiterates many of these points, emphasizing that, in a worldwide perspective, the affirmation of human rights "in distinguished international assemblies is merely a futile exercise of rhetoric, if we fail to unmask the selfishness of the rich countries which exclude poorer countries from access to development." This encyclical (like others) also draws on biblical teaching, especially the example of Jesus and his commands to love one's neighbor and serve those in need, stressing what liberation theologians have called the "option for the poor."[22] Gospel themes elucidate the meaning of "solidarity," a concept of social unity and responsibility that the pope introduced in his first social encyclical, *Laborem Exercens*, and that serves as a key to much of his thinking about the common good.[23]

Despite the fact that after Vatican II, papal encyclicals increasingly rested their moral appeals on religious and biblical foundations, a basic framework of "natural law" has never been abandoned.[24] The idea that moral values and norms are at a basic level shared by and in principle recognizable to all human societies is the premise that allows the Catholic social tradition to speak in the public sphere, and to urge social, political, and economic changes that will better serve the universal or global common good. Neither morality nor the public order is relative to cultural practices or majority opinion, but is instead grounded in "an objective moral law which, as the 'natural law' written in the human heart, is the obligatory point of reference for civil law itself."[25] Prescriptions supposedly based on the natural have in some areas of morality (for example, sexuality and the taking of innocent life) been derived in an ahistorical, deductive, and rigid manner that does more to reveal the vulnerabilities of claims about "universal" morality than to demonstrate them. In social ethics, however, Catholic teaching has always been more inductive and flexible, outlining a general framework of justice, rights and duties, and the common good, but leaving to different eras and to concerned social analysts and political actors the task of applying it concretely.

On the topic of genetic research or engineering specifically, the Church has repeatedly denounced any interventions that deliberately destroy embryos, which it regards as having the status of protectable persons from the moment of conception.[26] Recent objections to cloning have also targeted the commodification of human life and procreation that they threaten. A statement from the Vatican's Pontifical Academy for Life affirmed its commitment to the relief of human suffering, but insisted that an embryo is a human life too, and hence a subject with rights. Taking aim at the broader social context in which stem cell research is encouraged, Bishop Elio Sgreccia, vice president of the academy, characterized the U.S. government as "yielding to the pressures of the industries that want to commercialize human health."[27] In an August 29, 2000 speech to transplant surgeons in Rome, Pope John Paul II applauded attempts to remedy organ failure, but excluded the growing of new tissue that had its origin in embryonic stem cells. Improved health is not the only criterion of medical morality, he argued, since all human endeavors must meet the broader and higher standard of "the integral good of the human person." Including the embryo in the category "person," the pope excluded human cloning, the destruction of embryos, and the use of embryonic cells as means to better medical treatment.[28]

Nonetheless, Catholic teaching has never retracted the essentially open attitude to "genetic manipulation" expressed by the pope in 1983. In an October speech of that year to the World Medical Association, he endorsed therapeutic measures as in principle desirable, provided that they tend to the "real promotion of the personal well-being of man, without harming his integrity or worsening his life conditions," and he did not exclude the possibility even of genetic enhancement.[29] Given the drift of the papal concerns about economic exploitation, however, perhaps the question of genetic engineering should today be placed more firmly within a common good framework that includes global market forces and the difficulty of regulation to ensure fair international participation and distributive justice.

These concerns have been joined by other Catholic authors and organizations addressing issues in genetics. Debates over genetically modified foods and the use of patents to inhibit the development of more nutritious food for the Third World occasioned a report by an international consortium of fifteen Catholic nongovernmental organizations (NGOs), International Cooperation for Development and Security, Brussels (CIDSE). The report advocates a socially responsible use of property and technology, calling attention to "the poorest and most vulnerable members of society," and amplifying the moral range of its appeal by referring to Gandhi as well as general notions of justice and human rights.[30]

CIDSE describes international biopatenting law as biased toward the interests of both the industrialized countries and companies big enough to defend their investments at a tremendous legal cost. It calls on countries hurt by patenting laws to take advantage of exceptions built into WTO regulations, and judges that "the global applications of the TRIPS Agreement is in danger of imposing on poor societies and communities an alien set of concepts of property in which their interests are far from the main emphasis."[31] Reflected in this analysis are the Catholic tradition's concern for a public conception of the common good that can operate internationally; its use of religious ideas to evoke solidarity and a preferential option for the marginalized; the use of the principle of subsidiarity both to urge legal and regulatory restraint of market activities and to encourage the empowerment and independent initiative of subordinate social groups; and a commitment to social change born of its conviction that reasonableness and cooperative action can and will prevail over injustice.

Reinhold Niebuhr and Christian Realism

Although Niebuhr never addressed genetics or bioethics, he was regarded even in his own day as an incisive critic of politics and society, since he took up current questions of war, class, racism, international relations, and technology. Writing after the optimism of the Protestant "social gospel" had been dashed by two world wars, Niebuhr eschewed "idealistic" ethical theories in favor of "realism" about humanity's moral prospects. As a Christian social ethicist, his operating premise was quite the opposite of the Catholic social tradition: "In principle, the Christian faith holds that human nature contains both self-regarding and social impulses and that the former is stronger than the latter. This assumption is the basis of Christian realism."[32] But like the Catholic tradition, Niebuhr saw human moral and political action as responsible to an objective moral order, illuminated most clearly by faith, but certainly not limited in either scope or intelligibility to any particular cultural or religious community. As he put it,

Reason . . . inevitably places the stamp of its approval upon those impulses which affirm life in its most inclusive terms. Practically every moral theory, whether utilitarian or intuitional, insists on the goodness of benevolence, justice, kindness and unselfishness. Even when economic self-seeking is approved, as in the political morality of Adam Smith, the criterion of judgment is the good of the whole.[33]

What leads to fundamentally irrational behavior against the good of the whole is described decisively by Niebuhr as sin. Expounded most eloquently in *The Nature and Destiny of Man*, his 1939 Gifford Lectures, Niebuhr's psychological explanation of sin locates it both against a transcendent horizon of human meaning and at the center of the evil pervading human institutions. For Niebuhr, the human propensity to wickedness results from the uneasy dialectic between human freedom and human finitude. Unable to realize that the reconciliation of these two sides of human nature rests only in trust in a divine, transcendent source of meaning, humans either deny finitude in the sin of pride or flee from freedom in the sin of "sensuality" (a term that for Niebuhr means immersion in any of the tasks, pleasures, accomplishments, or distractions of life that allow us to avoid our other or higher responsibilities).[34]

It is through his depiction and explanation of the social manifestations of sin that Niebuhr provides a compelling diagnosis of the transgressions of genetic engineering against human nature. The social side of sin most developed by Niebuhr and applied to politics is "tribalism" or "collective egotism," expressions of the sin of pride. Niebuhr believed that although individuals have some potential to overcome selfishness and the drive to dominate others by embracing the ideals of mutuality and love, social groups find it virtually impossible. "The sinfulness of man makes it inevitable that a dominant class, group, and sex should seek to define a relationship, which guarantees its dominance, as permanently normative."[35] The chief source of human "inhumanity" and "brutality" is the "tribal limits" of our sense of obligation to others. This limitation results in group boundaries separating "we" from "they"—usually on the basis of class, race, religion, or language—and the denial of "an obvious common humanity."[36] Collective egotism is Niebuhr's designation of the "group pride" that achieves authority over individuals and permits group loyalty to make unconditional demands on its members. Inequality, mostly rooted in property ownership and economics, becomes the basis of a class solidarity that is virtually impermeable to persuasions of reason and conscience. To the contrary, the privileged classes rationalize their status by speciously arguing either that their advantages are the reward of merit or that they work for the good of the whole. "Disinterestedness" as a purported motive for group behavior is ineffectual if sincere, and otherwise a disguise for self-serving aims.[37]

By identifying with a group that claims to advance transcendent and universal ideals, or that simply pursues its own survival as the ultimate aim, the individual can assert dominance over others to an extent that would never be claimed on behalf of the self. While Niebuhr saw the nation-state as a primary purveyor of collective egotism, political and economic conditions at the beginning of the twenty-first century also bear out the appropriateness of naming other collectivities, such as the ethnic group and its history, the corporation and its shareholders, the scientific community and its discoveries, and the disease constituency and its needs. In Niebuhr's view, modern technology particularly plays into greed as a form of the will to power, since it tempts "contemporary man" to overestimate both the value and the possibility of overcoming the insecurity of nature.[38]

On the other side, but in a complementary fashion, sensuality is a demonic commitment to the finite goods and goals of life through which we escape the human calling to exercise our freedom well. Niebuhr himself tends to focus his discussion of sensuality on the individual sinner, who seeks to avoid the anxiety of his or her real condition through devotion to mutable goods. Like many traditional authors, he finds sex to offer both the "most obvious" and the "most vivid" illustration of the self's fall from God into sensuality.[39] Christian ethicist Robin Lovin, however, comments that the individualization of sensuality trivializes it, and diagnoses in social groups as well as individuals "a desire to measure our contingent achievements by a standard easier to grasp and more to our own liking" than loyalty to God or truly ultimate values would demand.[40]

Echoing the philosopher Alasdair MacIntyre, Lovin clarifies how sensuality can lead to social injustice by describing social endeavors or practices that seem to absorb all one's energy and sense of purpose, and to discourage participants from expanding their moral vision any further than a given endeavor's internal criteria of success. "Anything serves the purpose which gives us a well-regulated set of activities that seem to justify themselves. We can then lose ourselves in doing what the system requires."[41] Examples might range from devotion to one's family, to being a poet or research scholar, to being a medical doctor, genetic scientist, corporate executive, or delegate to the WTO. Christian realists will be on the lookout for both "signs of institutional pride and the arrogance of power," and the identification of the moral life with the myopic mastery of practices designed to serve finite and ultimately tribalistic goals.[42]

Niebuhr was often eloquent on the intransigence of the finite loyalties that lie at the root of social injustice as well as the deceptions necessary to keep them in place. In his view, all the "great and good men of history," all the philosophers and kings, will be tempted "to hide their will-to-power behind their virtues and to obscure their injustices behind their generosities."[43] Growth in human knowledge and capacities, so definitive of the age of globalization, is evident, grants Niebuhr, in the sense that "history obviously moves toward more inclusive ends, toward more complex human relations, toward the enhancement of human powers and the cumulation of knowledge." But growth is not necessarily progress, since tribal animosities may simply be expressed on new levels of violence; practices that commandeer the individual conscience for the sake of self-perpetuating finite goals may be projected onto global institutions. The biblical figure or religious symbol that represents the incremental power of evil alongside that of good is the Antichrist.[44]

Because of the depth and inevitability of personal and social sin, Niebuhr was never convinced that moral persuasion could do much to change human nature or social arrangements. Rather than calling, with the Catholic popes, for more human reasonableness and trust, he noted that the privileged have historically proven themselves unwilling to give up power unless forced. Therefore coercion, sometimes representing the competing assertion of interest rather than a pure moral ideal, must remain part of the picture of social ethics if societies are to be able to move in any degree toward greater approximations of justice.[45] Race relations in the United States provide a paradigm case. In the aptly titled *Moral Man and Immoral Society*, Niebuhr calls it "sentimental and romantic to assume that any education or any example will ever completely destroy the inclination of human nature to seek special advantages at the expense of, or in indifference to, the needs and interests of others."[46] Disadvantaged groups must find ways to assert pressure against the elites or oppressors; a balance of power and interests must be maintained by rule of law and, when necessary, by corrective pressures on the system if social justice is to be established or sustained.

Niebuhr is not completely pessimistic about this possibility, realistic though he may be about the measures required to attain it. First of all, as Lovin notes, Niebuhr's theory that all human persons and communities stand under the judgment of an objective moral order, and finally under the law of love, engenders a critical attitude toward social arrangements and creates a "pull of obligation" to realize the possibilities that the moral imagination recognizes.[47] Further, in a retrospective work composed in 1965, Niebuhr follows a discussion of tribalism and inhumanity with an allusion to "common grace" and hope for social reform.

Human self-seeking, he says, is intricately related to self-giving—for instance, in the fact that self-giving ultimately contributes to self-realization. Self-giving is enabled, he believes, through natural human experiences of community, paradigmatically the family, that support the self's sense of security and enable generous relations to others. Such relationships are a vehicle of "common grace," an experience of redemption in or through the shared realities of human nature. Indeed, he applies the term to "all forms of social security or responsibility *or pressure* which prompt the self to bethink itself of its social essence and to realize itself by not trying too desperately for self-realization."[48] Although Niebuhr would not agree with Pope John XXIII that moral appeals to those of "good will" will be adequate to the task of realizing peace on earth, he does come close to the Catholic tradition's critical concept of the common good, and likewise understands an important function of civil law to be the balancing of needs and interests. Although he would certainly not reject the idea that the social and political leadership should make an "option for the poor," he would even more strongly endorse the insight of liberation theology that empowerment of the disenfranchised will require their own self-advocacy, and their initiative in defining and claiming their rightful social agency.

But Is It Possible?

Although Niebuhr adds a salutary dose of reality to the encyclical tradition's nonconflictual social optimism, the realities of the new global economy may likewise need to correct Niebuhr's hope for change. Are limitation and control of genetic engineering really possible, given the powerful financial and political interests invested in its development and sale?

The more radical critics of globalization have painted a dismal, yet rather compelling picture of the gradual erosion of the nation-state, the national market, and the bargaining power of labor in a new "post-Keynesian" era in which the liberal welfare state has been dismantled in favor of the internationalization of capital under monetarist policies free of political interference.[49] When and if the global market is controlled at the global level (for example, by transnational institutions such as the World Bank, the International Monetary Fund, or the WTO), it ultimately will be in the interests of business. Indeed, although the "free market" is the philosophical linchpin of economic globalization, actual competition is highly circumscribed and, for the most part, limited to major trading blocs and relatively independent economic powers (for instance, the European Union, the United States, and Japan), and to "certain giant corporations, cartels, or oligopolies over world market share—in automobiles or pharmaceuticals, for example."[50] This analysis seems borne out by such phenomena as the international patent rights regime enforced by the WTO and the difficulty experienced by South Africa in obtaining drugs according to national legislation governing production or imports.

On the other side, however, these and similar examples may be indicating that lesser powers (including NGO's, nations, regional coalitions, and even internationally organized labor) can fight back. According to a more optimistic analysis, a new global civil society is taking shape, "made up of nonprofit organizations and voluntary associations dedicated to civic, cultural, humanitarian, and social causes."[51] The most prominent of these are Amnesty International, Greenpeace, Oxfam, and the International Committee of the Red Cross. During the past decade, these groups promoted treaties to limit global warming, establish an international criminal court to try human rights violations, outlaw land mines, cancel Third World debt, and gain regulations on bioengineered food products. Although these aims have been furthered with uneven success, the efforts behind them and the publicity they have engendered may mark a serious challenge to the new economic world order.[52] Nations, states, and regional associations can also be considered as agents in civil society, if and to the extent that they are nonparticipants in formulating the global policy authorized by the international financial institutions. Former *New York Times* chief Washington economic correspondent David Sanger opines that the really noteworthy aspect of the fracas over the WTO meetings in Seattle in 1999 was not the street demonstrations but "a remarkable rebellion against American primacy" that took place behind the scenes as developing nations (supported by bigger powers who saw their own interests at stake) resisted what they viewed as an "onslaught to reshape the world economy on Washington's terms."[53]

The chair of Cipla—as mentioned earlier, the Bombay pharmaceutical company that defied the transnationals to put cheap AIDS drugs on the South African market—expressed motives mixed of altruism and self-interest. On the one hand, he said, India had just experienced a devastating earthquake in 2001, and aid workers and volunteers from around the world were rushing in to help distribute donated goods and assist with rescue efforts. This was an inspiration. At the same time, he expressed the hope that Cipla's aggressive move would help make manufacturers of generic drugs in the developing world part of World Health Organization talks to involve multinational companies in offering drugs at reduced prices, and thus "break the stranglehold of the multinationals."[54] When Oxfam joined the campaign to force multinational drug price cuts and override patent laws against low-cost generics, it specifically voiced the intention to pressure the companies by attacking them on Wall Street and in London, in the hope of discouraging investment through bad publicity aimed at shareholders. Oxfam's spokesperson drew parallels to effective attacks on Shell for environmental policies in the Niger Delta and on Nestle for promoting infant formula to poor women.[55] Oxfam also suggested ways in which transnational drug companies could adopt a more socially responsible stance, similar to the "benefit-sharing" proposals that have elsewhere been recommended as part of a solution to distributive justice in genetics research.[56]

If countries like India, Brazil, Thailand, and South Africa are now banding together against big biotech companies with the help of well-placed NGO's, they can look to precedents already set by China in restricting access to desirable indigenous genetics research populations, following several scandals in the 1990s. For over a decade, U.S., French, and German research institutes have collaborated with Chinese organizations to collect genetic samples from isolated ethnic populations in China. The research was intended to help develop testing and genetics-based treatments for a number of disorders, including obesity, asthma, and cancer. Human subjects violations were reported to have occurred in a number of cases, including incomplete information about the risks and benefits, local political pressure to participate in studies, and reneging on promises of medical care to research subjects. Moreover, nationalist sentiment in China was stirred by the fact that foreign researchers were removing genetic samples for the benefit of Western research projects likely to result in sizable profits. In 1998, China's State Council issued a law requiring stricter approval of foreign-funded genetic research, signed consent from subjects, and tighter controls on sending genetic information abroad. Recently, Health Ministry bioethics adviser Qiu Renzong urged China to be more vigilant in protecting intellectual property rights to its DNA, and has rallied support from several national organizations, including China's Academy of Sciences and the Health Ministry.[57]

William Greider, a critic of global capitalism whose analysis converges in interesting ways with that of Niebuhr, tenders the hope that the pull of self-interest and the push of market and political pressures might work together to bring off a renewed sense of the common good among all of society's stakeholders, a general understanding that "we are all in this together." He contends that

with a little imagination, one may glimpse the possibility that a new version of the "virtuous circle" might emerge, a mutuality of interests in which the returns are shared in different ways, including as personal satisfaction for defending the common good. But in order for firms to ever reach that happy condition, they must be able to see a market that rewards their responsible behavior.[58]

In the developed world, this requires a reordering of tastes and priorities, and most especially a drastic qualification of our cherished political absolute of personal freedom, now extended to entrepreneurial corporations. To get there, we need a more sustained and democratic social and political dialogue about the role of economics and consumerism in our national culture, the distribution of biomedical resources, and the promises and perils of genetic manipulation. But this conversion must and no doubt will be pushed along by pressures from outsiders whose economic and social interests are entwined with ours, but who up to now we have been free to ignore, except as cheap labor or potential markets to enhance the opportunities of U.S. business (if not necessarily of U.S. workers). Some "realists" might interpret this scenario as just the latest phase in the ceaseless and more or less violent struggle for resources and power that has always characterized the relations of human societies, both internally and externally. But hopeful theorists of the common good, religious and otherwise, will be sobered by a dose of realism before undertaking the serious job of subjecting genetic engineering to critical analysis and gradual, limited, and full participatory implementation.

To the degree that a process of political participation results in the disproportionate influence of elites or even "majority rule," the problem of collective egotism about which Niebuhr worried does not disappear. Some safeguards against it are suggested by the struggle over patented drugs in South Africa. Among them are the inclusiveness of mechanisms and institutions of participation; the replacement of centralized control over the process by a pluralism of avenues and strategies of participation and influence, among which there will be some friction; and—the ultimate test—the incorporation of the interests of the most vulnerable into the social outcome. While inclusiveness, pluralism, and some friction signal that self-interest does not control the political process absolutely, improvement in the status of the most vulnerable signals that the process has been effective in achieving greater equality and justice in social life.

Notes

1. Aristotle, *Nicomachean Ethics*, trans. Terence Irwin (Indianapolis: Hackett Publishing, 1985), 1169b18–19.

2. Ibid., 1095a17–18, 1095b5.

3. Margaret Jane Radin, *Contested Commodities* (Cambridge, MA: Harvard University Press, 1996), 9, 71–72.

4. Margaret Talbot, "A Desire to Duplicate," *New York Times Magazine*, February 4, 2001, 68. See also Nancy Gibbs, "Baby, It's You! And You, and You . . . ," *Time*, February 19, 2001, 48.

5. Talbot, "A Desire" 45. See also Cathy Booth Thomas, "Copydog, Copycat," *Time*, February 19, 2001, 57.

6. Office of Communications, National Conference of Catholic Bishops, "USCC Official Urges Congress Adopt 'Meaningful' Ban on Human Cloning," February 2, 1998, www.nccbuscc.org/com/archives.

7. See James M. Gustafson, "Genetic Engineering and the Normative View of the Human," *Ethical Issues in Biology and Medicine*, ed. Preston N. Williams (Cambridge: Schenkman, 1972), 46–58; reprinted in James M. Gustafson, *Theology and Christian Ethics* (Philadelphia: Pilgrim Press, 1974) 272–296.

8. For basic information on patenting, see U.S. Department of Energy Office of Science, "Genetics and Patenting," 2000, www.ornl.gov/hgmis/elsi/patents.html; Susan Cartier Poland, "Genes, Patents, and Bioethics: Will History Repeat Itself?" *Kennedy Institute of Ethics Journal* 10, no. 3: 265–281; and Bartha Maria Knoppers, "Status, Sale, and Patenting of Human Genetic Material: An International Survey," *Nature Genetics* 22 No. 1 (May 1999): 23–25.

9. See Andrew Pollack, "Double Helix with a Twist: Do Fewer Genes Translate into Fewer Dollars?" *New York Times*, February 13, 2001, C1, C4.

10. For a more detailed and extensive account of this case, see David Barnard, "In the High Court of South Africa, Case No. 4138/98: The Global Politics of Access to Low-Cost AIDS Drugs in Poor Countries," *Kennedy Institute of Ethnics Journal* 12 (2002) 159–174; and Lisa Sowle Cahill, "Biotech and Justice: Catching Up with the Real World Order," *Hastings Center Report* 33 (2003) 34–44.

11. See Donald G. McNeil Jr., "Indian Company Offers to Supply AIDS Drugs at Low Cost in Africa," *New York Times*, February 7, 2001, A1, A10.

12. See Donald G. McNeil Jr., "Oxfam Joins Campaign to Cut Drug Prices for Poor Nations," *New York Times*, February 13, 2001, A5.

13. See "From the U.N. Statement on AIDS: 'Prevention Must Be the Mainstay,' " *New York Times*, June 29, 2001, A8.

14. See Tina Rosenberg, "Look at Brazil," *New York Times Magazine*, January 28, 2001, 26, 28–31, 52, 58, 62–63.

15. Leo XIII, *Rerum Novarum: On the Condition of Labor* (Boston: The Daughters of St. Paul, 1991), No. 27.

16. For a history of modern papal social teaching, see John A. Coleman, ed., *One Hundred Years of Catholic Social Thought: Celebration and Challenge* (Maryknoll, NY: Orbis Books, 1991); and David J. O'Brien and Thomas A. Shannon, eds., *Catholic Social Thought: The Documentary Heritage* (Maryknoll, NY: Orbis Books, 1998).

17. O'Brien and Shannon, *Catholic Social Thought*, 129.

18. See Quadragesimo Anno, cited in O'Brien and Shannon, *Catholic Social Thought*, 53.

19. See John XXIII, *Mater et Magistra: Christianity and Social Progress* (NJ: Panlist Press, 1968), nos. 53–54.

20. In fact, John Paul II's 1991 encyclical, *Centesimus Annus (On the Hundredth Anniversary of Rerum Novarum)*, written after the fall of socialist governments in Eastern Europe, seems to back off from the sharper critique of *Sollicitudo Rei Socialis* 1988 (see *Centesimus Annus*, nos. 35, 42).

21. John Paul II, *On Social Concern* (1987), in O'Brien and Shannon, *Catholic Social Thought*, nos. 28, 33.

22. John Paul II, *The Gospel of Life* (1995), in O'Brien and Shannon, *Catholic Social Thought*, nos. 18, 40–41.

23. John Paul II, *On Human Work* (1981), in O'Brien and Shannon, *Catholic Social Thought*, no. 8. See also John Paul II, *Evangelium Vitae*, in O'Brien and Shannon, *Catholic Social Thought*, no. 6.

24. See John XXIII, *Pacem in Terris*, in O'Brien and Shannon, *Catholic Social Thought*, nos. 5–9.

25. John Paul II, *Evangelium Vitae*, no. 70.

26. On infertility therapies, see the 1987 Congregation for the Doctrine of the Faith's *Donum Vitae* (*Instruction on Respect for Human Life*) February 27, 1987. See also John Paul II, *Evangelium Vitae*, nos. 37, 53, 60, 63.

27. Elio Sgreccia, cited in John Thavis, "Church Leaders Criticize Decisions on Human Embryo Research," *Catholic News Service*, August 28, 2000.

28. John Paul II, "Address to the 18th International Congress of the Transplantation Society," August 29, 2000, <http:///www.vatican.va/holy-fathor/john.paul_ii,speeches/2000/jul_sept/documents/hf_jp–ii_spe_2000829_trawsplnats_en.html> (January 26, 2004).

29. John Paul II, "The Ethics of Genetic Manipulation," *Origins* 13, no. 23 (November 17, 1983): 388.

30. CIDSE Task Group on the European Union, Trade, and Food Security, *Biopatenting and the Threat to Food Security*, February 2000, www.cidse.be/pubs.

31. Ibid.

32. Reinhold Niebuhr, *Man's Nature and His Communities* (New York: Charles Scribner and Sons, 1965), 39.

33. Reinhold Niebuhr, *Moral Man and Immoral Society* (New York: Charles Scribner and Sons, 1932), 27.

34. Reinhold Niebuhr, *The Nature and Destiny of Man*, vol. 1, *Human Nature* (New York: Charles Scribner and Sons, 1941), 178–297.

35. Ibid., 282.

36. Niebuhr, *Man's Nature and His Communities*, 84–87.

37. Niebuhr, *Moral Man and Immoral Society*, 117, 268.

38. Niebuhr, *Nature and Destiny of Man*, 1:191.

39. Ibid., 239.

40. Robin W. Lovin, *Reinhold Niebuhr and Christian Realism* (Cambridge: Cambridge University Press, 1995), 144.

41. Ibid., 145.

42. Ibid., 152.

43. Niebuhr, *Nature and Destiny of Man*, 1:227.

44. Reinhold Niebuhr, *The Nature and Destiny of Man*, vol. 2, *Human Destiny* (New York: Charles Scribner and Sons, 1943), 315, 316.

45. Niebuhr, *Moral Man and Immoral Society*, 272.

46. Ibid., 197.

47. Lovin, *Reinhold Niebuhr*, 83, 89, 91.

48. Niebuhr, *Man's Nature and His Communities*, 107, 125 (emphasis added).

49. See Gary Teeple, *Globalization and the Decline of Social Reform: Into the Twenty-First Century*, 2nd ed. (New York: Prometheus Books, 2000), 76–77.

50. Ibid., 87.

51. Richard Falk and Andrew Strauss, "Toward Global Parliament," *Foreign Affairs* 80 (January/February 2001): 212.

52. Ibid. These authors note that "patients who need medicines pay prices influenced by WTO-enforced patent rules, which allow pharmaceutical companies to monopolize drug pricing. Most of the 23 million sub-Saharan Africans who have tested positive for the AIDS virus cannot afford the drugs most effective in treating their illness. They will die much sooner as a consequence" (213).

53. David E. Sanger, "A Grand Trade Bargain," *Foreign Affairs* 80 (January/February 2001): 66.

54. Cited in McNeil, "Indian Company," A1.

55. See McNeil, "Oxfam Joins Campaign," A5.

56. See Bartha Maria Knoppers, "Biotechnology: Sovereignty and Sharing," in *The Commercialization of Genetic Research: Ethical, Legal, and Policy Issues*, ed. Timothy Caulfield and Bryn Williams-Jones (New York: Kluwer Academic, 1999), 1–11. See also The Human Genome Organization Ethics Committee, *Statement on Benefit Sharing*, April 2000, www.humgen.umonreal.ca.

57. See Noah Smith, "Chinese Media Warn of 'Stolen Genes,'" Japan Economic Newswire, December 5, 2000, web.lexis-nexis.com/universe/docum.

58. William Greider, *One World, Ready or Not: The Manic Logic of Global Capitalism* (New York: Simon and Schuster, 1997), 461, 462.

13

Human Genetic Intervention: Past, Present, and Future

LeRoy Walters

This chapter discusses human gene transfer research, primarily in the United States but also in Europe. It examines the most successful gene transfer study to date, considers in depth the issue of public oversight for human gene transfer research, and looks at issues for the future, particularly the brain, enhancement, and the germ line.

I will begin with a proposal about terminology. The phrase "human gene therapy" was always in danger of seeming to overpromise benefits to the participants in the early clinical trials of human gene transfer. Especially in light of the meager results of human gene transfer studies from 1990 to the present, it seems more accurate and honest to use a neutral phrase that simply describes the procedure that is undertaken. In English, this more neutral phrase is "human gene transfer." The phrase parallels a term like *transplantation*, which also describes the movement of cells or tissues from one individual to another but does not run the risk of unduly raising the expectations of recipients. In this chapter, then, I will employ the wording human gene transfer research except in cases where the alternative language appears in the original document.

Human Gene Transfer Research in the United States, 1988–2003

Between 1988 and June 2003, approximately 569 human gene transfer protocols had been submitted to the Office of Recombinant DNA Activities at the U.S. National Institutes of Health (NIH) (I say "approximately" because a few protocols were withdrawn and a few consolidated.) Table 13.1 shows the number of protocols submitted by year.[1]

Table 13.1
Human gene transfer protocols submitted to the Office of Recombinant DNA
Activities, U.S. National Institutes of Health, 1988–2003

Year	Protocols
1988	1
1989	0
1990	2
1991	9
1992	24
1993	31
1994	31
1995	44
1996	28
1997	56
1998	51
1999	91
2000	71
2001	73
2002	51
2003*	18

* Through June 10

The variations in the numbers of research protocols submitted
annually to the NIH are displayed graphically in Figure 13.1. These
research protocols can be subdivided into various categories:

By major type
• Disease-oriented studies: 523
• Gene-marking studies: 41
• Nontherapeutic studies: 5

By disease target in the disease-oriented studies
• Cancers of various kinds: 367 (70.2 percent)
• Single-gene disorders: 57 (10.9 percent)
• Other diseases or disorders: 60 (11.5 percent)
• Infectious diseases: 39 (7.5 percent)

By disease, among the most frequently targeted single-gene disorders
• Cystic fibrosis: 23
• Severe combined immunodeficiency: 6
• Hemophilia: 5

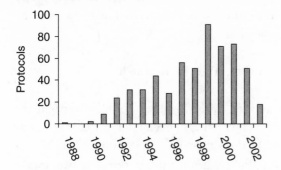

Figure 13.1
Variations in the number of human gene transfer protocols, 1988–2003.

The major conditions targeted in the "other diseases or disorders" category
  • Peripheral artery disease: 20
  • Coronary artery disease: 19
By type of infectious disease studied
  • HIV infection or AIDS: 37

The Most Successful Gene Transfer Study to Date

Despite the extensive efforts of U.S. researchers in more than five hundred disease-oriented gene transfer protocols, the clearest example so far of success in a human gene transfer clinical protocol occurred in France, where Doctor Alain Fischer and his colleagues at the Necker Hospital in Paris treated several young male children who had inherited X-linked severe combined immunodeficiency. In this disorder, neither of the two major components of the immune system functions properly. In Fischer's study, the children received their own genetically modified bone marrow cells, presumably including bone marrow stem cells. The modified cells seemed to have a competitive advantage over the native, malfunctioning cells, and produced positive results in all but one child. Fischer and his colleagues reported their positive results in *Science* in April 2000, and the *New England Journal of Medicine* in April 2002.[2] Much to everyone's regret, news reports from early October 2002 and additional information published in January 2003 indicated that two of the first nine children given gene transfer in this protocol had developed T cell leukemias. The retroviral vector used in Fischer's study activated an oncogene (LMO2) in some of the cells that were transferred into the children after genetic modification.[3]

Public Oversight for Human Gene Transfer Research

Three stages can be distinguished in the history of public oversight for this field in the United States. The first stage began in the 1980s and continued through the first half of the 1990s. From 1983 through 1995, the public oversight system for human gene transfer research was established. The second stage began in 1996 and continued through 1999; during this time, the existing public oversight system was substantially weakened. A third stage was triggered by the death of a research subject in a gene transfer trial in September 1999. From the time of Jesse Gelsinger's death forward, and especially from the years 2000 to 2002, an effective oversight system for gene transfer research was restored.

In the United States, there was an effective, though somewhat unstable, national oversight system in place for human gene transfer research between 1990 and 1995. During the early 1990s, every interested citizen and policy maker in this country and the world as a whole knew exactly what was happening in the field of human gene transfer research in the United States. In fact, several other countries established advisory committees that paralleled the NIH's Recombinant DNA Advisory Committee (RAC) in its public review of human gene transfer clinical research protocols.

The public oversight system established in the United States was an important precedent. Although it followed by several years the premature attempts by Martin Cline of the University of California at Los Angeles to perform human gene transfer, it was nonetheless an anticipatory system.[4] In fact, those of us who helped to develop the guidelines for research in this field in late 1984 and early 1985 were concerned that we might not conclude our work before the first research protocol was submitted. The first gene-marking study was proposed to RAC in 1988, however, and the first gene transfer study aimed at the treatment of subjects came forward only in early 1990.

There were weaknesses and ambiguities in the public oversight system, to be sure. The most critical weakness, in retrospect, was the failure of the NIH and the Food and Drug Administration (FDA) to establish precise, complementary roles in the review of gene transfer protocols. With the benefit of hindsight, one can also ask why the NIH, a funding agency, was involved in the regulation of research that it funded? Even more problematically, why was the NIH attempting to regulate clinical research being conducted by private-sector biotechnology and pharmaceutical companies? The short answer to these latter two concerns is that the NIH had developed a model in the mid-1970s by taking the initiative in reviewing recombinant DNA research proposals for the entire nation.[5] The NIH and the researchers that the agency funded preferred this mode of self-regulation to the possibly less flexible regulatory proposals that members of Congress were suggesting in 1976 and 1977.

Other questions also confronted RAC and the NIH during these years. Among them were the following:

• How high a standard should be set for the scientific merit of human gene transfer protocols?

• How much time and effort should be devoted to reviewing the consent forms for such trials?

• How could RAC and the NIH avoid having their approval of human gene transfer studies construed as a Good Housekeeping Seal that companies could then use to attract investors?

• How could RAC and the NIH counteract the hyperbole that researchers and companies sometimes employed in publicizing what seemed to be modest research successes?

• Could an advisory committee that was comprised primarily of academics and that met only once each quarter keep pace with a rapidly evolving field like human gene transfer research?

Despite the ambiguities in its role, RAC performed a creditable job in keeping pace with an accelerating number of research protocols from 1990 to 1995. Thanks to the insight and creativity of the late Brigid Leventhal, a pediatric oncologist from Johns Hopkins University, RAC devised a system that asked researchers to report annually on serious adverse events that had occurred to subjects in their gene transfer studies. In June 1995, RAC conducted a comprehensive audit of all U.S. human gene transfer research to date, noting the numbers of protocols reviewed, the various applications of gene transfer, and the target diseases in the studies that aimed to treat patients for a variety of genetic and nongenetic diseases. This comprehensive review constituted one of the finest moments in the history of RAC.[6]

In 1996 and 1997, this oversight system was substantially weakened by policy makers at the NIH and the FDA. Between 1994 and early 1996, opposition to RAC's role in reviewing human gene transfer research began to be expressed by some members of the biotechnology and pharmaceutical industries, AIDS activists, and academic researchers. The opposition ostensibly was based on the notion that RAC, meeting only quarterly, could not respond in a timely manner to new developments in a fast-moving arena of research. Suddenly, draft legislation appeared that, in the course of reforming the FDA's regulatory practices, would have abolished RAC oversight of the field. This provision was never adopted, but a warning about RAC's unpopularity in some quarters had clearly been sent by an antiregulatory Congress. For its part, Congress was responding to advocates for the biotechnology and pharmaceutical industries.

The grounds for this opposition to RAC's role were based in part on the ambiguities cited above. In other respects, however, the amount of hostility engendered by RAC during this time remains puzzling even now. One can only speculate about the motives of the opponents. They surely wanted to avoid unnecessary duplication and delay in the oversight system for this important field. Other critics may have concluded that RAC's quasi-regulatory review function should be located at a regulatory agency, the FDA. And one factor in the opposition of at least some private companies may have been the desire for the more confidential, and therefore less transparent, mode of regulation that occurs in the interactions between companies and FDA regulators.

Whatever the background for his decision, NIH director Harold Varmus announced his plans for the future of RAC in a May 1996 speech given at Hilton Head, South Carolina. No text of the speech is available, but on the basis of reports on the speech and an interview with Varmus, Eliot Marshall of *Science* published an article on the director's plans to "scrap the RAC."[7]

Varmus's speech was followed in June 1996 by attempts by NIH officials to explain the rationale for his new plan to members of Congress and their staff members. In July 1996, the *Federal Register* published the formal NIH proposal to abolish RAC and turn over virtually all public oversight responsibility for human gene transfer research to the FDA.

Between June and August 1996, substantial opposition to the NIH plans for RAC was expressed by four members of Congress and a majority of letters written in response to the *Federal Register* notice, including several authored by prominent figures in the field of bioethics.[8] Meanwhile, RAC skipped its March, June, and September 1996 meetings—in part, it was said, because there was an insufficient number of novel protocols requiring review. The director of the Office of Recombinant DNA Activities, which supported RAC's activities, departed the NIH for an academic position at the end of June 1996, thus further complicating RAC's situation.

In November 1996, February 1997, and October 1997, three further proposals for the new public oversight system were published in the *Federal Register*. The upshot of this long process was the following compromise:

• RAC would continue to discuss, at its quarterly meetings, gene transfer protocols that raised novel issues, used new vectors, or aimed to treat new diseases.

• There would, however, no longer be RAC approval or disapproval of human gene transfer protocols; approval or disapproval (more technically, permission to proceed) belonged solely to the FDA.

• The size of RAC was reduced from twenty-five to fifteen members.

• A new type of forum, the Gene Therapy Policy Conferences, would be associated with RAC's work and would discuss a theme—for example, in utero gene transfer—rather than a particular protocol. This innovation was, in my view, an excellent addition to RAC's role.

The most immediate and obvious effects of the 1996–97 changes were the loss of transparency in the oversight system, and the weakening of RAC's role in reviewing research protocols and monitoring the state of the art in the field. A University of Pennsylvania proposal to study gene transfer in subjects who had ornithine transcarbamylase (OTC) deficiency can perhaps serve as a paradigm case for the new situation that emerged in early 1996. RAC had discussed this protocol in detail at its December 1995 meeting and had provided the researchers with several suggestions for changes that might, in the committee's view, improve the study. Yet with RAC's missed meetings in March, June, and September

1996, and the ongoing debate about both the continuation and the proper role of RAC, the OTC deficiency protocol simply disappeared from public view. Here are several questions about the Penn protocol for which there were no clear answers in the years 1996 through 1999:

• Had the FDA given Penn approval to proceed with the OTC deficiency protocol in response to Penn's Investigational New Drug Application?
• Had the design of the study been changed after public RAC review?
• Had the consent form been changed after RAC review?
• Had the clinical trial been initiated?
• If so, had any serious adverse events occurred?

In fairness to the NIH, I should note that the new guidelines published in the *Federal Register* on October 31, 1997 did require researchers to report to the NIH and RAC all post-RAC-review changes and serious adverse events.

There was also more general evidence that RAC's role had been weakened and the national oversight system was less effective from 1996 on. There was no annual audit of the human gene transfer field conducted in 1996, 1997, 1998, or 1999. Thus, policy makers, the public, and researchers around the world lost the kind of comprehensive overview that RAC had provided in June 1995. Such an audit would have been difficult to conduct during these years for at least three reasons. No senior person (PhD or MD) was appointed to direct the staff that served RAC for more than two years after the former director's departure at the end of June 1996. Second, in 1995, the FDA had withdrawn its agreement to cooperate with the NIH and RAC in developing a public, online database to track serious adverse events in human gene transfer trials; NIH efforts to create such a database alone proceeded slowly and had not borne fruit four years later. Third, as noted above, the size of RAC was reduced from twenty-five to fifteen members early in 1997; thus, the shared workload that allowed the 1995 audit to be performed was more difficult to achieve.

In 1998 and 1999, the refusal by one researcher and one company to provide public disclosure of serious adverse events in their gene transfer trials was symptomatic of additional problems in the public oversight system. In preparation for their September 1999 meeting, RAC members were asked to sign a confidentiality agreement stating that they would be able to review serious adverse event reports from two protocols, but that they would not be permitted to discuss the adverse event reports in the public meeting. Some members of RAC were clearly not comfortable with this lack of transparency and drafted language, approved by a majority of RAC members, that sought to clarify the existing RAC policy—namely, that no adverse event reports were to be considered confidential. Press stories about these refusals to disclose serious adverse events also began to appear.

During 1997 and 1998, there was also a parallel development that has not been as widely reported; a few academic researchers and companies began recruiting subjects into novel gene transfer research protocols before RAC review had occurred, but after the FDA had given the researchers permission to proceed with their Investigational New Drug Applications. To their credit, the RAC chair, RAC's staff, and the NIH general counsel stood firm, ultimately threatening the academic institutions collaborating with the private companies in these protocols with the termination of all NIH grant and contract funding to those academic institutions if they did not wait until after RAC review before beginning the actual conduct of their trials.

The most dramatic event in the history of human gene transfer research occurred in September 1999. As mentioned above, Gelsinger died while participating in a gene transfer study. The death of this eighteen-year-old, relatively healthy research subject and the subsequent investigation revealed fundamental flaws in the oversight system and led to an agonizing reappraisal of clinical research involving human gene transfer.

As noted earlier, researchers at the University of Pennsylvania submitted an OTC deficiency protocol to the NIH and RAC in fall 1995. The director of the university's Institute for Human Gene Therapy (IHGT), James Wilson, took the lead in presenting the protocol to RAC. Yet the principal investigator for the protocol was Wilson's associate, Mark Batshaw, a pediatrician. In brief, OTC deficiency is a single-gene disorder that causes the buildup of excessive levels of ammonia in the liver. According to the protocol design, six cohorts, each comprised of three subjects, were to receive increasing doses of an adenoviral vector and an inserted gene. The protocol was designated a phase 1 study; that is, the goal of the study was to investigate the potential toxicity of the vector and the transgene rather than to provide a treatment for the subjects' underlying disease.

The OTC deficiency protocol disappeared from public view after the December 1995 RAC review, during which RAC voted to recommend several changes in the study design. The protocol did not become visible again until the June 1999 meeting of the American Society for Gene Therapy, for which Wilson and his colleagues prepared an abstract reporting results from their first four cohorts of subjects. Most members of the public and most RAC members did not attend this meeting, however, and were thus unaware of the study's progress. From the public record of the study compiled in late 1999 and 2000, we now know that this clinical trial proceeded through several stages between early 1996 and September 1999, the month during which a study participant died.

From February through December 1996, the FDA reviewed the OTC deficiency protocol. In December, the agency permitted the study to proceed. Recruitment of subjects began early in 1997, and in April the first subject in the first cohort completed her participation in the protocol. During the remainder of 1997, 1998, and the first nine months of 1999 the trial continued; three subjects were recruited into each of the first three cohorts, four were recruited into the fourth cohort, three into the fifth, and two into the sixth. The second subject in the sixth cohort, Gelsinger, died as a result of his participation in the trial.

There are contextual factors related to this trial that deserve more detailed review. The first set of factors concerns the local level—that is, actions taken and policies adopted by the researchers and the University of Pennsylvania. In June or July 1995, a funding arrangement was entered into by the IHGT, the University of Pennsylvania, and Genovo, a company that had been founded by IHGT's Wilson in 1992. According to the terms of the five-year agreement, Genovo would provide funding for IHGT's research in exchange for the exclusive right to license patents resulting from Wilson's human gene therapy research. This financial arrangement supplied approximately $4.7 million per year to IHGT, or approximately 20 percent of the institute's budget. The arrangement was approved by the University of Pennsylvania's Conflict of Interest Standing Committee.[9]

During late 1996 and the following year, there were two instances of miscommunication between the Penn researchers and the FDA. As both the IHGT and the FDA agree, in November 1996 the Penn research group failed to submit Protocol Version 1.0 to the FDA after the protocol was reviewed by Penn's Institutional Review Board. According to the FDA, nine months later, in August 1997, the Penn research group raised the permissible ammonia level for subjects entering the trial from fifty to seventy micromolar in Protocol Version 2.0 without listing this alteration in the summary of changes for the revision that was sent to the FDA.[10]

It would be possible to dismiss these omissions as failures to file routine paperwork with a regulatory agency. In retrospect, though, the next instance of miscommunication was potentially more important. According to the FDA, in October and November 1998, Grade 3 (moderately serious) laboratory toxicities in two subjects at the fourth dose level were not reported immediately to Penn's Institutional Review Board or the FDA, and the study was not placed on clinical hold. In response, the Penn research group agreed with the FDA's assertions, but replied that it did report these Grade 3 toxicities to the FDA in a January 1999 letter and a March 1999 annual report. The research group also summarized the toxicities in a table prepared for an annual review by the Penn Institutional Review Board on August 9, 1999.

There was also a breakdown in communication about parallel animal studies that were being conducted in 1998 by the Penn research group. From October through December 1998, the group conducted a preclinical study with three monkeys using adenoviral vectors. According to the FDA, two monkeys had serious reactions to early versions of the vector and were therefore euthanized; a third had milder symptoms in response to the third-generation vector that was simultaneously being used in the OTC deficiency trial. In reviewing the tragic events of September 1999, the FDA contended that the results of this preclinical study should have been reported to the agency because they were directly relevant to the OTC deficiency study. The Penn researchers agreed that the results of this study should have been communicated to the FDA in the annual report of March 2000, but argued that the doses of vector in the preclinical study were seventeen times higher than those used in the clinical trial. The researchers also noted that the response of the monkey that received the third-generation vector was less severe than that of the monkeys receiving the earlier-generation vectors.

In September 1999, patient 019, Gelsinger, was infused with the vector and the inserted gene even though his ammonia level was ninety-one micromolar on the day before he received the infusion. (The permissible level was either fifty or seventy micromolar, depending on the version of the protocol.) The Penn researchers replied that Gelsinger's ammonia levels were within the stated range when he was screened for possible participation in the trial in June 1999, that he was given a drug to reduce his ammonia levels, and that they had made a clinical judgment that an ammonia level of ninety-one would not be harmful to the subject.

In addition to the foregoing questions at the local level, the tragic history of the Penn OTC deficiency protocol revealed serious problems in the national oversight system for human gene transfer research. As noted above, there was a long period of uncertainty that stretched from May 1996 to October 1997, at least. During this time, there were multiple proposals about the role and the very existence of RAC. There were also multiple versions of the NIH guidelines. Researchers received quite clear signals from the NIH: "You in the research community will be dealing primarily with the FDA from now on." The net effect of these developments was confusion and an undermining of RAC's authority.

Perhaps the most important system problem was the failure of most gene transfer researchers to report serious adverse events to the NIH and RAC in a timely fashion. A December 21, 1999, letter from NIH director Varmus to Congressman Henry Waxman contains this sobering concession: "Of the 691 serious adverse events reported [in trials using adenoviral vectors], 39 had been previously reported as required by the *NIH Guidelines.*"[11] Thirty-nine out of 691 is 5.6 percent.

The great unknown at the national level is how the FDA was exercising its oversight responsibilities for the Penn OTC deficiency protocol and other human gene transfer protocols between 1996 and 1999. One would like to know the answers to honest questions such as the following:

• How many FDA medical officers and reviewers were involved in overseeing the OTC deficiency protocol?
• How carefully did they read correspondence and annual reports on this and other Investigational New Drug applications?
• What types of database capabilities did they have?

• Did they see patterns of serious adverse events in trials involving adenoviral vectors?

The follow-up to the death of Gelsinger was arduous for his family, the federal government, and the research community. In December 1999, the RAC meeting was devoted to reviewing what had caused Gelsinger's death and how the oversight system could be modified to prevent similar tragedies in the future. In January 2000, the FDA sent the Penn research group a series of inspectional observations and placed a clinical hold on the OTC deficiency trial. One month later, Senator Bill Frist convened a hearing on the oversight of human gene transfer research at which Gelsinger's father, Paul, and I testified. The FDA sent a formal warning letter in March to Wilson and the IHGT at Penn. Two months later, an external review committee chaired by former senator John Danforth reported its findings to University of Pennsylvania president Judith Rodin, who in response, decided to discontinue all clinical research at the institute.[12]

During the summer of 2000, the University of Pennsylvania decided not to renew its agreement with Genovo. According to published reports in the *Wall Street Journal* and the *Philadelphia Inquirer*, Genovo was sold to Targeted Genetics for newly issued shares of stock valued at $89.9 million. The newspapers also disclosed that Penn had owned a 3.2 percent equity stake in Genovo, for which it received Targeted Genetics stock valued at $1.4 million, and that Wilson had owned a 30 percent nonvoting equity stake, for which he received Targeted Genetics stock valued at $13.5 million. Biogen was to receive $50 million worth of Targeted Genetics stock in exchange for its stake in Genovo.[13]

In September 2000, the Gelsinger family sued the University of Pennsylvania for the wrongful death of Jesse Gelsinger. After six weeks of negotiation between the parties, the case was settled without going to trial. The terms of the settlement were not disclosed.[14]

The tragic death of Gelsinger in 1999 has had a decisive impact on the public oversight of human gene transfer research in the United States. Since October 2000, there have been several promising developments at the NIH and the FDA. One of the most encouraging developments of late 2000, 2001, and early 2002 has been the step-by-step restoration of RAC's traditional role. An October 2000 *Federal Register* notice stipulated that RAC review and subsequent local institutional approval must be completed before a clinical trial of human gene transfer can begin.[15] In December 2000 and again in November 2001, the NIH proposed the establishment of a Human Gene Transfer Safety Assessment Board to evaluate adverse events in gene transfer trials in an organized, systematic manner and to report regularly to RAC.[16] This board received final approval from the Office of Management and Budget in January 2002, and the revision of the guidelines that authorizes its establishment was published in the *Federal Register* in May 2002.[17] Moreover, in September and December 2001, RAC engaged in an extended discussion about the serious adverse events that had occurred in two clinical trials designed to study gene transfer in subjects with hemophilia. In response to the adverse events in the French trial of gene transfer for severe combined immunodeficiency, RAC provided detailed public analyses in December 2002 and February 2003. Finally, the number of RAC members has been expanded beyond fifteen so that more areas of scientific and clinical expertise can be represented on the committee.

For its part, the FDA announced in January 2001, during the waning days of the second Clinton administration, its intention to make public "certain data and information related to human gene therapy and xenotransplantation."[18] Public comments on this proposal will be considered before the new policy is enacted. The death of a healthy volunteer in an asthma study being conducted at Johns Hopkins University in June 2001 reminded researchers and the public alike that research subjects can be at serious risk even in seemingly innocuous trials.[19] Several months after this volunteer's death, the FDA established a new Office for Good Clinical Practice within the Commissioner's Office "to improve the conduct and oversight of clinical research and to ensure the protection of participants in FDA-regulated research."[20] Like RAC, the FDA has also analyzed the leukemias that occurred in the French gene transfer trial—at public advisory committee meetings held in October 2002 and February 2003.

Issues for the Future

When we look to the future, it is quite clear that the most critical issues involving human gene transfer research will involve the brain (especially behavioral traits), enhancement by genetic means, and the human germ line. I should add a caveat: in my view, it is probably too early to know what the relative contributions to human health will be of gene transfer, cell transplantation (including human embryonic stem cell transplantation), and drugs. A recent article suggests that a combination of factors may be involved.[21]

The Brain

In this arena, one can imagine that the brain, which has until now been off-limits except in efforts to treat diseases like glioma, will become a legitimate target for gene transfer research. A foretaste of things to come could be a recent gene transfer study that attempted to introduce the dopamine D2 receptor into rats, in an effort to decrease alcohol consumption.[22]

Enhancement

An obvious physical enhancement that also would be disease related would be a fine-tuning of the human immune system, so that it is much less likely to go awry either in attacking an individual's own body in the event of autoimmune diseases or in overreacting to environmental allergens. A candidate for intellectual enhancement would be the preservation of memory during the process of aging, in contrast to the dementia that afflicts so many elderly people. Important theoretical questions with regard to enhancement will be, What is enhancement? What is remediation of an undesirable condition? And can we draw a clear line between these two categories?[23]

Germ Line Intervention

To many people, the final and most forbidding frontier in genetics may seem to be deliberately attempting to transmit particular genes to our children and grandchildren. This may be a case in which incremental steps will lead to a point where each major industrial society will need to pause and consider what it wants its future policy on human germ line intervention to be. Here are several foreseeable steps that could be leading us toward this decision point:

• Germ line changes as unintended side effects of somatic cell gene transfer.

• Nuclear transfer in human eggs, to prevent mitochondrial disease.

- The genetic "repair" of sperm or egg cells to prevent disease.
- The genetic "repair" of preimplantation embryos to prevent disease.[24]

Conclusion

There are no easy answers to these breathtaking technological possibilities—either in one or a hundred chapters. Perhaps what we will need to do is commit ourselves to *procedures* and *modes of deliberation* that allow us to be prepared for such possibilities when they become actual. The first step will be both academic and political; it is exemplified by this volume. It involves calm, rational, anticipatory, and interdisciplinary discussion—discussion that also involves members of the public. The second step will be primarily political, but one hopes that it will not lose touch either with academia or the will of the general public. In order to be ready for and to cope with the genetic technologies of the future, we will need transparent, flexible, and vigorous oversight systems.

Notes

An earlier version of this chapter was presented in March 2001 in Berlin, Germany, at the international conference on "The Impact of Genetic Knowledge on Human Life," cosponsored by the Deutsches Referenzzentrum für Ethik in den Biowissenschaften. See LeRoy Walters, "Genforschung und Gesellschaft: Erwartungen, Ziele und Grenzen," in Ludger Honnefelder, et al., eds., *Das genetische Wissen und die Zukunft des Menschen* (Berlin: Walter de Gruyter, 2003), 152–166.

1. These data were derived from the Web site of the Office of Biotechnology Activities at the NIH. (www.od.nih.gov/oba/).

2. Marina Cavazana-Calvo, Salima Hacein-Bey, Genevieve de Saint Basile, et al., "Gene Therapy of Severe Combined Immunodeficiency (SCID)–X1 Disease," *Science* 288, no. 5466 (April 28, 2000): 627–629; and Salima Hacein-Bey-Abina, Francoise Le Deist, Fredoriove Carlier, "Sustained Correction of X-Linked Severe Combined Immunodeficiency by *ex vivo* Gene Therapy," *New England Journal of Medicine* 346, no. 16 (April 18, 2002): 1185–1193.

3. See, for example, Sheryl Gay Stolberg, "Trials Are Halted on a Gene Therapy Experiment," *New York Times*, October 9, 2002, A1, A20; Salima Hacein-Bey-Abina, Christol von Kalle, Manfsed Schmidt, "A Serious Adverse Event after Successful Gene Therapy for X-Linked Severe Combined Immunodeficiency," letter to the editor, *New England Journal of Medicine* 348, no. 3 (January 16, 2003): 255–256; and Rick Weiss, "Second Boy Receiving Gene Therapy Develops Cancer," *Washington Post*, January 15, 2003, A9.

4. See Larry Thompson, *Correcting the Code: Inventing the Genetic Cure for the Human Body* (New York: Simon and Schuster, 1994), 230–267.

5. For a fascinating study of this process, see Donald S. Fredrickson, *The Recombinant DNA Controversy: A Memoir* (Washington, DC: American Society for Microbiology, 2001).

6. The audit was published as "Gene Therapy in the United States: A Five-Year Status Report," *Human Gene Therapy* 7, no. 14 (September 10, 1996): 1781–1790.

7. Eliot Marshall, "Varmus Proposes to Scrap the RAC," *Science* 272, no. 5264 (May 17, 1996): 945.

8. On the opposition by members of Congress, see David Pryor, Mark Hatfield, Ron Wyden, and Henry A. Waxman, "A Word to Varmus," letter to the editor, *Hastings Center Report* 26, no. 4 (July–August 1996): 46–47.

9. See Scott Hensley, "Targeted Genetics Agrees to Buy Genovo," *Wall Street Journal*, August 9, 2000, B2; Scott Hensley, "Targeted Genetics' Genovo Deal Leads to Windfall for Researcher," *Wall Street Journal*, August 10, 2000, B12; and Andrea Knox and Huntley Collins, "Rival to Buy Local Biotech Pioneer Genovo," *Philadelphia Inquirer*, August 10, 2000, A1.

10. The communications are warning letters to James M. Wilson, March 3, 2000, http://www.fda.gov/foi/warning letters/m3435n.pdf (January 26, 2004) and July 3, 2000 http://www.fda.gov/foi/warning letters/m3897n.pdf (January 26, 2004), one warning letter each to Mark L. Batshaw and Steven E. Raper, November 30, 2000, http://www.fda.gov/foi/warning letters/m4911n.pdf (January 26, 2004) and http://www.fda.gov/foi/warning letters/m4912n.pdf (January 26, 2004) and a notice of initiation of disqualification proceeding and opportunity to explain letter to James M. Wilson, November 30, 2002 http://www.fda.gov/foi/nidpoe/n121.pdf (January 26, 2004). Unfortunately the replies of the University of Pennsylvania researchers are not part of the public record.

11. Letter from Harold Varmus to Henry Waxman, December 21, 1999 http://www.house.gov/waxman/issues/health/issues health gene therapy.htm/ (January 26, 2004).

12. For the information in this paragraph, see Deborah Nelson and Rick Weiss, "Penn Ends Gene Trials on Humans," *Washington Post*, May 25, 2000, A1.

13. Hensley, "Targeted Genetics"; Hensley, "Genovo Deal"; and Knox and Collins, "Rival."

14. See Deborah Nelson and Rick Weiss, "Penn Researchers Sued in Gene Therapy Death," *Washington Post*, September 19, 2000, A3; and Rick Weiss and Deborah Nelson, "Penn Settles Gene Therapy Suit," *Washington Post*, November 4, 2000, A4.

15. Office of Biotechnology Activities, "Recombinant DNA Research: Action under the NIH Guidelines; Notice," *Federal Register* 10, no. 65 (October 10, 2000): 60327–60332.

16. Office of Biotechnology Activities, "Recombinant DNA Research: Action under the NIH Guidelines," *Federal Register 65*, no. 239 (December 12, 2000): 77655–77659; and Office of Biotechnology Activities, "Recombinant DNA Research: Proposed Actions under the NIH Guidelines," *Federal Register 66*, no. 223 (November 19, 2001): 57970–57977.

17. Office of Biotechnology Activities, "Recombinant DNA Research: Notice under the NIH Guidelines," *Federal Register 67*, no. 101 (May 24, 2002): 36619–36620.

18. Food and Drug Administration, "Availability for Public Disclosure and Submission to FDA for Public Disclosure of Certain Data and Information Related to Human Gene Therapy or Xenotransplantation," *Federal Register 66*, no. 12 (January 18, 2001): 4688–4706.

19. See Jonathan Bor and Gary Cohn, "Research Volunteer Dies in Hopkins Asthma Study," *Baltimore Sun*, 14 July 2001, A1.

20. Food and Drug Administration, press release, October 26, 2001 (no longer available).

21. See William M. Rideout III, Konrao Hochedlinger, Michael Kyba "Correction of a Genetic Defect by Nuclear Transplantation and Combined Cell and Gene Therapy," *Cell 109*, no. 1 (April 5, 2002): 17–27.

22. See Panayotis K. Thanos, Nora D. Volkow, Paul Freimuth, "Overexpression of Dopamine D2 Receptors Reduces Alcohol Self-Administration," *Journal of Neurochemistry 78*, no. 5 (September 2001): 1094–1103.

23. On this topic, see LeRoy Walters and Julie Gage Palmer, *The Ethics of Human Gene Therapy* (New York: Oxford University Press 1997), 99–142.

24. On the topic of germ line intervention, see Walters and Palmer, *The Ethics of Human Gene Therapy*, 143–153.

14

Resistance Is Futile: The Posthuman Condition and Its Advocates

Langdon Winner

Twentieth-century philosophers skeptical about "progress" have sometimes argued that the quest to dominate nature for the benefit of humanity was likely to backfire. Eventually, the same techniques and powers used to dam the rivers, split the atom, and adapt plants and animals for our consumption would be focused on human beings themselves, leading to a thorough modification and, perhaps, the elimination of the human altogether. This prospect was sometimes upheld as the ultimate horror involved in the thoughtless proliferation of sciences and technologies in modern society—an impression echoed in hundreds of science-fiction novels and motion pictures from the 1950s to the present.

Concerns of this kind appear in the concluding pages of two notable works that explore the deeper roots and broader prospects of our civilization. In the final chapter of *The Technological Society*, French sociologist and theologian Jacques Ellul ponders the future of what he describes as "the monolithic technical world that is coming to be." "The new order," he writes, "was meant to be a buffer between man and nature. Unfortunately, it has evolved autonomously in such a way that man has lost all contact with his natural framework and has to do only with the organized technical intermediary which sustains relations both with the world of life and the world of brute matter." Ultimately, Ellul believes, this will lead to "a new dismembering and a complete reconstitution of the human being so that he can at last become the objective (and also the total object) of techniques."[1]

Similar musings appear at the end of Lewis Mumford's last great work, *The Myth of the Machine: The Pentagon of Power*. The book explores several centuries of philosophical, scientific, technical, industrial, and military developments that have gone into the making of what he calls "the megamachine." Trying to anticipate the future trajectory of a system that had given the world Hiroshima, the Apollo program, and the Vietnam War, Mumford observes, "On the terms imposed by technocratic society, there is no hope for mankind except by 'going with' its plans for accelerated technological progress, even though man's vital organs will all be cannibalized in order to prolong the megamachine's meaningless existence."[2]

In light of these bleak, seemingly overwrought warnings from decades ago, it is astonishing to see that in our time, the nightmare of the philosophers is now widely embraced as a fascinating, plausible, desirable, and perhaps even necessary project in biotechnology and information technology. For many of our contemporaries, the "abolition of the human" is no longer regarded as a distasteful possibility, much less a manifestation of evil. As the new millennium begins, projects in this genre—variously called posthuman, metahuman, transhuman, ultrahuman, or cyborg—are widely cherished as a marvelous intellectual challenge, a path to future profits, an opportunity for artistic fulfillment, and an occasion for exquisite personal transcendence. Although sentiments of this kind are increasingly common in writings about science, technology, and humanity, they remain minority views among intellectuals and within the world's populace. Nevertheless, they may signal the emergence of a climate of opinion that could influence policy choices in years to come. This climate, much like a weather front moving in from the west, stands in contrast to the elaborate, detailed arguments about the ethics of biotechnology and other policy debates about possible modifications to the human species. Yet it may be that a shift in the overall climate of prevailing views, a long-term change in the weather of beliefs, will prove more decisive than the outcome of particular debates in moral philosophy and public policy.

Scientific Enthusiasts of Posthumanism

One does not have to look far to find statements by those who are either engaged in speculation about prospects for the creation of posthumans or who propose programs of research to advance the cause. A number of prominent scientists and publicists for science are willing to lend their imprimatur to this quest. In his flamboyant essay *Metaman: The Merging of Humans and Machines into a Global Superorganism*, Gregory Stock presents a series of brash claims.

Both society and the natural environment have previously undergone tumultuous changes, but the essence of being human has remained the same. Metaman, however, is on the verge of significantly altering human form and capacity.

As the nature of human beings begins to change, so too will concepts of what it means to be human. One day humans will be composite beings: part biological, part mechanical, part electronic. By applying biological techniques to embryos and then to the reproductive process itself, Metaman will take control of human evolution.

No one can know what humans will become, but whether it is a matter of fifty years or five hundred years, humans will eventually undergo radical biological change.[3]

Stock's PhD in biophysics from Johns Hopkins University as well as an MBA from Harvard have helped give him a clear-eyed view of what lies ahead. As director of the Center for the Study of Evolution and the Origin of Life at the University of California at Los Angeles, Stock has outlined the changes he believes the future holds in store, including the conquest of aging. "The human species," he remarks, "is moving out of its childhood. It is time for us to acknowledge our growing powers and begin to take responsibility for them. We have little choice in this, for we have begun to play god in so many of life's intimate realms that we probably could not turn back if we tried."[4] In Stock's hyperinflated burlesque of ethical reasoning, taking "responsibility" involves recognizing the "inevitability" of Metaman and seizing each opportunity to use genetic engineering to move the human organism beyond what he depicts as its present decrepit condition. While he acknowledges that such developments will generate "stresses within society," he argues that moral deliberation and decisions about public policy are irrelevant. "But whether such changes are 'wise' or 'desirable' misses the essential point that they are largely not a matter of choice; they are the unavoidable product of the technological advance intrinsic to Metaman."[5]

Another colorful spokesperson for the posthuman future in the scientific community is molecular biologist Lee Silver. His book *Remaking Eden: Cloning and Beyond in a Brave New World* surveys near and distant prospects for biotechnology in various fields of medicine, especially those involved with control of human reproduction. In his view, ongoing developments in scientific laboratories will produce a revolution in society, an upheaval whose consequences will include the radical division of the species into superior and inferior genetic classes. Imagining conditions that he believes will characterize the United States in the year 2350, he writes:

> The GenRich—who account for 10 percent of the American population—all carry synthetic genes. . . . The GenRich are a modern-day hereditary class of genetic aristocrats.
>
> All aspects of the economy, the media, the entertainment industry, and the knowledge industry are controlled by members of the GenRich class. . . . In contrast, Naturals work as low-paid service providers or as laborers.[6]

Silver speculates that by the end of the third millennium, the two groups will have become "entirely separate species with no ability to cross-breed, and with as much romantic interest in each other as a current human would have for a chimpanzee."[7] For those who think his vision of the future resembles a bizarre sci-fi screenplay, Silver notes that his scenario "is based on straightforward extrapolations from our current knowledge base." It is "inevitable" that the use of repro-genetic technologies will change the species in fundamental ways. "There is no doubt about it. For better *and* worse, a new age is upon us."[8]

When statements of a similar sort were made in earlier decades, the horrified response would often be: "Aren't the scientists preparing to 'play God'?" And until recently, the common tendency among scientists was to reassure the public by saying, in effect, "No, we do not intend to play God at all. What we're actually doing is far more modest." Today, however, it appears that a number of scientists—not just zealots like Stock and Silver but also figures central to the development of biotechnology—are willing to own up to the godlike implications of their proposals for human bioengineering. Thus, James Watson, codiscoverer of the DNA double helix, announced at a scholarly symposium in 1998: "And another thing, because no one has the guts to say it, if we could make better human beings by knowing how to add genes, why shouldn't we do it? What's wrong with it?"[9] Addressing members of the British Parliament in May 2000, Watson exclaimed, "But then, in all honesty, if scientists don't play God, who will?"[10]

Scientific advocates for the radical retailoring of the human species and "progress" toward a posthuman successor species are not limited to the field of biotechnology. With his familiar eloquence, physicist Freeman Dyson has written about the branching of humanity into several distinct, deliberately created new varieties, some of which are superior to existing humans and destined to live on the moons of Jupiter and other homes in outer space.[11] The fields of computer science and robotics have spawned a number of posthuman visionaries including Marvin Minsky, Raymond Kurzweil, Hans Moravec, and Kevin Warwick. In their projections of where research and development in information technology will lead, thinkers of this stripe make it clear that humans are no longer the ultimate beneficiaries of technological development and are probably destined to obsolescence. In the larger picture, "progress" in the hot fields of computer science and robotics is truly *for* something else.

On the scale of outrageous fantasy, robotics engineer Hans Moravec clearly outdistances anything the biotechnology-oriented theorists of posthumanity have proposed to date. In *Robot: Mere Machine to Transcendent Mind*, he writes, "Today, as our machines approach human competence across the board, our stone-age biology and information age lives grow ever more mismatched." The growth of increasingly "intelligent" computerized robotic devices, he believes, points to the creation of both new, superior, artificial beings and new worlds to house them. "Our artificial progeny will grow away from and beyond us, both in physical distance and structure, and similarity of thought and motive. In time their activities may become incompatible with the old Earth's continued existence."[12]

Moravec sees the eventual replacement of humans as foreshadowed by ongoing innovations in the business world—changes propelled by the quest for better service at lower prices. Phone calls are handled by intelligent systems of voice mail; automated teller machines take care of much of the work of banking; automated factories increasingly handle the work of production as the contribution of human labor subsides. He expects developments of this variety to spread, absorbing all significant areas of economic activity before long. Even the belief that the owners of the means of production are the ones who will guide these changes and benefit from them is, in Moravec's view, woefully mistaken. Before long, he argues, "owners will be pushed out of capital markets by much cheaper and better robotic decision makers."[13]

Moravec imagines generations of robots in the distant future that look less like the clunky machines we see today, and more like artificial, self-reproducing organisms. One has the shape of "the basket starfish"; another model, "the Bush Robot," features a stem, treelike branches, balls attached to its limbs like fruit, and microscopic fingers that "might be able to build a copy of itself in about ten hours." Eventually, super-intelligent creatures of this kind, "Ex-humans" or "Exes," would grow weary of the limitations of Earth, seeking their fortunes elsewhere in the universe. The question of what will become of ordinary humans in this brave new world is for Moravec of little concern. It is clear that his sympathies lie with the smarter, more resourceful, more powerful successors to our pathetically weak and incompetent species. At one point, he suggests that when robots end up producing all foods and manufactured goods, "humans may work to amuse other humans."[14] In the longer term, however, this pattern is likely to prove unstable. "Biological species," Moravec writes, "almost never survive encounters with superior competitors." He speculates that generations of robots who leave Earth may eventually return with aggressive intentions. "An entity that fails to keep up with its neighbors is likely to be *eaten*, its space, materials, energy, and useful thoughts reorganized to serve another's goals. Such a fate may be routine for humans who dally too long on slow Earth before going Ex."[15]

Unstated in visions of this kind, but clearly implied by the drift of discussion, is the conviction that God's original creation was inadequate. With the knowledge available to them now and in the future, scientists can do better than the Creator, that bumbling old fool, who gave us such a terribly inadequate world and equipped us with such a decrepit physique (especially the brain). Surely, we the enlightened can do far better, designing new beings and new worlds based on the power of rapidly advancing technologies. If one prefers a story that sidesteps the theological dimensions and relies on theories of evolution, a common prediction among posthumanists is that science will create the means to channel evolution along marvelous new paths, ones that will, alas, eventually lead to human extinction. In either context, though, the belief that somehow progress is "for us" needs to be discarded; at this juncture it is merely an outmoded prejudice.

Enthusiasts of Posthumanism in Popular Culture

What is it that attracts people to speculations about the creation of posthumans and to projects that seem to lead in that direction? Clearly, there are many motives at work. For some contemporary scientists, the goal of "improving" or transcending humanity is appealing simply because it is there to be done. Why not use the same knowledge and techniques that we apply to the cloning of Dolly and Polly the sheep or the creation of genetically modified foods and apply them to our own species? Why not produce generations of superartifacts that expand intelligence far beyond anything mere humans could ever hope to achieve? Because it is possible to accomplish powerful, unprecedented effects, the impulse for doing so seems irresistible to some people. Indeed, the default setting on the moral compass of technological choice in our time seems to be, "Hell, why not?" As a science undergraduate in a colleague's philosophy class recently explained, "If I had the opportunity to make the first cloned human, would I do it? Hell yeah!"

Even projects in this genre that have little likelihood of success may seem highly appealing because they hold out possibilities of great wealth and instant fame. Support from venture capital in Silicon Valley and other centers of high technology already awaits biotech entrepreneurs who can spin plausible tales about the eventual payoff of cutting-edge research. Expectations of enormous profits surround corporations jockeying for position in the emerging field of genomics. Meanwhile, the prospect that someone might actually achieve results worthy of mention in the *Guinness Book of Records* inspires a good many to give it a shot. Each morning I read the newspaper, expecting to find the headline "Science Clones First Human Being" or perhaps "Science Clones First Bioethicist." That story has not appeared yet, but I'm told it's just a matter of months.[16]

Beyond these familiar passions, other powerful desires lend support for ambitious schemes in posthumanism. Many people who are neither scientists nor businesspeople enjoy the excitement involved in the race to new frontiers and identification with developments that promise the latest and greatest in technological change. Sentiments of this kind, regularly displayed in *Wired* and other magazines hawking high-tech boosterism, have inspired a number of small but highly visible organizations that demand the rapid augmentation of humans and/or their replacement by superior, well-fabricated beings. Several international organizations of this stripe are affiliates of the World Transhumanist Association, whose statement of purpose explains, "Humanity will be radically changed by technology in the future. We foresee the feasibility of redesigning the human condition, including such parameters as the inevitability of ageing, limitations on human and artificial intellects, unchosen psychology, suffering, and our confinement to the planet Earth."[17] The association's electronic, peer-reviewed *Journal of Transhumanism* includes articles by leading figures in transhumanist research, including Moravec.

For the time being, the posthumanist, transhumanist movement is fairly small—a few hundred to a few thousand internationally at most—comprised of colorful, publicity-seeking artists and visionaries and their followers who have had good luck winning the attention of journalists and radio talk show hosts. In Marina del Mar, California, the Extropy Institute, headed by Max More and Natasha Vita-More, regularly organizes conferences and workshops to promote the Extropian vision. "We're at the early transhuman stage now," Vita-More told a reporter for *L. A. Weekly*. "Then we'll get to the mid-transhuman stage, where we start shedding more and more of our biology, start interfacing more and more with machines, prosthetics, implants, and transplants. It's a process, and it's becoming more rapid all the time."[18]

Perhaps an extreme reflection of the California desire to remain forever young in the sun, the Extropians are obsessed with the quest for perpetual beauty, longevity, and the avoidance of death. As Max More observes, "I think people will look back on the twentieth century and think, 'Why didn't more people see that there was a possibility now of actually doing something about aging and death, and why didn't people do something."[19] His wife is even more explicit about the elements of transhumanism that derive from upper-middle-class consumerism and hedonism. "I love fashion," Vita-More asserts. "Our bodies will be the next fashion statement; we will design them in all sorts of interesting combinations of texture, colors, tones, and luminosity."[20]

The Mores draw inspiration from an earlier prophet of transhumanism, F. M. Esfandiary, renamed FM–2030 to highlight his belief that anyone who lived to the year 2030 would be able to live forever. Esfandiary attracted a small but enthusiastic following of scientists, engineers, and others during the 1970s and 1980s, offering courses through the extension program of the University of California at Los Angeles. His book *Are You a Transhuman?*, published in 1989, spells out both personal strategies and paths for scientific research that will help people achieve immortality.[21] Regrettably, FM–2030 died of pancreatic cancer in 2000, cursing the pancreas as a "stupid, dumb, wretched organ." Following his last wishes, FM–2030's body has been cryogenically preserved and could be defrosted if research on extended longevity bears fruit.[22]

Another group in the vanguard of posthuman publicity is the Raelian movement, a cult founded by French journalist Claude Villion, who calls himself Rael. Its several hundred members in Canada and the United States are attracted by a message Rael received from a friendly extraterrestrial in 1973—the revelation that intelligent life on Earth had been created long ago by a visit from space aliens. In the Raelian view, it is now the duty of humankind to continue the work of those beneficent forebears, improving the species through cloning, genetic manipulation, and other techniques. To that end, the Raelians have organized Clonaid, Inc., "the first human cloning company." Based in the Bahamas where cloning is still legal, the firm hopes to make a variety of reproductive services, including human reproductive cloning, available to the market. Spokespeople for the Clonaid company indicate that some one hundred women have offered to help produce the first artificially cloned child, a result they expect to accomplish very soon.[23]

Of course, one can dismiss groups like the Extropians and Raelians as fringe movements whose ideas cannot be taken seriously. But when the U.S. Congress took up the question of whether to allow or ban human cloning in the United States in hearings held in March 2001, among the first witnesses called were none other than Rael himself and the "scientific director" of Clonaid, Brigitte Boisselier. "They say we're a cult," Rael told reporters before testifying. "But we're not a religion. Our God is science." Several Congresspeople who heard their testimony appeared shocked by the claims of Rael, Boisselier, and other witnesses who promised they were well on the way to cloning humans. Rael explained that the long-term goal was to enable adults to make clones of themselves just before their deaths. "We would transfer, or download, or upload, your personality and your soul into this new being."²⁴ As the hearings ended, the chair of the Committee on Energy and Commerce, Rep. Billy Tauzin, promised legislation to ban the practice altogether. While lobbying by the likes of Rael and Boisselier may generate negative reactions in the short term, today's posthumanists may be remembered as bold opinion leaders of a movement in which the combined fascination with UFOs, alien abductions, cyborg fashions, age-old yearnings for transcendence, and the promise of life-enhancing biomedical breakthoughs began to seem like an entirely reasonable, highly marketable package.

From Toolmaking Animal to Cyborg

Beyond the extravagant pronouncements of zealots from the community of scientists and the dreams of posthuman publicists, one finds that ideas that are at least highly compatible with projects of posthumanism are now very much in vogue in the social sciences and the humanities. Among prominent scholars and writers, the view that humans are stable, coherent natural entities has gone out of fashion. At the same time, the once commonsense view that there is an important distinction to be drawn between human beings and the technical implements they use has begun to fade, replaced by the conclusion that humans and their tools have finally merged.

The rise of this way of thinking can be traced through a sequence of three perspectives on humans and technology that have focused scholarly debates in recent decades. One persuasion widely endorsed by educated people in the middle of the twentieth century held that humans are toolmaking animals. This conception, formulated by Benjamin Franklin and creatively expanded by Karl Marx, took on renewed significance with twentieth-century archaeological evidence of protohumans and their evolution. Thus, anthropologist Sherwood Washburn, among others, argued that the chance discovery or haphazard creation of sharpened stones used in hunting enabled Australopithecus to increase the amount of animal protein in its diet, and this in turn led to the evolution of a larger brain and more robust physical features. In this view, toolmaking and tool use, especially the ability to perfect tools over time, was the ability that distinguished humans from other species and established their dominance. From this foundation, the complex structures of social organization and cultural life arose as a consequence of the tool-making, tool-using abilities of Homo sapiens.

A common moral and political lesson from the homo faber, "tool-making animal," theory was that the projects of modern technology—including nuclear weapons, the space program, and computers—were manifestations of humanity's most basic urges. As celebrated in numerous World's Fair exhibits, television documentaries, and the famous ape scene in Stanley Kubrick's movie *2001: A Space Odyssey*, tools make us who we are. So prominent was this point of view in the 1950s and 1960s that the skeptical Lewis Mumford chose to attack it directly in the first volume of *The Myth of the Machine*, subtitled *Technics and Human Development*.[25] Mumford argued that the development of symbols, language, and ritual both preceded the contribution of material tools and was far more influential in generating the intellectual, economic, and political accomplishments of human beings in prehistoric and historical times than anything tools had made possible. The myth of the machine, in his view, was the worshipful obsession with technology, a pathological obsession that deflects people from recognizing other, more hopeful dimensions of human creativity.

Although toolmaking animal conceptions stress the centrality of technology in human evolution and history, the underlying assumption is that humans are still distinct from the tools they fabricate and employ. Our instruments are available to us, ready to be used when needed. And certainly, the conditions of their use changes the activities and productivity of individuals and social groups, affecting how different populations flourish and how power is distributed among them. But this viewpoint takes for granted that a firm, reliable boundary exists between humans as organisms and tools regarded as material aids to their activity.

A second idea that has often been used to frame discussions of humans and artificial means—one that is greeted in some quarters as an important advance beyond simple notions about tools and humans—is the claim that technologies are powerful extensions of human organs. Although it had been suggested by earlier thinkers, this perspective attracted considerable attention in the late 1960s and early 1970s as the writings of Marshall McLuhan gained a widespread audience.[26] An obvious appeal of the extensionist position is that it finds power for individuals within the very complexes of electronic media and other sophisticated technologies of modern life that might otherwise seem overwhelming. Thus, the telephone extends a person's ability to hear and speak; television extends the effective perceptual range of one's eyes and ears; automobiles, trains, ships, airplanes, and so forth, are an extension of the mobility provided by human legs. The happy lesson that the extensionist vision inspires is that enormous technological systems developed for corporate and military purposes eventually come to benefit everyday folks. During the so-called space age and era of multimedia spectacles, many found it thrilling to imagine themselves enlarged and augmented by guided missiles and satellite communications. For many, this was good news because it suggested individuals could overcome the limitations of biological forms and abilities received at birth. Hence, during the era of Richard Nixon, Gerald Ford, and Jimmy Carter, McLuhanesque fantasies of the "global village" along with dreams of the colonization of space gave hope to technophiles, especially in the United States.[27] By the 1990s, such dreams had by and large shifted to a new technical template, the Internet.

But despite the insistence that "technology is humanity extended," despite the growing sense that humans and technical systems are intimately connected, extensionist renderings of the story still assume that electronic and other technologies are to a considerable degree distinct from the human organism itself. Yes, one frequently attaches new media to one's limbs and sense organs. But these devices are not in themselves regarded as intrinsic features of human beings; they are long links that could at any moment be disconnected and replaced with extensions of another variety, or by none at all. It remained for another turn in thinking about the relationship between humanity and technology to take a further step, affirming that there is actually no meaningful boundary between humans and technology at all.

Within prominent fields of social theory today—science studies and cultural studies, for example—commonly used categories point to a continual, pervasive blending of nature and artifice. Among the more popular names for these blended entities are "hybrid," "quasi-object," and "cyborg," with events that bring such creations into being called "implosions" and "boundary crossings." The initial stimulus for notions of this kind came from a growing sense that the objects studied by social scientists and humanists should be regarded as social and cultural constructions. Rejecting positivist notions that science obtains knowledge through neutral observation of what happens in nature, many scholars assert that knowledge is to a large extent constructed rather than "discovered." From this belief it becomes possible to reexamine or "interrogate" objects in the world once regarded as purely natural, and find them to be intricate combinations of cultural, social, and physical features. An eagerness to identify and interpret social constructs and blended entities now extends to the names of the activities and institutions once called "science and technology," but now renamed "technoscience" to acknowledge that, if one looks carefully, the two realms continually flow into and through each other.

There are a number of ways in which terms like hybrid and cyborg, and the intellectual strategies associated with them, have been useful to scholars. This terminology and perspective makes it possible to account for the interactions of scientific knowledge, technological change, and social practice in ways not limited by conceptions of nature and society inherited from earlier times. Thus, discussions of power and how it works—including power derived from natural sources—can be depicted in a new light, as a set of hybrid creations whose description enables us to propose new strategies for dealing with sources of power. Similarly, discussions of various knowledge claims about the natural realm need not commit us to judgments that naturalize things that are better regarded as social and cultural constructions, as the history of biological taxonomy and medical definition of various diseases, to cite two examples, clearly reveals. By looking at products, institutions, and living inhabitants of modern society as hybrids, elaborate mixes of elements from culture and nature, social theorists sidestep the badly mistaken identifications and explanations inherited from earlier generations.

Approaches of this kind have played a significant and, in my view, largely positive role in helping historians, philosophers, and social scientists reexamine the concepts, theories, research programs, political ideologies, and social policies that have surrounded science and technology in modern society. There have been many fruitful debates about when and how distinctions among animals/humans/machines have been drawn, and about the practices involved in drawing them.[28] Inquiries in this vein also have interesting political implications, for it is evident that projects in Western science and technology frequently have imposed categories on groups of people and natural things that contained highly suspect, often flagrantly unjust assumptions, ones frequently implicated in relationships of domination. A positive first step is to call into question these inherited categories and to rethink the beings and situations involved. In this way, a wide variety of prejudices can be dispelled, opening the way (in theory at least) for renegotiation of who and what has standing, and which practical steps are most promising. Thus, science studies and cultural studies about technoscience sometimes present themselves as radical, not just in an intellectual sense, but also as a force for progressive political change.[29]

For many writers in science studies and cultural studies, the methods of interpretation and explanation that they employ to study things like bacteria and quarks, also demand a new vision of what human beings are and might become. As anthropologist David Hakken notes, "Cyborg anthropology extends anthropological holism by positioning humans as entities in technology actor networks, thereby reconceptualizing them as bio-techno-cultural entities."[30] Hakken draws inspiration from the theory of actor networks developed by Michel Callon and Bruno Latour in which social systems are described as hybrids composed of "actors" and "actants," living and nonliving agents, arranged in complex combinations. Latour argues that an unacknowledged crisis in modern social thought is that "the proliferation of hybrids has saturated the constitutional framework of moderns." Owning up to this crisis requires a new understanding of humanity altogether since people mistakenly believe that being human is a narrowly bounded condition. "The expression 'anthropomorphic,'" Latour writes, "considerably underestimates our humanity. We should be talking about morphism. Morphism is the place where technomorphisms, zoomorphisms, phusimorphisms, ideomorphisms, theomorphisms, sociomorphisms, psychomorphisms, all come together. Their alliances and exchanges, taken together, are what define the *anthropos*."[31]

Attempts to deny that relevant creatures, objects, systems, and situations are hybrids and to insist that significant varieties of nature and culture be recognized in their former simplicity is a move Latour calls "the work of purification."[32] With insights available to us now, however, we can set aside such purifying labors and confront the world of hybrids directly. In this light, Latour notes that some people seem "threatened by machines." But he advises that such fears are groundless, since human beings have by now thoroughly merged with mechanical devices in wide-ranging conditions of hybridity. "Where does the threat come from?" he asks. "From those who seek to reduce it to an essence and who—by scorning things, objects, machines and the social, . . . make humanism a fragile and precious thing at risk of being overwhelmed by Nature, Society or God."[33]

Even more explicit as an advocate of ideas about the condition of humanity as thoroughly infused with the projects and products on contemporary technoscience is Donna J. Haraway, whose writings have inspired a vast literature on cyborgs and what she calls "promising monsters." Humans, in her view, are merely one of a vast range of entities that have finally been removed from anything resembling their original biological condition and are now subject to powerful, intellectually challenging acts of "transgressive border-crossing." Her category "cyborg" includes much more than the human/machine creations described in cold war research documents and depicted in sci-fi films such as *Terminator*. Haraway writes that "cyborg figures—such as the end-of-the-millennium seed, chip, gene, database, bomb, fetus, race, brain, and ecosystem—are the offspring of implosions of subjects and objects and of the natural and artificial."[34] Needed today, in Haraway's grand narrative (which she terms a "modest-witness"), are wide-ranging, feminist deconstructions that reveal the character of these "implosions" and give us ways of thinking about their products unbiased by benighted programs of scientific and philosophical discourse received from previous generations.

To focus on cyborgs and their histories, in Haraway's view, is merely to recognize things that already exist and/or are rapidly coming to be. Yes, their features sometimes strike many people as grotesque. But rather than recoil in horror at even the most unsettling hybrids produced by contemporary technoscience, one must seek to find kinship with the cascade of synthesized, recombinant entities and creatures that increasingly populate the world. She asks, "Who are my kin in this odd world of promising monsters, vampires, surrogates, living tools, and aliens? What kinds of crosses and offspring count as legitimate and illegitimate, to whom and at what cost?" One of the beings she recognizes as kin, for example, is the genetically modified OncoMouse—bred explicitly for research that seeks cures for cancer—a creature she calls "my sister."

"Whether I agree to her existence and use or not, s/he suffers, physically, repeatedly, and profoundly, that I and my sisters may live."[35]

In Haraway's elusive, endlessly beguiling way of writing, the method-ological commitments of contemporary science studies and cultural studies begin to generate a collection of moral sentiments—ones offered as interpretive insights, but never fully argued as explicit ethical com-mitments. Thus, her expressions of kinship with cyborgs and hybrids stem from the view that "technoscience as cultural practice and practi-cal culture, . . . requires attention to all the meanings, identities, materi-alities, and accountabilities of the subjects and objects in play. That is what kinship is about in my 'ethnographic' fugue."[36] An important con-sequence of this approach is to discredit beliefs that things in nature have distinctive integrity, wholeness of being, or harmony with their sur-roundings that deserve emphasis in considerations about where techno-science and global corporations can properly move. In Haraway's view, beliefs of this kind predicate a world that no longer exists, if indeed it ever did. What we must focus on now are the circumstances in which a culturally created nature confronts us with things that are only partly identifiable by origins and conditions that existed prior to the arrival of modern civilization. She writes:

Located in the belly of the monster, I find discourses of natural harmony, the nonalien and purity unsalvageable for understanding our genealogy in the New World Order, Inc. Like it or not, I was born kin to PU239 and to transgenic, transspecific, and transported creatures of all kinds; that is the family for which and to whom my people are accountable. It will not help—emotionally, intel-lectually, morally, or politically—to appeal to the natural and the pure.[37]

One can, however, appeal to the weird, the transgressive, and the disharmonious. In her vision of the world, nature is reduced to a kind of comic puzzle. The category that now merits our attention, indeed our awe, is technoscience, the new buzzword of science studies, which she continually reifies in all of its colorful, shape-shifting perversity.

One of Haraway's concerns, a legitimate one, is that the names and the theories produced by science in the past have helped inspire and justify racist policies and institutions in both the North and the South. Using her methods to witness "implosions of nature and culture" and undermine racist strategies and their rhetorics of "purity," she feels she must also dismiss contemporary arguments that applications of biotechnology violate the natural order, for ideas of that kind have gotten us into trouble in the past. She recognizes that, unfortunately, this stance puts her at odds with many of her colleagues in progressive movements around the globe that deploy arguments about purity and danger to resist forceful intrusions of global capitalism. She laments, "Perhaps it is perverse for me to hear the dangers of racism in the *opposition* to genetic engineering and especially transgenics at just the moment when national and international coalitions of indigenous, consumer, feminist, environmental, and development nongovernmental organizations have formed to oppose 'patenting, commercialization and expropriation of human, animal and plant genetic materials.'"[38] But this is a perversity that Haraway decides she can live with. She opposes the patenting of many life-forms, including human genes, because the practice commodifies genetic resources and also excludes the participation of indigenous people, who have a right to decide how these resources are used. But she rejects all contentions that affirm the need to protect species boundaries as a primary good, for such policies are at odds with her belief that the primary responsibility of feminist theory and the new science studies is to call all such boundaries into question, and to deconstruct and thereby reject all claims about wholeness.

Many of Haraway's personal political commitments are laudable ones. She hopes that her work will support efforts by a host of local groups to make "claims rooted in a finally amodern, reinvented desire for justice and democratically crafted and lived well-being." But her approach forbids producing arguments that could make these "claims" evident as coherent and persuasive positions to illuminate personal and policy choices. What she calls for instead are ongoing "contestations"—"contestations for possible, maybe even liveable, worlds of globalized technoscience."[39] In a world in which many of the plans and strategies of global corporations are hatched in secret with little public awareness or debate, one can only hope that such contestations spread and flourish. But Haraway's perspectives on these matters offer little in the way of guidance for those with specific causes to advance or battles to carry to those in power. "We must cast our lot with some ways of living on this planet, and not with others," she suggests.[40] Yet other than observing that ways of living are endlessly contestable (which they certainly are), her writings offer no tangible suggestions about where, when, how, and in which direction particular lots ought to be cast. In Haraway's postmodernism/posthumanism, moral and ethical sentiments are always emotive and personal, expressed on the fly rather than rigorously argued. In an odd way, the philosophy of science in this mode echoes the prejudices of the logical positivists decades earlier for whom moral judgments were little more than expressions of personal taste.[41]

In the end, as Haraway describes the ongoing mergers of natural and artificial things, she clearly sides with the artificial. Her books and writings take delight in depicting and deconstructing the projects and products of corporate technoscience, modestly witnessing a flow of laboratory and corporate concoctions that will leave indelible marks on the future. At the same time, she derides attempts by others to uphold some things as "natural" as a risible blunder. Indeed, the valence of her writings lends support to the radical restructurings of natural creatures and their habitats, including measures that involve obvious acts of violence. A similar disposition seems to have taken hold within the new subdisciplines of science studies, cultural studies, and technology studies: a kind of bemused indifference when confronted with a world filled with artificial devices, artificial systems, and now, artificially produced living beings. Scholars began with a methodological affirmation that the world for us is composed of social and cultural constructs. Perhaps it is no surprise that they ended up embracing things that most clearly are constructs, hybrid entities that are the products of engineering broadly conceived. In this way, the new scholarship meshes nicely with the work of radical reconstruction and recapitalization at stake in today's technical and corporate realms. In fact, many scholars enjoy the work of ethnography and theory that places them elbow to elbow with the scientific researchers and business leaders who move and shake with initiatives in globalization. Overlooked in this approach is a haunting memory: that most of the world still consists of things and creatures that neither scientists, business people, nor social theorists had any hand in making.

Conclusion

Will the prevailing winds in the three arenas of discussion I have described eventually come together to produce a change in climate in society's view of the prospects for posthumanism? It is too soon to tell.

There are signs, however, that the borders between theory in the social sciences and the humanities and the advocacy of scientific zealots and posthumanist social movements has begun to blur. Haraway's writings, for example, are often cited not only as aids in thinking about the world of cyborgs and posthumans but also as a justification for plowing ahead in that direction as rapidly as possible. Thus, James Hughes's manifesto for the radical modification of the human species, "Embracing Change with All Four Arms: A Post-Humanist Defense of Genetic Engineering," cites Haraway as "the principal touchpoint for post-humanism." From now on, Hughes contends, true social progress depends on "faith in the potential unlimited improvability of human nature and expansion of human powers far more satisfying than a resignation to our current limits."[42]

As the old millennium drew to a close, enthusiastic speculation about cyborgs and their ways of living became a popular topic of discussion among supposedly radical voices in the U.S. and European academy. A five-hundred-page compendium of views of this kind, *The Cyborg Handbook*, edited by Chris Hables Gray with a foreword by Haraway, explores the exhilarating joys and perils of living in a world mutually constructed by modern technology and theoretical discourse—a world in which cyborgs rapidly proliferate. Indeed, for some several writers in the collection, describing oneself as a cyborg has finally become a badge of honor. Chela Sandoval, for example, writes that "colonized peoples of the Americas have already developed the cyborg skills required for survival under techno-human conditions as a requisite for survival under domination over the past three hundred years."[43] At the book's conclusion, Gray and Steven Mentor look back on their colleagues' cyborg discourses and find much to celebrate. "There is no choice between utopia and dystopia, Good Terminator or Evil Terminator—they are both here. We are learning to inhabit this constructed, ambiguous body (and explore who constructs it). . . . Perhaps, after all, we just need to learn cyborg family values—good maintenance, technical expertise, pleasures dispersed and multiple, community research and development, improved communication."[44] Cyborg family values?[45] Oh, good; something to look forward to.

The vogue of posthumanism reflects a basic disagreement in modern political philosophy about what radical, progressive thinking involves.

One understanding of its purpose seeks freedom and social justice for all human beings, with people regarded as being fundamentally equal. During the past two centuries, thinkers who began from that standpoint saw the key challenge as that of justifying and working to realize the social, economic, and political conditions that would foster human liberation. Always key to these efforts was the elimination of oppressive institutions and the creation of better ones. Approaches of this kind are to be found in the writings of a host of reformers and revolutionaries from the eighteenth century to the present day—such as Jean-Jacques Rousseau, Thomas Jefferson, the utopian socialists, Marx, John Dewey, and the like.

A quite different path for radicalism, however—one characteristic of some nineteenth-century romantic visionaries, twentieth-century sci-fi novelists, and today's prophets of posthumanism—is one that aspires to the transcendence of the human shell in quest of more exquisite ways of being. The possibility that fascinates many here, is that a vastly improved person, a Nietzschean *Übermensch* or other superior creature, is an accomplishment well worth seeking. Hence, the focus of revolutionary aspirations no longer rests on cumbersome institutions so notoriously difficult to change, but rather on the physical composition of the body one inhabits. The recent shift in social theory away from concerns about justice and the retailoring of human institutions toward narcissistic concerns about achieving a revolution in the body points to a definite weariness about the strategies for change advocated in earlier decades—organizing unions and resistance movements, for example. In its place is a renewed willingness to affirm the transformative powers of science and technology while overlooking the sometimes unsavory workings of the complex of institutions recently dubbed technoscience.

Whether they intend to or not, social theorists fascinated with hybrids and cyborgs could end up playing a significant role in upcoming debates about practical initiatives to achieve posthuman dreams in tangible form. More eloquently than the scientists who have embraced posthumanist projects, they express a weariness about identifying oneself as merely human at all. That label and all it implies seems to many thinkers so badly outmoded or so badly stained by histories of violence and injustice that it would be just as well to renounce it altogether. Rather than persist in the failed project called humanity, let's find something new and improved. In fact, let's junk this worn-out theme, the human, altogether and come up with a better trope. Much of contemporary social theory has this message as an explicit subtext. Such sentiments dovetail nicely with visions like that of cyberneticist Kevin Warwick, a British scientist who now implants computer chips in his own body as a way to augment his nervous system and who often proclaims his fervent desire to become a cyborg. "I was born human," he wrote in *Wired*. "But this was an accident of fate—a condition merely of time and place. I believe it is something we have the power to change."[46]

For anyone who wanted to argue that there exist fundamental boundaries that should not be crossed in biotechnology, robotics, and other engineering projects, the response of cyborg social theorists is perfectly clear: Face it, folks, the relevant boundaries have already been breached. Thousands of ingenious boundary crossings are already evident in the creation of hybrids of every conceivable description. Mixes of things formerly given in nature along with new things from laboratories, design shops, and marketing agencies have already filled our world. How can anyone suggest this should not continue as it already has for some time now? At the very least, no one can claim any longer that such boundary crossings and their progeny are unprecedented.

As should be clear from the tone of my observations so far, I find the themes and projects of posthumanism a bizarre way of imagining the choices we face. Within three prominent domains of contemporary posthumanism—the natural sciences, social movements, and social theory—one finds levels of self-indulgence and megalomania that are simply off the charts. The greatest puzzle about this fin de siècle fad is how tawdry notions could have attracted such a large audience at all.

Fortunately, there is an appealing alternative to today's frenzy about cyborgs, hybrids, transhumans, extropians, and the like—rethinking what it means to be human in the first place. Far from being an exhausted concept or failed project, being human is a question whose possibilities are very much open to intellectual inquiry and practical realization. The relevant category, in my view, is perhaps less that of "human nature" than of the "human condition." To face this condition squarely involves, for example, the recognition of mortality as a basic fact of human existence. It also entails acknowledging that we are creatures whose history and prospects for survival are indelibly rooted in the circumstances of a blue planet that revolves around the Sun. Yes, it is possible to rebel against fundamental conditions of this kind, for instance, by seeking a vastly extended longevity or by rocketing away from Earth into cold, inhospitable corners of the universe. But such attempts are haunted by the question, Why would anyone want to take such steps other than as an expression of sheer hubris?

It is perfectly true that our ways of being human in the modern world are deeply connected to scientific knowledge and technological devices of all kinds. As I proofread this paper, I am helplessly dependent on the eyeglasses that help me see. But pondering this situation, does one emphasize the glasses or the person viewing, the package of technical equipment in the mix or the distinctive organism that puts it to use? The penchant for placing the technical hardware before the human (and it has come to that in much of contemporary thinking) is to my mind a terrible blunder, the perfect operational definition of a condition long feared in modern society—dehumanization.

One serious consequence of the move to abandon a vital concern for humans and their condition and to search for more exotic, posthuman ways of being is to remove the foundations on which some crucial moral and political agreements can be sought—an appeal to our common humanity. Thus, at the beginning of World War II, Franklin Delano Roosevelt argued that the central issue in the conflict was not merely the victory of the United States and its allies over the Fascists but the victory of democracy and its "simple principles of common decency and humanity." From this simple but persuasive standpoint, Roosevelt announced that "the objective of smashing the militarism imposed by war lords upon their enslaved peoples; the objective of liberating the subjugated nations; the objective of establishing and securing freedom of speech, freedom of religion, freedom from want, and freedom from fear everywhere in the world."[47] The creation of the United Nations after the war and the affirmation of the Universal Declaration of Human Rights by the UN General Assembly offered hope that the principles of "common decency and humanity" might be realized. And while it is obvious that practice has fallen far short of this idealistic affirmation, the concern for a shared humanity and the desire to alleviate the suffering of one's fellow humans remains perhaps the most powerful anchor for ethical conduct and wise policy in global politics, even among those who disagree on specific steps. Are there similar anchors in today's inflated rhetoric about posthumans—moral lessons derived from "our common cyborgity" perhaps? I think not. Indeed, most of the benefit from such discourse appears to be career development for well-heeled intellectuals in Paris, Santa Cruz, Cambridge, and other R & D hubs.

What can one say about the actual condition of the humans living on Earth at present? For anyone who cares to examine them, the data are chilling. According to the 2001 edition of the UN *Human Development Report*, 1.2 billion people on the planet suffer in extreme poverty, surviving on less than $1 a day, while a total of 2.8 billion (roughly half the world's population) live on less than $2 a day. Some 2.4 billion people are without access to basic sanitation. Of the world's children, 325 million are out of school at the primary and secondary levels. For children under the age of five, 11 million die annually from preventable causes.[48] Perhaps those now enthralled with cyborgs, hybrids, extropians, and posthumans will find such information insufficiently novel or thrilling to deflect their ambitious philosophical and research agendas. But the rest of us should take notice.

It is interesting to imagine what humanity as a whole might become if the best of moral understandings, personal sympathies, and practices of democracy were universally applied. One promising approach has never been tried—evening out the wealth available to human individuals, including redistributing worldwide much of the wealth now commanded by the most prosperous states of Europe and North America. If undertaken with sufficient concern for the health of the world's ecosystems and the diverse species that coinhabit the planet with us, this seems a far more promising policy than that of breeding exotic posthuman hybrids. In fact, it is well overdue for scientists and intellectuals in the North to focus strongly on all present and future members of human species, seeking to improve understandings of and connections with them—matters that have, by all accounts, remained woefully underappreciated with the creation of a modern, industrial society and today's global economy. To set aside this effort may be simply the latest stage of colonization, even among those who label themselves postcolonialist thinkers. Yet many seem eager to announce to persons living on less than one dollar a day that their bodies, abilities, and identities have been superseded by new products, new hybrids, produced in European and U.S. high-tech labs and social theory seminars.

In the decades ahead, a climate of opinion centering on posthumanism could well emerge to inform debates about crucial points of departure in public policy. Within this mood, initiatives of bioengineering will be regarded as perfectly normal and endlessly fascinating. By the same token, any resistance to innovations in human reproductive cloning and human germ line modification could appear regressive, reactionary, and outmoded. Within this "forward-looking," "progressive" climate of opinion, one might still debate which specific models of cyborgs, posthumans, transhumans, and the like should be engineered. These are the matters that we can "interrogate,"—matters that are still wonderfully "contestable." But to deny that any such projects should be launched at all will likely be rejected as simply out of touch with contemporary trends. For you see, dear friends, the boundaries have already been breached, the precedents established, the work of innovation set in motion, and the "promising monsters" all introduced at the cyborg-feminist/science studies debutante ball. What fascinates us now is the lovely and, oh, so wonderfully frightening dance of "transgressions" performed to the currently fashionable "ethnographic fugue."

Hence, as we look forward to pending discussions on the posthuman prospect, contemporary social theorists may have something consequential to add. For those who propose that it would be a grand idea to erase biological boundaries and embark on a wide range of radical and untested adventures in the reengineering of humankind, scholars in "the humanities" can happily say, "Haven't you heard? It's already well under way!"

Notes

1. Jacques Ellul, *The Technological Society*, trans. John Wilkinson (New York: Alfred A. Knopf, 1965), 428, 431.

2. Lewis Mumford, *The Myth of the Machine: The Pentagon of Power* (New York: Harcourt Brace Jovanovich, 1970), 435.

3. Gregory Stock, *Metaman: The Merging of Humans and Machines into a Global Superorganism* (New York: Simon and Schuster, 1993), 150, 152, 164, 168.

4. Gregory Stock, "Human Germline Engineering: Implications for Science and Society," introduction, http://research.mednet.ulca.edu/pmts/Germline/bhwf.htm.

5. Stock, *Metaman*, 168.

6. Lee M. Silver, *Remaking Eden: Cloning and Beyond in A Brave New World* (New York: Avon Books, 1997), 4, 6.

7. Ibid., 7.

8. Ibid., 11.

9. James Watson, cited in Gregory Stock and John Campbell, ed., *Engineering the Human Germline: An Exploration of the Science and Ethics of Altering the Genes We Pass to Our Children* (New York: Oxford University Press, 2000), 79.

10. James Watson, cited in Steven Connor, "Nobel Scientist Happy to 'Play God' with DNA," *Independent*, May 7, 2000, 7.

11. Freeman J. Dyson, *The Sun, the Genome, and the Internet* (New York: Oxford University Press), 99–113. Dyson exclaims, "To allow the diversification of human genomes and lifestyles on this planet to continue without restraint is a recipe for disaster. Sooner or later, the tensions between diverging ways of life must be relieved by emigration, some of us finding new places to live away from the Earth while others stay behind. In the end we must travel the high road into space, to find new worlds to match our new capabilities. To give us room to explore the varieties of mind and body into which our genome can evolve, one planet is not enough" (113).

12. Hans Moravec, *Robot: Mere Machine to Transcendent Mind* (New York: Oxford University Press, 1999), 7, 11.

13. Ibid., 130, 133.

14. Ibid., 152, 132.

15. Ibid., 146.

16. Shortly after I wrote these words, a biotechnology business firm, Advanced Cell Technology, announced that it had successfully cloned human embryos, which died after no more than eight cells. See Gina Kolata, "Company Says It Produced Human Embryo Clones," *New York Times*, November 26, 2001, A1.

17. World Transhumanist Association, "The Transhumanist Declaration," http://www.transhumanism.org/declaration.htm.

18. Natasha Vita-More, cited in Brendan Bernhard, "The Transhumanists," *L.A. Weekly*, January, 19–25 2001, 3.

19. Max More, cited in ibid., 6.

20. Natasha Vita-More, cited in Brian Alexander, "Don't Die, Stay Pretty: Introducing the Ultrahuman Makeover," *Wired* 8, no. 1 (January 2000) 6.

21. FM–2030, *Are You a Transhuman? Monitoring and Stimulating Your Personal Rate of Growth in a Rapidly Changing World* (New York: Warner Books, 1989).

22. Myrna Oliver, "Futurist Predicted Immortality," obituary, *Los Angeles Times*, July 1, 2002, B6.

23. Clonaid's claims can be found on the company's Web site, http://www.clonaid.com.

24. Claude Villion, cited in "We're Ready to Clone Humans, Raelian Founder Tells Panel," *Ottawa Citizen*, March 29, 2001, A8.

25. Lewis Mumford, *The Myth of the Machine: Technics and Human Development* (New York: Harcourt Brace Jovanovich, 1967).

26. See Marshall McLuhan, *Understanding Media: The Extensions of Man* (New York: McGraw-Hill, 1964), *The Gutenberg Galaxy: The Making of Typographic Man* (Toronto: University of Toronto Press, 1962), and *The Mechanical Bride* (New York: Vanguard Press, 1951).

27. See, for example, Stewart Brand, ed., *Space Colonies* (New York: Penguin Books, 1977).

28. See, for example, Erica Fudge, Ruth Gilbert, and Susan Wiseman, eds., *At the Borders of the Human: Beasts, Bodies, and Natural Philosophy in the Early Modern Period* (New York: St. Martin's Press, 1999).

29. A useful review of these discussions can be found in David Hess, *Science Studies: An Advanced Introduction* (New York: New York University Press, 1997).

30. David Hakken, *Cyborgs@cyberspace? An Enthnographer Looks to the Future* (New York: Routledge, 1999), 78.

31. Bruno Latour, *We Have Never Been Modern* (Cambridge, MA: Harvard University Press, 1993), 50–51, 137.

32. Ibid., 30.

33. Ibid., 138.

34. Donna J. Haraway, *Modest_Witness@Second_Millennium: FemaleMan©_Meets_OncoMouse™: Feminism and Technoscience* (New York: Routledge, 1996), 12.

35. Ibid., 52, 79.

36. Ibid., 82.

37. Ibid., 62.

38. Ibid.

39. Ibid., 267, 270.

40. Ibid., 270.

41. See, for example, Alfred Jules Ayer, *Language, Truth, and Logic* (New York: Dover Publications, 1952).

42. James Hughes, "Embracing Change with All Four Arms: A Post-Humanist Defense of Genetic Engineering," *Eubios: Journal of Asian and International Bioethics* 6.4 (1996): 94–101.

43. Chela Sandoval, "New Sciences: Cyborg Feminism and the Methodology of the Oppressed," in *The Cyborg Handbook*, ed. Chris Hables Gray with

Heidi J. Figueroa-Sarriera and Steven Mentor (New York: Routledge, 1995), 408.

44. Chris Hables Gray and Steven Mentor, "The Cyborg Politic: Version 1.2," in *The Cyborg Handbook*, ed. Chris Hables Gray with Heidi J. Figueroa-Sarriera and Steven Mentor (New York: Routledge, 1995), 465.

45. See also Chris Hables Gray, *Cyborg Citizen: Politics in the Posthuman Age* (New York: Routledge, 2002).

46. Kevin Warwick, "Cyborg 1.0," *Wired* 8, no. 2, (February 2000) 1. See also Kevin Warwick, "I Want to Be a Cyborg," *Guardian*, January 26, 2000, www.guardian.co.uk/comment/story/0,3604,238778,00.html (accessed January 20, 2004).

47. Franklin Delano Roosevelt, "Annual Message to Congress," January 6, 1942, in *The Public Papers and Addresses of Franklin D. Roosevelt, 1942*, ed. Samuel I. Rosenman (New York: Harper and Brothers Publishers, 1950) 32–42.

48. United Nations Development Programme, *Human Development Report 2001: Making New Technologies Work for Human Development* (New York: Oxford University Press, 2001).

Contributors

Harold W. Baillie is Professor of Philosophy at the University of Scranton.

Lisa S. Cahill is the J. Donald Monan, S. J. Professor of Theology at Boston College.

Timothy K. Casey is Professor of Philosophy at the University of Scranton.

Jean Bethke Elshtain is the Laura Spelman Rockefeller Professor of Social and Political Ethics at the University of Chicago.

Diane B. Paul is Professor of Political Science at the University of Massachusetts, Boston.

Robert N. Proctor is the Ferree Professor of the History of Science at The Pennsylvania State University.

Paul Rabinow is Professor of Anthropology at the University of California, Berkeley.

Bernard E. Rollin is a University Distinguished Professor at Colorado State University, Fort Collins.

Mark Sagoff is a Fellow at the Institute for Philosophy and Public Policy at the University of Maryland.

Thomas A. Shannon is Professor of Religion and Social Ethics at the Worcester Polytechnic Institute.

LeRoy B. Walters is the Joseph P. Kennedy Professor of Christian Ethics at the Kennedy School of Ethics, Georgetown University.

Langdon Winner is Professor of Political Science at Ransselaer Polytechnic Institute.

Richard M. Zaner is the Ann Geddes Stahlman Professor Emeritus of Medical Ethics and Philosophy of Medicine at the Vanderbilt University Medical Center.

Index

Abortion, 144, 156, 162–164, 170, 171n3, 171n6, 172n11
Acheulean tools, 237, 241–248
Affectio commodi, 22, 290–292, 309
Affectio justitiae, 22, 290, 292–296, 309
Affirmative action, 340
Agriculture, 36–37, 70, 73, 85, 87–88
AIDS drugs, 348–349, 360
Alexander the Great, 317
Altruism, 282, 289, 310–311
Ancient science, 39, 41, 44, 60
Animal husbandry, 319–320, 322, 329
Animal nature, 321
Animal rights, 321
Antinori, Severino, 343
Aquinas, Saint Thomas, 85, 88, 178
Archaeology, 237
Arendt, Hannah, 100, 114, 224–225
Artificial selection, 73–74, 127, 130, 134–135, 322, 326, 331
Aristotelian science. See Ancient science
Aristotle, 19, 24–25, 36, 39, 41, 44–45, 57–58, 60, 62n13, 88, 135, 178, 213, 214, 304, 317–319, 321, 326–331, 336n3, 339
Augustine, Saint, 174n36, 278, 293
Autonomy. See Freedom

Bacon, Francis, 2, 53, 78, 192
Baltimore, David, 69

Barthes, Roland, 100
Bayertz, Kurt, 189
Behaviorism, 58
Bellamy, Edward, 129
Bellow, Saul, 45
Bernal, J. D., 64n40, 130, 133, 134
Bernard, Claude, 187
Bible, 61n3, 169, 329
Biodiversity, 74, 140
Bioengineering, 2, 61, 67–69, 70, 72, 74, 88, 102, 114, 147n24, 138, 155, 159, 162, 177, 335, 386–389, 400, 405, 407
Bioethics, 78, 102
Biological natures. See Essence
Biological solidarity, 274–275
Biologism, 59
Biology, 7, 55, 58–59, 64n34, 65n45, 103, 112, 114, 127, 130, 177, 317–319, 327–329
Biomedicine. See Medicine
Biopolitics, 175n43
Biotechnology. See Bioengineering
Birth, 17, 49, 76–73, 79–82, 167, 193–202, 223
Blish, James, 177, 179, 183, 191
Blumenberg, Hans, 118n1
Body, 14, 15, 50, 167, 178, 193, 201–202, 212, 216, 218–219, 223–224, 333
Bonaventure, Saint, 300, 307
Bonhoeffer, Dietrich, 156, 169–170
Brace, C. Loring, 235, 265n56

Brain, 304, 381
Breeding, 123–124, 127, 131, 134,
    326–327
Brenner, Sydney, 101, 103, 115
Buffon, Georges-Louis, 241
Burnett, MacFarlane, 178–179, 189
Butterfield, Herbert, 41, 62n7,
    62n9

Callahan, Daniel, 77
Callon, Michael, 398
Calvin, William H., 245–247,
    262n33
Calvinism, 89
Camus, Albert, 203
Capitalism, 37, 46–47, 49, 108–109,
    114–115, 120n30, 129, 191, 401
Capital punishment, 156, 175n44
Carson, Rachel, 136
Catholic social ethics, teaching and
    tradition, 26, 60, 270, 340,
    350–354
Cavalli-Sforza, Luigiluca, 275–278
Charles, Prince, 87–88
Children, 159–163, 168, 172n13,
    173n22, 229–230
Christian ethics, 339–340
Christian realism, 339, 354–359
Christian theological anthropology,
    155–156, 166, 168, 171
Christianity, 38–39, 47, 50, 60, 85,
    88, 127, 137–138, 155–156,
    168–171
Cipla Ltd., 27, 139, 194n51,
    348–349, 360
Clarke, W. Norris, 62n3
Clockwork universe. See Mechanistic
    metaphysics
Cloning, 35, 81, 89, 101–102, 137,
    164–167, 170, 177, 179, 184, 191,
    200–202, 343–346, 387, 391, 393,
    408
Cole-Turner, Ronald, 73, 85
Common good, 350–354
Computers, 56–57, 395
Computer science, 389

Confinement agriculture, 320–321,
    324, 327, 330
Coon, Carlton, 255
Copernicus, Nicolaus, 60, 68, 107
Cosmology, 45, 55, 107, 336n3
Crick, Francis, 270
Curran, Charles, 84
Cybernetic humanity, 29, 54, 61
Cybernetics, 56–61

Darwin, Charles, 55, 64n34, 89, 107,
    126, 135, 189, 241, 272
Dawkins, Richard, 22, 275, 281–282,
    286–288, 301–302, 305
Death, 77–78, 164, 194–195, 220,
    222–224, 322
Deep ecology, 59
Deism, 303
Derrida, Jacques, 184
Descartes, 5, 36, 41–46, 48, 54, 56,
    60, 62n11, 220
Cartesian dualism, 19, 36, 42, 45,
    50, 52, 54–56, 60, 318
Cartesianism, 231n6
Determinism, 36, 56, 61, 72, 200
Dewey, John, 404
Diffusionist model of tool design, 248
Disenchantment of nature, 57, 111
DNA, 10, 54, 70, 72, 85, 87,
    102–103, 114, 119–7, 124, 139,
    182, 193, 256, 270, 274–275,
    277–278, 284, 300
Dolly, 391
Dorff, Elliot N., 86
Down syndrome, 14, 160–161, 334
Drosophila, 99–101, 103, 120n35
Dostoyevsky, Fyodor, 192–193
Duns Scotus, John, 22, 289–296,
    309–311
Dwarfism (achondroplasia), 179–183,
    188, 197–199
Dyson, Freeman, 143, 389, 409n11

Eaves, Lindon, 23, 298–300,
    307–308
Eccles, John, 178–179, 189, 200

Ecofeminism, 59
Ecology, 59, 85, 89
Ehrenreich, Barbara, 191
Ehrlich, Paul, 306, 308–310
Eldridge, Niles, 239
Eliot, T. S., 193
Ellul, Jacques, 385
Elshtain, Jean Bethke, 140, 202
Embodiment, 156–158, 163–164,
    169–170, 190
  body as property, 155
  perfecting the body, 155–156, 160,
    163–164, 170
Empathy, 310–311
Empedocles, 326
Engelhardt, H. Tristram, Jr., 193
Energeia (Activity), 216–219,
    221–224
Enlightenment, 11, 106, 107, 108,
    111, 113, 117, 120n30
Entelecheia (actuality), 216–219,
    223–224, 337
Environmental ethics, 74, 89, 326
Environmentalism, 85
Environmentalists, 87, 136
Essence, 88, 214, 218
  bionatures, 321
  natures, 317–318, 329
Eugenics, 11, 86, 123–28, 130–132,
    135, 137, 139–140, 142–145, 159,
    165–166, 172n13, 175n43, 179,
    186, 333
Euthanasia, 164, 170, 175–43
Evolution, 21, 44, 58–59, 64n41,
    67–68, 72, 79, 84–85, 103, 123,
    126, 128–129, 131–133, 135–136,
    177, 189–190, 235, 249, 272–274,
    326, 387, 390, 394–395
Evolutionary psychologists, 245
Extropians, 392–393, 405, 407

Factory farming, 321
Failure, 224, 225
Faust (Faustian), 70, 175n39
Feminist philosophy of science, 54, 59
Finalcause. *See* Telos

Fisher, Alain, 369
Fletcher, Joseph, 137
Food and Drug Administration, 27,
    370, 373–380
Foucault, Michel, 99
Frank, William, 293–295
Frankenstein, 69, 72, 87, 230
  foods, 99, 175n89
Franklin, Benjamin, 394
Freedom, 13, 19, 42–44, 47, 48, 51,
    53, 58, 61, 84, 90, 133, 138, 141,
    144–145, 156–157, 161, 165–169,
    190, 195, 212–213, 215, 219,
    280–282, 292–296, 299, 309, 321,
    329, 331, 335
Frere, John, 240–243
Freud, Sigmund, 9, 64n42, 104–108,
    112, 115–117, 119n13
Friedman, Thomas, 64n43
Fukuyama, Francis, 125
Future generations, 59, 61, 86, 136,
    141, 190, 407

Galen, 178–179
Galileo, 36, 40–41, 43–44, 55, 60
Galton, Francis, 127–128, 132–
    133
Gattaca, 159–160
Gelsinger, Jesse, 370, 375–379
Gene therapy, 35, 70, 79, 86,
    172n13, 179, 210, 211
  somatic therapy, 84 (*see also*
    Genetic enhancement)
Genetically modified food, 61, 391
Genetic counseling, 144
Genetic engineering, 12, 19–20, 23,
    30, 35–36, 53, 56, 59, 67, 69–70,
    74, 79, 84, 87, 89–90, 99, 115,
    123–126, 134, 137–140, 142–144,
    145n3, 149n56, 155, 158–160,
    162–163, 175n43, 177, 181, 185,
    191, 193, 210, 220, 223–224, 226,
    322–327, 330–331, 333–339,
    341–342, 381, 387, 393, 401, 403,
    408
  and the environment, 86–89

Genetic enhancement, 5, 58, 78–79,
    84–86, 158–159, 172n13, 210,
    214, 227–229, 335, 381
    research, 2
Genetic essentialism, 71–72
Genetic manipulation. *See* Genetic
    engineering
Genetic medicine. *See* Medicine
Genetics, 68–70, 100, 102, 115, 155,
    158, 165, 174n31, 178–183, 185,
    188–191, 196, 272–275, 334, 391
Gene transfer protocols, 369
Genomes, 101–103, 115
Genomics. *See* Genetics
Genomism, 159, 160
Genovo, 376
Germ line intervention, 79, 84, 210,
    381
Gilbert, Walter, 178, 190, 193, 200
Gilman, Charlotte Perkins, 127
Givenness of nature, 83, 163,
    167–169, 194, 229
    and ethics, 195
    human life as a gift, 163, 168, 195,
    201
Globalization, 359, 402
Glover, Jonathan, 139
God, 155–156, 168–170, 174n36,
    296, 301, 303, 304
Gore, Al, 85
Gould, Stephen Jay, 63n34, 239, 250,
    255
Grace, 23, 299
Great leap forward, 239, 260n9, 306,
    308
Greider, William, 361–362
Gross, Lora, 23, 298–300, 307–308
Guttenberg, Johannes, 40

Habermas, Jürgen, 113, 115, 125
Hakken, David, 398
Haldane, J. B. S., 125, 130–132, 134,
    137, 143, 147–24, 147n31
Hamilton, William, 283
Hand axes. *See* Acheulean tools,
    Oldowan tools

Happiness, 218
Haraway, Donna, 399–403
Haring, Bernard, 82–84
Harvey, William, 62n12
Hayes, Zachary, 300
Hegel, G. W. F., 47, 100, 214
Heidegger, Martin, 6, 36, 45, 49–54,
    59–60, 113, 178, 332
Heredity, 123, 127–129, 133, 166
Hippocrates, 77–78, 189
History, 35, 52, 55, 60–61, 69, 73,
    83, 90, 100, 105–108, 117, 124,
    126, 130, 139, 185, 195, 203, 331,
    395
Hobbes, 217, 320
Holland, Alan, 89
Hominid bushiness (Hominid
    phyletic diversity), 22, 238,
    252–254, 258
Horgan, John, 63n34
Hotchkiss, Rollin, 137, 145n3
Howard, Ted, 138, 149n51
Hubris, 52, 203
Human condition, 53, 61, 112, 157,
    164, 179, 192, 203, 392, 398–399,
    405–406
Human essence. *See* Human nature
Human gene transfer, 367, 370, 380.
    See also Genetic engineering
Human genome, 35, 58, 67, 69,
    70–72, 76, 78, 81–83, 87, 90,
    100–101, 136, 140, 178, 183, 197,
    200, 409n11
Human genome project, 67, 91, 102,
    158, 178–179, 183, 190, 193, 197,
    200, 269–271, 289
Humanism, 1, 57
Human nature, 7, 9, 12–13, 15, 17,
    20, 55, 58, 67–98, 106, 116, 125,
    128, 130, 134, 137–138, 140,
    149n56, 157, 167–170, 178,
    193–195, 201–202, 213, 220, 222,
    235–237, 267n73, 271–272, 279,
    291, 297, 306, 321, 327–331, 339,
    341–342, 345, 385–386, 389, 394,
    403, 405

Humanness, 35, 53, 166, 193,
  201–202
Human recency, 239, 248, 253
Human value, 48–49
Humans as a standing reserve, 53, 58
Human will, 290, 292–296
Hume, David, 43, 73
Husbandry, 24
Husserl, Edmund, 194, 206n37
Huxley, Aldous, 130, 132, 331
Hylomorphic psychology, 19,
  214–220, 225 ff.

In vitro fertilization (ectogenesis),
  130, 132–133, 140, 182, 198, 200
Individuality, 274–278
Industrial agriculture, 320. *See also*
  Factory farming
Information technology, 389
Ingelfinger, Franz J., 205n26
Institute for Human Gene Therapy,
  375–376
International Cooperation for
  Development and Security, (CIDS),
  354

Jacob, François, 115
Jakabson, Roman, 100
Jefferson, Thomas, 404
Jonas, Hans, 55, 57, 60, 65n45, 166,
  192–193, 228, 232n12
Judaism, 85–86, 139, 168
Justice, 46, 143, 156–157, 199, 329

Kant, 43, 106, 112, 178
Kass, Leon, 77, 138, 149n56, 167,
  168, 206n34, 196, 201
Katz, Jay, 187–188
Kinesis (motion), 216, 221
King, Martin Luther, 174n32
Kolata, Gina, 165
Koyré, Alexandre, 44
Kubrick, Stanley, 57, 395

Lacan, Jacques, 100
Laing, R. D., 193

Lamarckism, 129–130
Lander, Eric, 67, 72, 76
Latour, Bruno, 190, 398, 399
Lederberg, Joshua, 178–179
Leonardo da Vinci, 40
Levi-Strauss, Claude, 100, 184
Lewis, C. S., 59, 64n42
Lovin, Robin, 157, 356–357
Lucretius, 78
Luddites, 159
Luther, Martin, 155–156
Lyell, Charles, 263n35

McKibben, Bill, 125
McLuhan, Marshall, 395
Man the toolmaker, 46
Marx, Karl, 6, 36, 45–52, 55, 100,
  134–135, 169, 214, 394, 404
  humanization of nature, 46–49
Material cause, 217, 218, 223
Matter, the transcendent potential of,
  297–301
Mawer, Simon, 16, 179–183, 187,
  196, 198
Maxim to Respect Telos, 322–325
Mechanistic metaphysics, 37–38,
  41–45, 317–319, 328
Medicine, 77–79, 136, 189, 192,
  198. *See also* Restorative
  medicine
Medieval industrial revolution,
  36–39, 41
Medieval science, 39–41
Medieval technology, 36–39
Mendel, Gregor, 179, 180, 182–183
Messerich, Valerius, 295–296
Metaman, 387
Metaphysics, 35, 41, 43, 45, 56, 60,
  89, 99, 211–212, 318. *See also*
  Mechanistic metaphysics
Middle Ages, 36–39, 90, 334
Mill, John Stuart, 8, 75–76, 89,
  330–331
Modern Industrial Revolution,
  62n5
Modern political philosophy, 404

Modern science, 34, 40–42, 44, 52, 54, 57–59, 64n34, 70, 89, 104–121, 131, 185, 187–192. See also Technoscience

Modern technology, 37, 48, 50–53, 56, 82, 87, 89–90, 105, 124–125, 136, 141, 191, 192, 333

Molecular anthropology, 238, 255–257

Molecular biology, 55–56, 99, 111–112, 114, 137, 145n3, 186, 190, 318

Molecular medicine. See Medicine

Moore, G. E., 73

Moravec, Hans, 389–390, 392

Morton, Peter, 124–125

Muller, H. J., 132–137

Mullis, Kerry, 119n7

Mumford, Lewis, 38, 385, 395

National Institutes of Health, 27, 91, 102, 190, 367–368, 372, 374

Natural selection, 36, 55, 58–59, 126, 128, 189, 324, 326
and capitalism, 129

Natural vs. artificial, 69, 73, 75, 87

Nature, 7, 37, 40, 42, 44, 46, 48–60, 62n11, 64n37, 35–65, 76–98, 126, 139, 157, 163, 166, 168–170, 171n5, 171n6, 318–319, 385, 387–388, 397–400, 402, 405

Nature as a standing reserve (Bestand), 50–53

Nature vs. culture, 75, 184, 189, 200

Natures. See Essence

Nazism, 86, 104, 123, 142, 159, 165, 170, 175n43, 185, 240, 251, 253, 255

Neanderthal, 235, 255, 258, 265n50, 306

Neoplatonism, 60

Newton, Sir Isaac, 44

Newtonian mechanics, 76

Newtonian revolution, 317

Niebuhr, Reinhold, 26, 339–340, 354–359, 362

Nietzsche, Friedrich, 48, 50–51, 112, 116, 404

Nihilism, 116

Oldowan tools, 237, 242, 247

Office of Recombinant DNA Activities (RAC), 367–368, 373

Oncomouse, 399–400

Ornithine transcarbamylase (OTC) deficiency, 373–376, 378

Orwell, George, 17n20

"Out of Africa," 239, 256–258

Oxfam, 27, 348, 360

Owens, Joseph, 220

Paleontology, 238, 240–241

Patented drugs, 348–349, 362, 365

Patenting human genes, 347–348, 401

Pence, Gregory, 125, 141–142

Perthes, Jacque Boucher de, 241, 244

Person, 19, 340

Personhood, 9, 211, 227

Peters, Ted, 142

Physician-assisted suicide, 171n6, 174n34, 175n43

Physics, 37, 48, 55, 75–76, 112, 114, 177

Plato, 77, 178, 317

Playing God, 74, 99, 118n1, 128, 139, 198

Political theories, 340

Politics, 191–193

Pope John XXII, 351, 358

Pope John Paul II, 26, 169, 171n2, 300, 351–353

Pope Leo XIII, 26, 350

Positivism, 35, 43, 174

Posthumanism, 386, 390–392, 394, 402, 405, 408

Posthumanity, 28, 389, 391, 403, 406–408

Postmodernism, 402

Preferential option for the poor, 340, 359

Progress, 385

Prometheus, 125, 131
Proteomics, 103
Public oversight, 370

Race, 238–239, 240, 275–277
Racism, 400–401
Radin, Margaret Jane, 342
Raelians, 29, 343, 393
Rahner, Karl, 8, 82–83, 298, 307
Ramsey, Paul, 67, 137
Rawls, John, 227
Recombinant DNA Advisory
    Committee, 27, 370–374
Reinders, Hans S., 161–162
Religion, 260–9, 296, 301–311
Ressourcement, 22, 270, 289
Restorative medicine, 181, 183, 186,
    189
Rheinberger, Hans-Jörg, 184–185,
    190–191, 196
Rifkin, Jeremy, 88, 124, 138–139
Robotics, 389–390, 405
Rollin, Bernard, 65n45, 88–89
Roosevelt, Franklin Delano, 406
Rothman, Barbara Katz, 136, 143
Rousseau, Jean-Jacques, 19,
    212–214, 404

Sarich, Vince, 236
Sartre, Jean-Paul, 169, 195
Scheler, Max, 194
Schutz, Alfred, 194–195, 200–202
Science as value neutral, 54–55, 60,
    188, 306
Scientific materialism, 296–297
Second Vatican Council, 82, 351
Self-identity, 193–203
Serendipity, 19, 219, 223, 227,
    229–230
Sexual selection, 128, 130, 135
Shattuck, Roger, 175n39
Shelley, Mary, 230, 332
Silver, Lee, 125, 134, 140, 143,
    387–388
Sin, 14, 26, 39, 340, 355–356
Singer, Peter, 321

Single-species hypothesis, 249–254
Sinsheiner, Robert, 85, 137, 165
Slippery slope, 187–188, 193,
    202–203, 211
Sloterdijk, Peter, 125, 134, 143
Smith, Adam, 37, 49
Snow, C. P., 114
Social constructs, 396–397, 402
Social ethics, 340
Social injustice, 357–358. *See also*
    Justice
Socialism, 46–47, 49, 132
Sociality, 17
Sociobiology, 271, 275, 279–289
Soul, 212, 214, 216, 218
Spencer, Herbert, 129, 135
Spiegelberg, Herbert, 197, 199
Spinoza, Benedict de, 318
Stapledon, Olaf, 131
Stem cell research, 164
Sterilization, 124–125, 127, 131,
    141, 159
Sterilization laws, 189
Stock, Gregory, 125, 387
Szasz, Thomas, 333

Tämmsjö, Torbörn, 140
Taylor, Charles, 158
Technoscience, 45, 49, 53–54, 99,
    397–402, 404
Teleology, 42, 57, 318–319, 327–
    328
Telos, 24–25, 88–89, 214, 304,
    317–329, 334
Theology, 39, 40, 67, 80, 82–86
Thompson, Judith Jarvis, 171n6
Tode ti, 214–215
Tool use, 6, 49, 394–395
    design, 248–249
    vs. language, 395
Toth, Nicholas, 244, 247–248
Toulmin, Stephen, 45, 54–55
Trade Related Aspects of Intellectual
    Property Rights (TRIPS), 347
Tragedy, 61, 209
Tragic, 210

Transgenics, 401
Transhumanism, 392–393
Tribalism, 55
Trotsky, Leon, 134

UNESCO Statement on Race, 21,
    236, 238, 240, 253, 255–256, 258
University of Pennsylvania, 373–379
U.S. Department of Energy, 102, 190
U.S. National Conference of Catholic
    Bishops, 344
Ussher, Archbishop James, 241

Varmus, Harold, 372
Vonnegut, Kurt, 178

Wallace, Alfred Russel, 128–129,
    133, 135
Warwick, Kevin, 389, 405
Washburn, Sherwood, 394
Watson, James D., 143, 190, 200,
    388
Waxman, Henry, 378
Weber, Max, 9, 118n4, 108–114,
    116–117, 118n4, 120n30
Wells, H. G., 134
White, Lynn, Jr., 38, 39, 50, 62n4,
    62n5
Will, The, 290, 292–296
Wilmut, Ian, 178, 201
Wilson, Allan, 236
Wilson, E. O., 22, 275, 280–
    286, 288, 296–297, 302–
    304
Wilson, James, 375–376, 379
Wired, 391, 405
Wissenshaft. See Modern Science
Wissmann, Gerard A., 205n27
Wolpoff, Milford, 256
Wolter, Allan B., 290–292, 295,
297
World Council of Churches, 84
World Health Organization, 349, 360
World Trade Organization, 347–349,
    354, 359

Worldview. *See* Mechanistic
    metaphysics; Metaphysics

Young Hegelians, 134

Zallen, Doris T, 158–159
Zavos, Panos, 343